Moral Dilemmas in Community Health Care

Cases and Commentaries

Becky Cox White, PhD
Department of Philosophy
California State University, Chico

Joel A. Zimbelman, PhD
Department of Religious Studies
California State University, Chico

PEARSON
Longman

New York • San Francisco • Boston
London • Toronto • Sydney • Tokyo • Singapore • Madrid
Mexico City • Munich • Paris • Cape Town • Hong Kong • Montreal

This volume is dedicated to Kelly W. White
and Linda K. Zimbelman, who face moral
dilemmas in health care with equanimity
and determination.

Vice President and Publisher: Priscilla McGeehon
Executive Marketing Manager: Ann Stypuloski
Production Manager: Charles Annis
Project Coordination, Text Design, and Electronic Page Makeup: PrePress Company, Inc.
Cover Design Manager: Wendy Ann Fredericks
Cover Designer: Pema Studio
Cover Art: Russell Thurston/Photodisc Green/Getty Images, Inc.
Senior Manufacturing Buyer: Dennis J. Para
Printer and Binder: R. R. Donnelley and Sons Company
Cover Printer: Phoenix Color Corp.

Cataloging-in-publication Data on file at the Library of Congress

Please visit our website at http://www.ablongman.com

ISBN 0-321-13355-2

1 2 3 4 5 6 7 8 9 10—DOC—07 06 05 04

Contents

uncooperative. The staff increasingly turn to the son to make decisions as a more efficient decisional strategy.

CHAPTER 3

The Not-So-Golden Years • 62

An elderly Navajo woman needing assistance with activities of daily living begins to decline. Her neighbor suspects her son, the caregiver of record, is taking financial advantage of her and eliciting her silence.

CHAPTER 4

Patients We Love to Hate: The Noncompliant • 80

When a diabetic refuses to comply with dietary and medication regimens, and transfer to other providers is practically impossible, may her physician discontinue the relationship?

CHAPTER 5

I'm Doing the Best I Can • 95

A nurse practitioner in an isolated small community is asked to guard the confidentiality of a patient raped by her minister and to provide psychiatric support for the victim—a service that exceeds his skills.

CHAPTER 6

Must Health Care Professionals Always Tell the Truth? • 111

A nurse in the only accessible emergency room accidentally gives an infant an overdose of morphine. The staff debate whether to tell family members the real reason the baby stopped breathing.

CHAPTER 7

Who Makes Decisions in Family-centered Health Care? • 130

A pregnant African-American woman with herpes consents to a caesarean section, but requests that her health care providers not notify her partner of her infection. The unknowing partner requests that he be told the reason for the C-section.

CHAPTER 8

Border Crossings • 145

The family of a Hmong child objects to emergency room treatment. The family insists that they be allowed to remain

in the room, and to have a Hmong healer present and
consulted about treatment.

PART 2

Your Money or Your Life! Dilemmas in Paying for Health Care •

CHAPTER 9

Why Should We Have to Shoulder This Burden Alone? • 167

Too poor to buy insurance or pay out of pocket, but too
rich for Medicaid, a woman visits the emergency room
whenever her asthma flares. The hospital administrator
requests of local physicians that one of them make her a
pro bono patient.

CHAPTER 10

Dollars or Drugs? • 185

A pharmacist dispensing drugs to a recent organ transplant
recipient is alarmed by the patient's request to stop taking an
expensive prescription, putting his own health and the
statistical outcomes of a newly established transplant
center at risk.

Introduction, 187 • A Transplant Team's Analysis, Andrea D. Hoso, RN, CCTC, and Roblee P. Allen, MD, 191 • An Ethicist's Analysis, Laura Siminoff, PhD, and Richard E. Morse, MA, 194 • A Pharmacist's Analysis, Brian L. Kaatz, PharmD, 196 • Further Reflections, 198

CHAPTER 11

Who Defines "Enough"? • 200

When the young Amish parents of a seriously ill premature infant for whom prognosis is guarded refuse health care for financial reasons, what are the moral obligations of the caregivers?

Introduction, 202 • A Parent's Analysis, Helen Harrison, 208 A Nurse Ethicist's Analysis, Jennifer Girod, PhD, RN, 213 • A Neonatal Intensive Care Unit Analysis, Elizabeth Catlin, MD, Margaret Doyle Settle, RNC, MS and Mary Martha Thiel, MDiv, 215 • An Ethicist's Analysis, Eric H. Gampel, PhD, 219 A Philosopher and Disability Advocate's Analysis, Anita Silvers, PhD, 221 • Further Reflections, 224

CHAPTER 12

Patients We Love to Hate: The Obese • 226

A seriously obese patient taxes the emotional and physical resources of the staff of a small community hospital.

Introduction, 228 • A Nurse's Analysis, Janet Brown, RN, MSN, CNS, 232 • A Philosopher and Disability Advocate's Analysis, Anita Silvers, PhD, 234 • An Ethicist's Analysis, David Resnick, JD, PhD, 237 • Further Reflections, 239

CHAPTER 13

Professional Promises in the "Real" World: Skilled Nursing Facilities (SNFs) • 241

When inadequate resources and lack of referral opportunities in a small rural community obstruct the professional commitment to patient welfare, what are a nurse's moral obligations?

CHAPTER 14

Are We Our Patients' Keepers? • 256

Physicians in a small rural community refuse, for financial reasons, to sign a contract with the only HMO available in the area.

PART 3

HARD CHOICES FOR SOCIETY: DOES THE GOOD OF THE MANY OUTWEIGH THE GOOD OF THE INDIVIDUAL PATIENT? •

CHAPTER 15

You're Just His Doctor; I'm His Boss! • 275

When an employee whose duties include hazardous tasks is admitted to his small town's emergency room, the open-bay structure results in several local residents hearing the physician order a blood alcohol and a drug screen. His employer arrives and insists on being informed of the test results.

CHAPTER 16

Daddy Dearest • 289

An elderly Puerto Rican male, comatose and with profound
brain damage from a stroke, has a Power of Attorney for
Health Care (PAHC) requesting all possible life-sustaining
treatment. His daughters insist that life-support be
discontinued.

CHAPTER 17

But You Need a Real Doctor • 306

A patient with chronic headaches requests a referral
to a chiropractor.

CHAPTER 18

To Feed or Not to Feed • 326

A family disagrees about a decision to withhold food and
fluids from an elderly, comatose patient who had verbally
requested not to be sustained with medical nutrition and
hydration, but who had not completed a PAHC. Her
physician and daughters consider secretly providing
inadequate treatment as the easiest solution, to deceive the
sons, who would never agree to "starve mom to death."

CHAPTER 19

Is My Obligation to My Clients or My Neighbors? • 343

The only pharmacist in a small, isolated town contemplates refusing to fill a Viagra (sildenafil) prescription for a known sex offender.

CHAPTER 20

When Bad Things Happen to Good Doctors • 355

When the physician in an isolated town appears increasingly irresponsible, what are the moral obligations of his colleagues?

CHAPTER 21

Do Health Care Professionals with HIV Disease Have a Duty to Warn Their Patients? • 372

In a small town setting where trained ICU nurses are rare, the supervisor of an ICU nurse with HIV Disease considers telling patients and colleagues of the nurse's HIV status and transferring the nurse from the ICU.

Preface

The editors of this volume were both educated in academic medical settings. Upon graduation, they were keen to apply their wealth of knowledge to "real life," and so they were delighted when invited to serve on various regional bioethics committees. Their colleagues in health care listened with interest to their suggestions. Then, more often than not, they explained politely why these solutions "wouldn't work *here*." And they were almost always right. No pediatric psychiatrist practiced "here"; the nearest burn unit was two hours away; the only rabbi was on vacation; no one spoke Farsi; attracting and retaining experienced critical care nurses was an ongoing challenge, and so on and so on. In the insights of these health care providers, in their keen appreciation of the ubiquity of moral dilemmas, and in their commitment to resolving them, the idea for this volume took root.

We have concentrated on analysis of case studies, believing that these typically provide the best portal to the study of clinical bioethics. Students are drawn into the discipline by the stories of everyday people in distress (the case studies) and come to appreciate the complexity of moral dilemmas and develop the skills of moral analysis, reasoning, and justification better when their decisions matter—that is, when their solutions can be applied immediately and meaningfully to concrete, authentic moral dilemmas in clinical situations.

This volume provides instructors, students, and practicing clinicians with an accessible tool that complements the more abstract and theoretical resources assigned in most classes and considered in many books of case studies. At the same time, this volume provides four distinct resources not found in most extant bioethics case study books.

First, this volume *emphasizes the importance of a rich appreciation of context for full moral insight*. It provides readers with principled analyses of the most salient characteristics of the dilemmas while emphasizing the particular and diverse professional, institutional, or community practice settings in which the dilemmas arise. This volume is animated and informed by one essential question: How do the geographical, social, cultural, and professional contexts of the participants and the often limited available resources inform the moral reflection required to address the challenges of these dilemmas? The messy details of the dilemmas and the presence of multiple, often contradictory, voices and perspectives realistically complexify the dilemmas in ways that provide readers with rich and authentic occasions for moral analysis.

Second, our volume *focuses on the sorts of dilemmas that arise outside of tertiary medical care settings*. While analysis and resolution of moral dilemmas in sophisticated health care settings are surely important, the majority of health care professionals do not spend the bulk of their careers in such environments. Our dilemmas are, for the most part, *set in contexts in which practitioners lack easy—or any—access to the plethora of resources found in large medical centers*. Thus, the dilemmas focus on the management of patients who have a limited choice of providers or institutions; whose family, economic, or professional identities complicate health care decision making; and whose social, cultural, and religious tenets are typically underrepresented and often unappreciated by health care professionals (HCPs). We demonstrate in the introductory comments on each case the distinct influences that attend these dilemmas *because of where they occur and who they involve*. The way in which moral dilemmas are encountered, experienced, construed, and ultimately resolved in community settings may seem less dramatic than the research-driven, education-oriented, or technology-centered dilemmas of tertiary or teaching medical complexes. However, their successful identification and resolution have daily import for the majority of health care practitioners and their patients.

Of course, many of the issues arising in these dilemmas—e.g., end-of-life care—also arise in sophisticated medical centers. Practitioners in those settings will find the dilemmas instructive because of the focus on the particularities of patients rather than on unavailability of resources (though, as the debate swirls around health care financing, perhaps in regard to resource-related issues as well).

Third, *analyses of the dilemmas incorporate perspectives other than those of physicians and ethicists*. Typically, a constricted range of perspectives obscures the interdisciplinary nature of moral dilemmas and the way in which discipline-specific training and clinical concerns too narrowly shape interpretations of the moral landscape. These dilemmas illustrate the importance of the perspectives of a broad range of HCPs—as well as of patients, families, and professionals in other disciplines—to successful resolution of moral dilemmas. Perspectives of professionals such as disability advocates, psychologists, religious counselors, lawyers, health care administrators, social workers, pharmacists, dietitians, emergency medical technicians, and health educators, as well as patients, parents, and children, enrich the analyses of these dilemmas.

Fourth, our volume *incorporates a thorough, useful method for honing (or developing) critical skills in moral awareness and reasoning that will help students and practitioners more fruitfully address moral dilemmas*. In the essay that is this book's introduction, "A Framework for Moral Reasoning," Eric Gampel, PhD, introduces readers to the Analysis and Justification (AJ) Method, a five-step framework for moral reasoning. The framework is designed to be portable and can be incorporated by readers across the various contexts in which they will encounter and need to grapple with moral dilemmas.

In the editors' introductions to each case study, the first three steps of the AJ Method are elaborated:

- In Step 1 (Information Gathering), the editors indicate some (though surely not all) facts that inform deliberations.
- In Step 2 (Creative Problem Solving), we suggest the form an alternative (though not the content of a particular or clear-cut) solution should take.
- In Step 3 (Listing Pros and Cons), we identify what each moral principle might contribute to the analysis of the dilemma. In this step we list issues that could be identified by a careful analysis as reasons for and against particular options. These issues are organized in terms of the major moral principles identified by Gampel—consequences, autonomy, rights, virtues, and equality, (justice) or fairness. These principles form a mnemonic—CARVE—that the reader may use to structure future considerations. For each principle, the names of commentators are inserted in parentheses, directing the reader to the particular concepts considered by individual commentators.

Note that the introduction focuses on those moral concepts that are seminal— rather than tangential—to the dilemma under consideration. Note, also, that we do not undertake Steps 4 or 5. Those steps—Analysis and Justification—are left for the reader, who will be aided by the explorations and analyses provided by commentators on each case.

A caveat: many commentators do not explicitly embrace the AJ method, per se. This is not surprising, as other systematic, AJ-like approaches to moral analysis are available and we urged commentators to follow those approaches that have historically served them well. For readers who have not yet developed a procedural preference, we offer the AJ—an approach we have found to be extraordinarily helpful in classrooms, bioethics committee meetings, and ethics consultations.

Following Gampel's essay, 21 case studies are presented. Introductions highlight a number of issues worthy of analysis and central to appreciating the moral challenges of each dilemma. Commentaries present distinct personal and professional perspectives on salient concerns raised in the introductions, together with discussions of relevant codes of professional ethics and/or important moral values central to the relevant profession or community perspective.

Our goal is to help readers to gain an appreciation for multiple theoretical and professional perspectives crucial to identifying, clarifying, and addressing the moral challenges of each dilemma. The discrete analyses of each commentary allow readers to focus, if desired, on those perspectives most relevant to the class in which this volume is used, or to professional needs and interests. Introductions and most commentaries are supported with bibliographies of relevant monographs, articles in the professional literature, and Web sites. Study questions at the end of each case study (grouped under Further Reflections) provide probing analyses of each dilemma, structured around the moral principles introduced by Gampel and incorporated into the introductions for each case study.

A final caveat: The volume devotes scant attention to legal aspects of the case studies presented here. While health care practitioners must surely be conversant with legal restrictions on practice, and while law often reprises themes developed in the ethics literature, law and ethics are distinct. In our experience, persons struggling with moral dilemmas too frequently believe they have achieved *moral* resolution upon determining *legal* obligations. However, even if one has determined what action is *legally* required, what action is *morally* required remains an open question. Still, as law and health care so frequently intersect, each introduction identifies several pressing legal issues raised by the dilemma, and directs readers interested in investigating legal aspects to relevant resources.

Several sorts of readers will benefit from our volume. Our case studies should appeal to faculty teaching (and students taking) interdisciplinary courses in the ethics of family, community, and geriatric medicine. Additionally, law students will benefit from the analyses provided here, which will help them discern the pivotal relationship between moral and legal obligations. Further, individuals embarking on careers in public policy and public administration will discover in these case studies the fundamental values—along with a perspective on interpersonal and institutional relationships—that lie at the heart of these disciplines.

Finally, faculty in university-based public and community health, philosophy, bioethics, nursing, social work, and counseling programs have in this volume a resource that emphasizes the sorts of dilemmas students are likely to face in their careers. While today's university-based ethics classes often leave students with the impression that they are likely to face the standard dilemmas of allocation of organs and ICU beds, cloning, active euthanasia, and technology's relationship to public policy (for example), it is equally helpful to introduce dilemmas where future patients have the chance to imagine themselves forgoing care they cannot afford, disagreeing with health care providers over treatment of an elderly parent, being caregivers and decision makers for an elderly, young, or chronically ill family member, or being forced to make personnel decisions based on medical needs of employees. This volume shifts the encounter with moral dilemmas and concerns in the direction of these sorts of mundane and ubiquitous dilemmas.

Acknowledgments

The idea for this volume developed out of our editorial responsibilities of the *Bioethics Bulletin*, a regional, case-based clinical ethics quarterly published under the aegis of the Bioethics Committee of Enloe and Chico Community Hospitals, Chico, California, and The Center for Applied and Professional Ethics (CAPE) at

California State University, Chico. During the nine years of the *Bulletin's* publication, we benefitted from the dedication and professional insights of its Editorial Board, including Nadine Bernica, MSW; Carol Blacet, RNC, MSN; Janet Brown, RN, MSN; Libby Buchwalter, MSW; Jerry Calbert, RN, BSN; Jannell Campbell, MA; Elise Debord, RNC; Laura Douglas, MICP; Jeanesse Fowkes-Hawkley, MFCC; Arlene Phalen-Hostetter, MSW; Robert Kellerman LCSW, Jeff Moo, MD; Donna Moore, MD; Bonnie Morgan, LUTCF; Linda Russell, RN, CCRN; Michael Sterling, RN; and Patrick Tedford, MD. To all of these colleagues, we give our thanks. Thanks, too, to Enloe Medical Center, Chico, California for allowing us to harvest ideas from volumes of the *Bioethics Bulletin* for several of the cases presented herein. Special thanks are due to Carol Blacet, RN, MSN, Director of Education at Enloe Medical Center, for her enthusiastic support and for making negotiations with Enloe MC painless.

We are also indebted to the professional insights and review of several early drafts of cases by Betsy Catlin and Anita Silvers (Who Defines Enough?); Andrew Flescher (Daddy Dearest); Jane Rysberg (Mommy Dearest); Kristin Lundberg and Bee Lo (Border Crossings); Laura Douglas, Lisa Emmerich, and Raymond Reid (The Not-So-Golden Years); Patrick Giammarsee, Joel Rothfeld, and Gerard Clum (But You Need a Real Doctor); and Richard Kronick (Why Should We Have to Shoulder This Burden Alone?).

We also wish to thank California State University, Chico for their support of this volume through sabbatical leaves and partial release from teaching responsibilities for us.

We would be remiss if we failed to thank our contributors. We continue to be amazed at the generosity of colleagues in both academic and health care professions who were willing to commit whole-heartedly to this project, adding yet another obligation to their overly full schedules. Our deepest appreciation goes to Eric Gampel for articulating a framework that is particularly helpful to those seeking to refine their skills in moral analysis.

Thanks are due, also, to Priscilla McGeehon, our editor at Longman, for her ceaseless, timely, and invaluable support and encouragement. We have, as well, a debt of gratitude to the eight blind reviewers whose suggestions have improved the volume in countless ways; and to Robin Gordon of Pre-Press Company, Inc. for her copyediting direction.

Finally, deep appreciation goes to our families—Linda, Lexie, and Lauren Zimbelman, and Kelly, Kathryn, and Cassi White—whose support for and patience with the efforts required for this project know no bounds.

Becky Cox White
Joel A. Zimbelman

Contributors

Roblee P. Allen, MD, is Professor of Clinical Internal Medicine, Division of Pulmonary and Critical Care Medicine, Department of Internal Medicine, School of Medicine, University of California, Davis. His research interests include photodynamic therapy of superficial malignancies, treatment for septic shock, and antifungal therapy in immunocompromised patients. He has published in *Journal of Bronchology*, *Journal of Respiratory Diseases*, *Transplantation Proceedings*, and *Journal of Surgical Investigation*. Email:roblee.allen@ucdmc.ucdavis.edu

John D. Banja, PhD, is Clinical Ethicist, Center for Ethics, and Associate Professor, Department of Rehabilitative Medicine, Emory University, Atlanta, Georgia. He is the coauthor of *Rehabilitation Medicine: Contemporary Clinical Perspectives* (Lea & Febiger, 1992). His research interests include work on professional ethics and truth telling. Email: jbanja@emory.edu

Tami Borneman, RN, MSN, is Research Specialist/Palliative Care Nurse Educator, Georgetown University Medical Center, Lombardi Cancer Center, Department of Oncology, Palliative Care Program, Washington, DC. Her research interests include pain management, end-of-life care, quality of life, and palliative care. She has published in *Cancer Practice*, *Journal of Palliative Care*, *Generations*, *Journal of Hospice and Palliative Nursing*, *Journal of Palliative Medicine*, and *Primary Care and Cancer*. Email: trb28@georgetown.edu

Sarah-Vaughan Brakman, PhD, is Director, The Ethics Program, and Assistant Professor, Department of Philosophy, Villanova University, Villanova, Pennsylvania. Her research interests include ethics of adoption, approaches to resolving moral dilemmas, and family responsibility in long-term care. She has published in *The Hastings Center Report*, *Generations*, *Tijdschrift voor Geneeskunde en Ethiek* (The Netherlands), and *Medisch Contact* (The Netherlands). Email: sarah.vaughan.brakman@villanova.edu

Howard Brody, MD, PhD, is Professor of Family Practice and Philosophy and Professor, Center for Ethics and Humanities in the Life Sciences, Michigan State University, East Lansing, Michigan. He is the author of *The Healer's Power* (Yale, 1991) and *Stories of Sickness* (Oxford, 2002). His research interests include medical ethics, the placebo effect, and the ethical and policy aspects of the relationship between the medical profession and the pharmaceutical industry. Email: Howard.Brody@ht.msu.edu

Janet Brown, RN, MSN, CNS, is Associate Professor, College of Nursing, California State University, Chico. Her research focuses on pain assessment and acute pain management. She has published in *Medical-Surgical Nursing Journal, Pain Management Nurses,* and *Clinical Nurse Specialist.* Email: jebrown@csuchico.edu

Diana Buccafurni, PhD(c), is a doctoral student, Department of Philosophy, University of Utah, Salt Lake City. Her research interests focus on understanding the relationship between personal identity and advance directives, and the relationship between selective abortion and attitudes toward disability. She has published in *Proceedings of the University of Utah Humanities Graduate Conference.* Email: db20@utah.edu

Robert A. Buerki, PhD, is Professor of Pharmacy Practice and Administration, The Ohio State University College of Pharmacy, Columbus. He is the coauthor of *Ethical Practice in Pharmacy: A Guidebook for Pharmacy Technicians* (American Institute of the History of Pharmacy (AIHP), 1997); *Ethical Responsibility in Pharmacy Practice* (AIHP, 2002); and editor of *The Challenge of Ethics in Pharmacy Practice* (AIHP, 1985). Email: Buerki@dendrite.pharmacy.ohio-state.edu

Courtney Campbell, PhD, is Professor and Chair, Department of Philosophy, Oregon State University, Corvallis. His research interests include philosophies of the body, religious warfare and terrorism, and faith communities and bioethics. He is coeditor of *Duties to Others* (Kluwer, 1994) and *What Price Parenthood: Ethics and Assisted Reproduction* (Dartmouth Publishing, 1992); and is the former Editor (1988–1990) of *The Hastings Center Report.* Email: ccampbell@orst.edu

Elizabeth Catlin, MD, is Chief, Neonatology Unit, MassGeneral Hospital for Children, Boston, and Associate Professor of Pediatrics, Harvard Medical School. She has published in *The New England Journal of Medicine, Neonatal Intensive Care, Pediatrics, Critical Care Medicine, Journal of Clinical Ethics,* and *Death Studies.* Her research interests include spiritual components of patient care, the place of prayer and theological thinking in the "survival" of families with infants in NICUs, and neonatal pathophysiology and management. Email: ecatlin@partners.org

Frank A. Chervenak, MD, is Given Foundation Professor and Chairman, Department of Obstetrics and Gynecology and Obstetrician and Gynecologist-in-Chief and Director, Maternal-Fetal Medicine, New York Presbyterian Hospital Weill Medical College of Cornell University, New York. His research interests include ultrasound, ethics, and clinical obstetrics. He is author, coauthor, or editor of 13 books, including *The Fetus as a Patient: The Evolving Challenge* (Parthenon, 2002); *Fetal and Neonatal Neurology and Neurosurgery,* 3d ed. (Churchill Livingstone, 2001); *Ultrasound Screening for Fetal Anomalies: Is It Worth It?* (New York Academy of Sciences, 1998); and *Ethics in Obstetrics and Gynecology* (Oxford, 1994). Email: fac2001@med.cornell.edu

Gerard W. Clum, DC, is President and Professor, Chiropractic Sciences Division, Life Chiropractic College West, Hayward, California. His research and professional interests include issues surrounding the Health Insurance Portability and Accountability Act of 1996 (HIPPA) and cultural and sociological trends affecting the chiropractic profession and health care. He has published in *The American Journal of Clinical Chiropractic, Alternative Healthcare Management*, and *Dynamic Chiropractic*. Email: gclum@lifewest.edu

David Edwin Damazo, MD, is board certified in emergency medicine and practices in the Oroville Medical Center, Oroville, California. His research interests focus on infectious diseases and diabetes. Email: bdamazo@csuchico.edu

Rebekah Damazo, RN, PNP, MSN, is Professor, School of Nursing, California State University, Chico. Her research interests include public health nursing assessment and international health. She has published in *Journal of Health Education, American Journal of Nursing*, and *The Journal of Continuing Education in Nursing*. Email: bdamazo@csuchico.edu

Milenne L. deLeon, MPH, RD, is Assistant Professor, Department of Nutrition and Dietetics, School of Allied Health Professions, Loma Linda University, Loma Linda, California. Her research interests include ethics and end-of-life issues, ethical issues in dietetics and health care, childhood obesity, and alternative therapies. She has published in the area of maternal-infant nutrition. Email: milennede@mac.com

Laura Douglas, EMT-P, is a member of the Enloe Medical Center Flight Crew, Chico, California. Her professional responsibilities focus on pediatrics, water safety, and flight transport of emergency and trauma cases. She has served as a member of the Enloe Medical Center Bioethics Committee and published in *Bioethics Bulletin*. Email:LDouglas91@aol.com

Theresa S. Drought, PhD, RN, is Co-Director, Northern California Ethics Department, Kaiser Permanente, Oakland. Her research interests include end-of-life care, bioethics and multiculturalism, and the challenges of implementing the California Health Care Decisions law. She is coauthor of *Ethical Dilemmas in Nursing Practice*, 4th ed. (Prentice Hall, 1997). Email: Theresa.Drought@kp.org

Tiffany Eskelson is Sexual Assault Prevention Coordinator, Wyoming Coalition Against Domestic Violence and Sexual Assault, Laramie.

Andrew Flescher, PhD, is Assistant Professor, Department of Religious Studies, California State University, Chico. He is the author of *Heroes, Saints, and Ordinary Morality* (Georgetown University Press, 2003). His research interests include religious ethics, the nature of altruism, the nature of evil, biomedical ethics, and contemporary Jewish and Christian thought. Email: Aflescher@csuchico.edu

Leslie Pickering Francis, PhD, JD, is Alfred C. Emery Professor of Law, College of Law, and Professor of Philosophy and Chair, Department of Philosophy, University of Utah, Salt Lake City. Her research interests include law, public policy, gender issues in health care, land use, and the distribution of social goods. She is the author, coauthor, or editor of nine books, including *Americans with Disabilities: Implications for Individuals and Institutions* (Routledge, 2000); *Date Rape: Feminism, Law, and Morality* (Pennsylvania State University Press, 1996); and *Ethical Issues in the Professions* (Prentice Hall, 1989). Email: Francisl@law.utah.edu

Eric H. Gampel, PhD, is Associate Professor, Department of Philosophy, California State University, Chico. His research interests are in medical ethics, political philosophy, and metaethics. He has published in *Philosophical Papers*, *Philosophical Studies*, and *Canadian Journal of Philosophy*. Email: egampel@csuchico.edu

Lisa Gannett, PhD, is Assistant Professor, Department of Philosophy, St. Mary's University, Halifax, Nova Scotia, Canada. She has published in *Biology and Philosophy*, *British Journal for the Philosophy of Science*, *Philosophy of Science*, and *Studies in History and Philosophy of Biological and Biomedical Sciences*. Her research focuses on the history and philosophy of genetics. Email: lisa.gannett@smu.edu

Jennifer Girod, PhD, RN, is a Research Associate, Poynter Center for the Study of Ethics and American Institutions, Indiana University, Bloomington. Her research interests include bioethics, sectarian religious groups and modern medicine, and narrative ethics. She has published in *Second Opinion* and *Journal of Medical Humanities*. Email: jgirod@indiana.edu

Susan Dorr Goold, MD, MHSA, MA, is Associate Professor of Internal Medicine and Director, Bioethics Program, University of Michigan Medical School, Ann Arbor. Her work focuses on the allocation of scarce health care resources, particularly the perspectives of citizens and patients. She has published in *The Hastings Center Report*, *Journal of Health Politics Policy and Law*, *Social Science and Medicine*, and others. Email: sgoold@umich.edu

Anthony Graybosch, PhD, is Professor, Department of Philosophy, California State University, Chico. His research interests include ethical issues in childcare, philosophy of love, epistemology, and American philosophy. He is the coauthor of *Ethics and Values in the Information Age* (Thomson Learning, 2002) and *The Philosophy Student's Writer's Manual and Guide to the Art of Philosophical Writing* (Prentice Hall, 1998, 2003). Email: agraybosch@csuchico.edu

Ginny Miller Hamm, JD, is Staff Attorney, Department of Veterans Affairs, Indianapolis, Indiana; Special Assistant United States Attorney; and Assistant Professor, Department of Behavioral Science, College of Medicine, University of Kentucky, Lexington. Her research interests include the management of medical mistakes, honesty in clinical encounters, and current issues in medicolegal practice. She has published in *Bioethics Forum*, *Annals of Internal Medicine*, and *VA Practitioner*. Email: Ginny.Hamm@mail.va.gov

Helen Harrison is the mother of a 27-year-old prematurely born son and a full-term 23-year-old daughter. She is the author of *The Premature Baby Book* (St. Martin's, 1983). She serves as a parent advisor to neonatal research projects and writes and speaks on perinatal medical and bioethical issues. Email: Helen1144@aol.com

Donald Heinz, PhD, is Professor, Department of Religious Studies, California State University, Chico. He is the author of *The Last Passage: Recovering a Death of Our Own* (Oxford University Press, 1999). His research interests include explorations of theology and culture, death and dying, and the uses of religious symbolism in contemporary society. Email: dheinz@csuchico.edu

Terry Hill, MD, is Medical Director, Laguna Honda Hospital and Rehabilitation Center and Assistant Clinical Professor, Department of Medicine, University of California, San Francisco. His research and service interests include improving care for the dying, nurse-physician communication, institutional change, and ethnogeriatrics. He has published in *Journal of Palliative Care*, *Journal of the American Medical Directors Association*, *Journal of the American Geriatrics Society*, and *Annals of Internal Medicine*. Email:terry.hill@sfdph.org

Benjamin E. Hippen, MD, is a Fellow in the Division of Nephrology, University of Alabama, Birmingham. His research interests focus on concerns surrounding procurement and allocation of organs for transplantation, humoral transplant rejection, and polyoma virus nephropathy. He is a member of the Editorial Advisory Board of the *Journal of Medicine and Philosophy* and a reviewer for the *American Journal of Transplantation*. Email: bhippen@uab.edu

Georgia E. Hodgkin, EdD, RD, FADA, is Associate Professor, Department of Nutrition and Dietetics, School of Allied Health Professions, Loma Linda University, Loma Linda, California. She has published in *Military Medicine* and *Topics in Clinical Nutrition*, and developed technical reports on vegetarian diets. Her research interests include nutrition care management, malnutrition and R.D. reimbursement, Parkinson's Disease and antioxidants. Email: ghodgkin@univ.llu.edu

Andrea D. Hoso, RN, CCTC, is Lung Transplant/Advanced Lung Disease Coordinator, University of California, Davis Medical Center, Sacramento. Her research interests include patient compliance and quality-of-life issues in lung transplant and pulmonary hypertension patients, and efficacy of treatment options in relation to functional status of pulmonary hypertension patients. She has published in *Chest, Journal of Investigative Medicine, American Journal of Respiratory and Critical Care Medicine, and Transplantation Society XVII World Congress*. Email: Andrea.Hoso@ucdmc.ucdavis.edu

Kenneth V. Iserson, MD, MBA, is Professor, Department of Emergency Medicine and Director, Arizona Bioethics Program, College of Medicine, University of Arizona, Tucson. He has authored more than 250 scientific articles and 20 books including *Ethics in Emergency Medicine*, 2nd edition (Galen Press, 1995), *Death to Dust: What Happens to Dead Bodies?* (Galen Press, 2001), and *Grave Words: Notifying Survivors About Sudden Unexpected Deaths* (Galen Press, 1999). Email: kvi@u.arizona.edu

Troy Jollimore, PhD, is Assistant Professor, Department of Philosophy, California State University, Chico. He is the author of *Friendship and Agent-Relative Morality* (Garland, 2001). His research interests include the justification of moral requirements; the role of impartiality in moral reasoning; the value of happiness, pleasure, and suffering; and the nature of evil. Email: tjollimore@csuchico.edu

Brian L. Kaatz, PharmD, is Dean and Professor, College of Pharmacy, South Dakota State University, Brookings. He has published in *South Dakota Journal of Medicine, American Journal of Health-System Pharmacy, Clinical Pharmacy, Annals of Emergency Medicine, American Journal of Pharmaceutical Education*, and *Drug Intelligence and Clinical Pharmacy*. His academic interests include biomedical ethics, roles for pharmacists, and health care policy. Email: Brian.kaatz@usdsu.sdbor.edu

Steve S. Kraman, MD, is Professor of Medicine, Division of Pulmonary and Critical Care Medicine, University of Kentucky College of Medicine, Lexington. He has published in *Critical Care Medicine, Chest, Annals of Internal Medicine, Lung, Pediatric Pulmonology, Archives of Internal Medicine*, and *Bioethics Forum*. His research and professional interests include pulmonary acoustics, patient safety, and medical risk management. Email: sskram01@uky.edu

Richard Kronick, PhD, is Professor and Chief, Division of Health Care Sciences, Department of Family and Preventive Medicine, School of Medicine, University of California, San Diego. His research interests explore whether and how markets work in health care, particularly for vulnerable populations. He is coauthor of *Medicare HMOs: Making Them Work for the Chronically Ill* (Health Administration Press, 1998). Email: rkronick@ucsd.edu

John M. Lincourt, PhD, is the Bonnie E. Cone Distinguished Professor of Teaching, Department of Philosophy, University of North Carolina, Charlotte. He has published in *Journal of Investment Consulting, HealthCare Ethics Committee Forum, Journal of Business*

Ethics, and is the author of *Ethics Without a Net: A Case Workbook in Bioethics*, 2nd edition (Kendall/Hunt Publishing, 1995). His research interests include health care ethics, computer ethics and privacy, and conflicts between the goals and expectations of professionals. Email: jmlincou@email.uncc.edu

Elizabeth Ann Lindberg, MD, is Assistant Professor of Clinical Emergency Medicine, Department of Emergency Medicine, University of Arizona College of Medicine and Medical Director, Urgent Care, University Medical Center, Tucson. Her research interests include clinical problem solving in the emergency room environment and ethical issues related to emergency care. She has published in *Annals of Emergency Medicine* and *American Family Physicians*. Email: blind@aemrc.arizona.edu

Bee Lo, ND, is a Naturopathic Practitioner in private practice with the La Crosse Natural Health Center, La Crosse, and the Natural Health Center, Onalaska, Wisconsin. He is active in community service and speaks frequently to academic and community groups on Hmong culture and medicine, and natural medicine; and has taught Hmong language and naturopathic/alternative medicine in the Extension Program of the University of Wisconsin, La Cross. Email: dr_bee_lo@yahoo.com

Kristin Lundberg, RN, MA, PhD(c), is a doctoral student, Department of Anthropology, University of Kansas, Lawrence. Her research interests include health and healing practices of Southeast Asian cultures, international development, and changing Western systems of health care. She holds a predoctoral fellowship through the National Institute of Nursing Research of the National Institutes of Health, and is conducting fieldwork research during 2003–2005 on the social reproduction of health in Lao women weavers and their families living in Vientiane, Laos. Email: lundberg@ku.edu

B. Andrew Lustig, PhD, is Director, Program on Biotechnology, Religion, and Ethics, and Research Scholar in Religious Studies, Department of Religious Studies, Rice University, and Baylor Center for Medical Ethics and Health Policy, Baylor College of Medicine, Houston, Texas. His research interests include philosophy of medicine, issues in palliative care, justice and health care allocation, and theological ethics. He is the editor of *Bioethics Yearbook, Vols. 1–5* (Kluwer Academic Publishers, 1991, 1992, 1993, 1994, 1997); coeditor of *Duties to Others* (Kluwer Academic Publishers, 1994); and the founding coeditor of *Christian Bioethics: A Non-ecumenical Journal*. Email: alustig@rice.edu

Stephen A. Magnus, PhD, MAE, MS, is Assistant Professor, Department of Health Policy and Management, University of Kansas School of Medicine, Kansas City. His research interests include the role of debt in not-for-profit hospitals and hospital policies regarding uncompensated care. He has published in *Research in Healthcare Financial Management*, *Journal of Health Politics, Policy and Law*, *Journal of Homosexuality*, *Health Care Management Review*, and *American Journal of Public Health*. Email: smagnus@kumc.edu

Laurence B. McCullough, PhD, is Professor of Medicine and Medical Ethics, Center for Medical Ethics and Health Policy, and Faculty Associate, The Huffington Center on Aging, Baylor College of Medicine, Houston, Texas. His research interests include obstetric ethics, autonomy of subjects in research, the history of medical ethics, and philosophy and medicine. Among the books he has authored or coauthored are *Medical Ethics: The Moral Responsibilities of Physicians* (Prentice-Hall, 1984); *Ethics in Obstetrics and Gynecology* (Oxford University Press, 1994); *Long-Term Care Decisions: Ethical and Conceptual Dimensions* (Johns Hopkins University Press, 1995); *Surgical Ethics* (Oxford University Press, 1998); and *Medical Ethics: Codes, Opinions, and Statements* (Bureau of National Affairs, 2000). Email: Mccullou@ bcm.tmc.edu

Ann E. Mills, MSc (Econ), MBA, is Assistant Professor and Director for Outreach Programs, Center for Biomedical Ethics, University of Virginia. Ms. Mills is coauthor of *Organization Ethics in Health Care* (Oxford University Press, 2000) and *Developing Organization Ethics in Healthcare: A Case-Based Approach to Policy, Practice, and Compliance* (University Publishing Group, 2001). Her research interests focus on organization ethics in health care institutions and clinical settings. Email: amh2r@Virginia.edu

Ezra Mirvish is a premedical and philosophy major at University of California, Berkeley. Email: emirvish@hotmail.com

Richard E. Morse, MA, is Senior Fellow, Institute for Ethics, American Medical Association, Chicago, Illinois. His areas of research interest include end-of-life decision making, physician-patient communication, and consent to organ transplantation. Email: richard. morse@cwru.edu

Alvita Nathaniel, DSN, APRN, BC, is Assistant Professor and Coordinator, Nurse Practitioner Track, School of Nursing, West Virginia University, Charleston. Her research interests include nursing ethics and moral distress in nursing. She is the coauthor of *Ethics & Issues in Contemporary Nursing*, 2nd edition. (Delmar, 2002). Email: anathaniel@ hcs.wvu.edu

Barbara B. Ott, PhD, RN, is Associate Professor, College of Nursing, Villanova University, Villanova, Pennsylvania. Her research interests include end-of-life decision making, spiritual support at the end of life, and surrogate decision making. She has published in *Pediatric Nursing, Nursing Outlook, Image: Journal of Nursing Scholarship, Archives of Internal Medicine, American Journal of Critical Care, Heart and Lung*, and *MedSurg Nursing*. Email: Barbara.ott@villanova.edu

Susan Parry, MA, is a PhD candidate in the Department of Philosophy and a Research Assistant, The Center for Bioethics, University of Minnesota, Minneapolis-St. Paul. Her research focuses on bioethics and the philosophy of science, patient desires, and the practice of medicine. She has published in *APA Newsletter on Philosophy and Medicine* and *South African Medical Association Continuing Medical Education*. Email: Parr0068@umn.edu

Elizabeth Peter, PhD, RN, is Assistant Professor, Faculty of Nursing, and a member of the Joint Centre for Bioethics, University of Toronto, Ontario, Canada. She has published in *Nursing Inquiry, Healthcare Ethics Committee Forum, Canadian Journal of Nursing Research, British Medical Journal, Hospital Quarterly*, and *Journal of the American Medical Association*. Her research interests include trust in clinical relationships and ethical issues in home care. Email: Elizabeth.peter@utoronto.ca

Lisa Rasmussen, PhD, is managing editor of the *Philosophy and Medicine* and Assistant Editor of the *Philosophical Studies in Contemporary Culture* book series for Kluwer Academic Publishers; and comanaging editor of *The Journal of Medicine and Philosophy*. Her current research interests include bioethics consultation, moral expertise, and role morality. She is coeditor of *Bioethics and Moral Content: National Traditions of Health Care Morality* (Kluwer Academic Publishers, 2002) and *Moral Expertise: A Critical Analysis* (Kluwer Academic Publishers, forthcoming 2004). Email: Lisaraz@hotmail.com

Lissa Rechtin, MD, PhD, is a psychiatrist with Kaiser Permanente, San Francisco, California. Her research interests include work in child and adolescent psychiatry. She has published in *Journal of Phenomenological Psychology and Psychiatry* and *Journal of the British Society for Phenomenology*. Email: admi@flash.net

Raymond Reid, MD, is Research Associate, Department of International Health, Center for American Indian Health, Johns Hopkins Bloomberg School of Public Health, Baltimore, Maryland. His research interests include the study and amelioration of H. influenzae diseases, pneumococcal infections, and infantile diarrheas. He has published in *Pediatrics, New England Journal of Medicine, Journal of Pediatrics, Pediatric Infectious Disease Journal, The Lancet, Archives of Internal Medicine*, and *International Journal of Epidemiology*. Email: rreid7@juno.com

David B. Resnik, JD, PhD, is Professor, Department of Medical Humanities, The Brody School of Medicine, East Carolina University, Greenville, North Carolina, and Associate Director, The Bioethics Center, University Health Systems of Eastern North Carolina. He is the author of *The Ethics of Science: An Introduction* (Routledge, 1998); *Human Germ-line Gene Therapy: Scientific, Moral, and Political Issues* (RG Landes Bioscience, 1999); *Responsible Conduct in Research* (Oxford, 2002) and *Owning the Genome: A Moral Analysis of DNA Patenting* (SUNY Press, 2003). His research interests include the ethical dimensions of human genetics, pain management, and intellectual property. Email: resnikd@ mail.ecu.edu

Susan M. Reverby, PhD, is Professor of Women's Studies, Wellesley College, Wellesley, Massachusetts. She is the author of *Ordered to Care: The Dilemma of American Nursing, 1850–1945* (Cambridge University Press, 1987) and the editor of *Tuskegee's Truths: Rethinking the Tuskegee Syphilis Study* (University of North Carolina Press, 2000). She is completing a book on memory and the different stories told about the Tuskegee Study. Email: sreverby@wellesley.edu

Joel Rothfeld, MD, PhD, is in private practice in Neurology and Neurorehabilitation in Chico, California. He has published in *Brain Research, Pharmacological Biochemical Behavior, Experimental Brain Research, Molecular Brain Research*, and *Medscape Neurology*. His current clinical and research interests include the care and treatment of individuals with a variety of neurological disorders, including the diagnosis and treatment of Alzheimer's Disease. Email: pardar@aol.com

Jane Rysberg, PhD, is Professor, Department of Psychology, California State University, Chico. She has contributed essays to such volumes as Kathleen Kendall-Tackett, ed., *Health Consequences of Abuse in the Family: A Clinical Guide for Evidence-Based Practice* (American Psychological Association, 2003) and Charles Figley, ed., *The Handbook of Women, Stress and Trauma* (Taylor and Francis, 2004). Her research focuses on life span development. Email: jrysberg@csuchico.edu

Suresh Sahadevan, MD, FRCP, DGM, FAMS, is Senior Consultant, Department of Geriatric Medicine, Tan Tock Seng Hospital, Singapore. He has published in *International Journal of Geriatric Psychiatry, Alzheimer Disease and Associated Disorder Journal, Age and Aging*, and *International Psychogeriatrics Journal*. His research and study interests include the ethics and economics of care for the frail elderly and organization ethics. Email: suresh_sahadevan@ttsh.com.sg

Lawrence Schneiderman, MD, is Professor, Department of Family and Preventive Medicine and Department of Medicine, University of California, San Diego School of Medicine, San Diego. His research interests focus on medical ethics (including futile treatment) and literature and medicine. He is the author of *The Practice of Preventive Health Care* (Addison-Wesley, 1981) and coauthor of *Wrong Medicine: Doctors, Patients and Futile Treatment* (Johns Hopkins University Press, 2000). Email: ljs@ucsd.edu

Margaret Doyle Settle, RNC, MS, is Nurse Manager, Perinatal/Newborn Intensive Care, Massachusetts General Hospital, Boston. Her research interests include the physiologic, psychosocial, and spiritual care of infants, families, and caregivers in NICUs. She has published in *Neonatal Network, Critical Care Nurse*, and *Childbirth Educator*. Email: msettle@partners.org

Cecilia Silva, PhD, is Professor, School of Education, Texas Christian University, Forth Worth. Her research interests include bilingual and multicultural education. She has published in *Bilingual Research Journal*, *Journal of Teacher Education*, *International Journal of Inclusive Education*, *Language Arts*, and *Teacher Education and Practice*. Email: c.silva@tcu.edu

Anita Silvers, PhD, is Professor, Department of Philosophy, San Francisco State University, San Francisco, California. She is the author, coauthor, or editor of *Disability, Difference, Discrimination: Perspectives on Justice in Bioethics and Public Policy* (Rowman and Littlefield, 1998); *Americans With Disabilities: Exploring Implications of the Law for Individuals and Institutions* (Routledge, 2000); *Medicine and Social Justice* (Oxford University Press, 2002); and *Physician Assisted Suicide: Expanding the Debate* (Routledge, 1998). Her research interests include rehabilitation ethics, genetic discrimination, social contract theory, and the ethics of trust. Email: asilvers@sfsu.edu

Laura Siminoff, PhD, is Professor of Bioethics, Family Medicine, and Oncology, Case Western Reserve University School of Medicine, and Co-Director, Program in Cancer Prevention, Control and Population Research, University Hospital of Cleveland, Comprehensive Cancer Center, Cleveland, Ohio. Her research interests include consent to organ and tissue transplantation, informed consent to clinical trials, and access to care. She has published in such journals as *Annals of Internal Medicine*, *The Hastings Center Report*, *Journal of Transplant Coordination*, *Journal of Clinical Oncology*, *Journal of the American Medical Association*, *New England Journal of Medicine*, and *Journal of the Kennedy Institute of Ethics*. Email: las5@po.cwru.edu

Martin L. Smith, STD, is Chief, Clinical Ethics Service and Associate Professor, Critical Care, The University of Texas MD Anderson Cancer Center, Houston. His research interests include ethical issues related to end-of-life care, institutional ethics committees, medical mistakes, pastoral care education, and ethical issues related to patients with epilepsy. He has published in *The Hastings Center Report*, *The Journal of Clinical Ethics*, *HealthCare Ethics Committee Forum*, and *Cambridge Quarterly for Healthcare Ethics*. Email: mlsmith@MDanderson.org

Edward M. Spencer, MD, is Director of Developing Healthcare Ethics Programs, Center for Biomedical Ethics, University of Virginia Medical Center, Charlottesville. He helped establish the Center's outreach activities through the VHEN (Virginia Healthcare Ethics Network). His educational and research interests include organization ethics and research ethics. He is the coeditor of *Organization Ethics in Health Care* (Oxford University Press, 2000). Email: ems2n@virginia.edu

Harriet Spiegel, PhD, is Professor, Department of English, California State University, Chico. Her research focuses on the lives and writings of Medieval women. She is the editor and translator of Marie de France's *Fables* (University of Toronto Press, 1987). Email: hspiegel@csuchico.edu

David Swanson, PhD, is Professor, Department of Physical Education and Exercise Science, California State University, Chico; and Co-Director, Research 50 Plus Fitness Association, Palo Alto, California. His research interests include exercise physiology (health and performance), health promotion in the elderly, and patient spiritual care. He is the coeditor of *Control of Breathing: A Modeling Perspective* (Plenum, 1989) and has published in *Journal of Applied Physiology*, *Computers in Biomedical Research*, and *Biology of Sport*. Email: dswanson@csuchico.edu

Anita J. Tarzian, PhD, RN, is a Research Associate for the Law and Health Care Program at the University of Maryland School of Law, Baltimore. She has published in *The Pain Clinic*, *Journal of Law, Medicine & Ethics*, *Journal of Clinical Ethics*, *The Journal of Nursing Scholarship*, *Western Journal of Nursing Research*, and *Journal of Nursing Administration*. Her research interests focus on health care ethics, end-of-life care/hospice, palliative care, multiculturalism, and underserved populations. Email: Atarzian@juno.com

Mary Martha Thiel, MDiv, is Director of Chaplaincy and Clinical Pastoral Education Supervisor, Massachusetts General Hospital, Boston. Her research interests include spiritual care at the end of life, spiritual distress in health care providers, and spiritual caregiving by health care professionals. She has published in *The Journal of Clinical Ethics* and *Journal of Perinatology*. Email: mthiel@partners.org

Louis D. Vottero, RPh, MS, is Emeritus Professor of Pharmacy, Ohio Northern University, Ada, where he taught Ethics of Professional Pharmacy Practice and History of American Pharmacy. He is coauthor of *Ethical Practice in Pharmacy: A Guidebook for Pharmacy Technicians* (American Institute of the History of Pharmacy, 1997). He is a member of the Ethics Committee of the Canadian Pharmacists Association and a former member of the Code of Ethics Revision Committee for the American Pharmacists Association. Email: Lou@Vottero.com

Suzanne M. "Mikki" Westbie is an undergraduate major in biology and ethics at California State University, Chico. Email: mwestbie@mail.csuchico.edu

Becky Cox White, PhD, is Professor of Philosophy at California State University, Chico. She is the author of *Competence to Consent* (Georgetown University Press, 1994). Her research interests include the role of emotions in moral decision making, competence to consent, and teaching ethics. Email: bcwhite@csuchico.edu

Joel A. Zimbelman, PhD, is Professor and Chair, Department of Religious Studies, California State University, Chico. His research interests include religious ethics; technology, religion, and culture; and assisted suicide. He has published in *The Journal of Professional Nursing, The Journal of Medicine and Philosophy, HealthCare Ethics Committee Forum, Christian Bioethics: A Non-ecumenical Journal,* and *Asia Hospital.* Email: jzimbelman @csuchico.edu

A Framework
for Moral Reasoning

Eric H. Gampel, PhD

This essay offers a systematic framework for reasoning about the kinds of ethical issues that come up in health care contexts. Following an introduction to the topic of ethics, we examine the major moral principles that are especially important to medical ethics. A five-step procedure for analyzing and resolving ethical issues that incorporates those principles is then described. The procedure offers a principled alternative to the appeals to gut instinct, tradition, and politics that all too often characterize ethical problem solving. Finally we discuss the fields of moral theory and moral philosophy—areas for further study that can also improve ethical decision making.

Ethics and Health Care

Ethical issues involve matters of right and wrong, good and bad, virtue and vice, rights and responsibilities. When we take the *moral point of view*,[1] we evaluate human actions and characters morally, making judgments such as "Sara was *wrong* to unplug Uncle John from the respirator before the rest of the family could arrive"; or "Steve has a *right* to a pay raise after all he has done for the company." We will refer to these as "moral" or "ethical" judgments.[2] Of course, the moral point of view is not the only point of view we can take: we can also consider whether something is cost-effective, legal, conducive to self-interest, in accord with applicable policy, beautiful, educational, interesting, and so on. But the moral point of view can be identified through four distinguishing features.

1

First, it is mostly about *how we ought to treat people*—including, in some cases, how we ought to treat ourselves. The moral point of view is especially concerned with whether actions or persons harm others, violate their rights, are unfair, or otherwise mistreat someone. Second, the moral point of view is *normative and prescriptive*; its primary task is not a description of what the world is like, but a prescription of what people ought to do (or what a person's character ought to be like). The purpose of the moral point of view is to guide action, not simply to describe how things are. Third, the moral point of view often *overrides* other considerations, especially those of self-interest. This does not mean that the moral point of view always prevails, only that we often judge that it *should* prevail.[3] Fourth, the moral point of view is *universalizable*, leading us to make moral judgments we expect others to share, even if they come from very different cultural or religious backgrounds. This is most clear in the case of very general moral claims, such as the wrongness of deliberate harm, or of not giving people what they deserve. Of course, there are also moral claims we take to be *subjective* or relative to a cultural context, such as whether honoring parents requires letting them choose your marriage partner, or whether to show respect through a handshake or by spitting at the ground. But there still seems a universal core: even if *how* we honor parents or show respect differs across cultures and communities, the importance of having *some* customary manner of doing so is a universal and uncontroversial human value.

For some ethical issues there is not much controversy at all—just about everyone agrees on what would be the morally right (or wrong) thing to do. These include most of the actions forbidden by criminal and civil law in all cultures—murder, theft, assault, negligence, fraud. In health care contexts, such actions sometimes involve physicians, nurses, or other health care professionals (HCPs) who have become clearly "corrupt"—stealing medications for personal use, providing inappropriate therapies for personal gain, writing ghost prescriptions to sell drugs on the black market, and so on. These kinds of ethical issues do not usually call out for analysis or careful reasoning—we know what is morally right, have passed laws to enforce it, and need only keep watch that any who violate the laws are prosecuted.

But other ethical issues are less clear-cut. Should the truth be told when it will do harm to tell it? Do the bonds of friendship mean we must protect a friend or colleague, even in his or her unethical behavior? How far must we sacrifice our own interests to help others, and in what ways? When our jobs seem to require acts about which we have ethical reservations, should we ignore the job's requirements and do what we believe to be morally right? Not everyone agrees about these kinds of ethical issues—they involve controversial questions about the shape of our ethical duties. Partly for that reason, it is common for there to be no laws, rules, or policies governing the more controversial ethical issues—or for there to be uncertainty regarding how to interpret, or whether to follow, any legal or institutional requirements. This is where clarity and careful ethical reasoning are important. We all must make choices involving ethical issues, and those choices stem from and help define our characters and our values. Moreover, the choices are often made in social contexts of friendships, families, and professional life, in ways that affect other people, are seen by others, and establish patterns of behavior for ourselves and others to follow. So how we resolve the less clear-cut ethical issues matters—to us as individuals, to those directly affected by our actions, and sometimes to a broader community as well.

Health care is filled with these less clear-cut ethical issues, where law, policy, and widely shared moral rules do not settle the question of what we should do. For instance, if family members of a dying woman disagree about whether it is time to unplug her from a respirator, how should the decision be resolved? If a patient does not consent to a beneficial treatment, should a nurse try to further inform and persuade the patient, or simply let the patient's decision stand? When not all can receive a scarce medical resource, such as an organ or simply a health professional's time and attention, what criteria should be used to select those who receive it? Such ethical issues saturate medicine, and they form the material for the cases in this book.

The Hippocratic tradition of medical ethics, beginning in ancient Greek times, sought to establish certain ethical principles and virtues that would help physicians navigate the less clear ethical waters. For instance, physicians were often told "above all, do no harm"—an important reminder in the days when little was known about how to cure and the use of untried and risky measures was a daily temptation. In general, the Hippocratic tradition handled ethical issues "in-house," with an emphasis on developing virtuous character and good general dispositions. Physicians trained students to follow the time-tested ways, developing the bedside manner and character traits of a virtuous physician: a dedication to helping patients, a devotion to medical learning, respect for patient confidentiality, and loyalty to fellow physicians. This approach worked well enough, perhaps, when most physicians were general practitioners, working with patients whom they knew intimately for long periods of time. But in modern medicine, the explosions of technology and specialization since the 1960s have meant that health professionals often work in teams, and meet their patients for the first time as referrals. In addition, patients now come from diverse cultural, religious, moral, and linguistic backgrounds, increasing the possibilities for misunderstanding and moral disagreement.

In this modern context of health care, the number and complexity of ethical issues has also increased, and has led to the establishment of health care ethics as a field of study in its own right. Since the 1960s, a regular stream of books and articles have been published, ethics committees have been formed, and policies have been developed, all to come up with better ways to handle the kinds of ethical issues that arise in modern medicine. Individual HCPs must still navigate by their own moral compasses, but there is a scholarly background of medical ethics that has been shaped by a self-conscious and wide-ranging ethical reflection.

Major Moral Principles

Modern health care is subject to a plethora of explicit laws, rules, and policies. For instance, only 20 years ago physicians just talked informally to the terminally ill about whether they would want ventilation support or other life-sustaining measures. Today, there are multipage advance directive forms, such as living wills and powers of attorney for health care, along with laws requiring that hospitals tell patients about the forms. As a result, most hospitals have implemented policies requiring staff to obtain patient signatures indicating they have been informed about the availability of advance directives.

Many such rules and policies were established in the name of ethics: to ensure that medical professionals treat patients well, acting with compassion and respect for individual rights. But the rules and policies are still not the "court of last appeal" when considering what it would be ethical to do. For one thing, the rules can change, even dramatically, as evidenced by the rise of advance directives. More significantly, the rules sometimes conflict with other moral ideas. For instance, one might question whether it is humane to insist on every patient's "right" to fill out a form about when he or she would like life-sustaining treatments withheld. What about a frightened patient facing a low-risk surgery, whose fear is exacerbated by considering the extremely unlikely situations addressed by advance directives? What about patients whose ability to think clearly is compromised by the anxiety of a medical emergency, by illness, or by medications? Might it be best not to worry about advance directives for such patients, at least low-risk ones? Should one perhaps "bend" legal or administrative rules, for instance getting signatures indicating patients have been informed about advance directives by simply offering the signature in a stack of paperwork, without explaining the nature or purpose of advance directives?

So HCPs cannot (and generally do not) just blindly follow the rules or the "standard" procedure: they reflect on the situation and evaluate what would be best, given the specific circumstances. For behind the rules and standard procedures, and behind the changes made in them over the years, are other, more fundamental moral ideas and values. The field of bioethics has developed a short and useful list of the kinds of fundamental moral principles significant to medical contexts.[4] The following list has been organized around the acronym CARVE as a memory aid:[5]

1. *Consequences* (C): promote the best possible consequences for all those affected by your action. This very broad moral principle includes three subprinciples regarding the health and well-being of persons:
   a. *The principle of nonmaleficence* (NM): refrain from causing unnecessary harm. This principle reminds HCPs to take due care not to subject patients to unnecessary risks, or to harm patients through their own negligence.

b. *The principle of positive beneficence* (B): take action to benefit others. This principle identifies the goal of medicine: to help improve the health and well-being of individual patients.

c. *The principle of utility* (U): act so as to produce the best possible outcome for the welfare of the group as a whole, when some people are harmed while others benefit. This principle directs HCPs to look beyond their individual patients, considering how a decision might be affecting other patients, family, and the general public. As a result, utility allows trade-offs in which an individual patient's well-being might be sacrificed for the greater good, as in quarantines, mandatory inoculations, and violations of confidentiality that are required to protect third parties.

2. *Respect for Autonomy* (A): respect and promote the self-determination of competent persons. This is the principle behind rules of informed consent and truth-telling, since both seek to help patients make their own decisions about the course of their health care. The principle requires both letting patients make their own decisions, and giving them the information about risks, benefits, and burdens that is relevant to their decisions.

3. *Rights* (R): respect individual moral rights, such as rights to freedom and confidentiality. This principle directs HCPs to consider not just the legal but the moral rights of patients.

4. *Virtues* (V): act in accord with good character, expressing such virtues as honesty, courage, fidelity, integrity, and compassion. This principle focuses on the character, motives, and intentions of HCPs and patients.

5. *Equality* (E): treat people with equal consideration and respect, being fair and not discriminating on the basis of morally irrelevant features (such as income, race, or gender).[6] Note that when equality and fairness are at issue, people often speak of "justice" and "injustice," as they do when important moral rights are at stake.

These principles as stated are completely uncontroversial, in the sense that everyone grants their relevance to the practice of medicine. Any controversy stems from the details of their interpretation, application, or relative priority. People have different views about how to define harms, benefits, competence, rights, virtue, and fairness, as well as about how to weigh those different considerations. But the principles provide a shared and systematic way of identifying the concerns important to health care ethics, a basis for further discussion and reflection. Even in today's diverse environments of care, with persons from widely different cultural and religious backgrounds, the principles can serve—with a few caveats—as common touchstones for reasoning about ethical issues.

What people agree on is *not* that the CARVE principles are exhaustive or absolute, but that they are *prima facie* obligations on practitioners—presumptive obligations that give moral reasons for action, though reasons that might be out-weighed by other considerations (including competing moral principles from the CARVE list). This distinguishes the principles from *absolute* obligations, which hold independently of context and may never be outweighed. Some people take the Ten Commandments to be morally absolute; what makes the CARVE principles differ-ent, and much less controversial, is that they are offered for health care contexts only as prima facie obligations that identify the kinds of moral considerations we should take into account.

The result is that when a moral issue comes up in a health care environment, progress can be made in discussions or in personal reflection by considering how the CARVE principles apply to the situation. (You will see examples of the use of these principles in this essay, and in the commentaries throughout this book.) The principles cannot serve as a litmus test or simple decision procedure, of course, and HCPs are quite often faced with too little time to engage in detailed ethical analy-sis. But in many cases there is time, and analysis can always be done in retrospect, as HCPs seek to understand and improve on how situations are handled. The CARVE principles help identify the major values at stake—a first step in under-standing a moral issue. Sometimes this is simple, as when a single CARVE principle is clearly the primary and decisive consideration to take into account. But often one is blind to aspects of a case that are important, and going through all the CARVE principles can bring the other aspects to one's awareness. Indeed, people tend to emphasize one or another principle in their own personal and professional ethical lives: some people pride themselves on their compassion, others on their respect for individual rights. Those long-standing emphases can function as biases, albeit well-intentioned ones, that blind people to the other moral considerations relevant to health care ethics. Going through CARVE, making sure one sees all the ethical dimensions of a case, can thus be a useful corrective device.

The use of CARVE can also help overcome other kinds of prejudices and biases learned from one's upbringing or training as a health care professional. For instance, until fairly recently physicians were trained under a paternalistic model, according to which physicians were to do what was best for the patient even if it meant protecting them from the truth, or not granting them full decision-making power. This model was based on a long-standing medical tradition, learned directly from one's teachers, and it was associated with a cluster of gut feelings: compassion for the vulnerable pa-tient, a sense of expertise, and feelings of authority, privilege, and integrity. This pa-ternalistic model has been overthrown in recent decades, mainly on the grounds that it conflicts with two CARVE principles: the rights and autonomy of patients. Many physicians resisted the change for quite a while, since it went against deeply rooted instincts about the nature of the compassionate, virtuous physician. But antipaternal-ists argued that true compassion requires being responsive to the patient's need for autonomy, and that true integrity requires respecting the patient's rights. The point is that a blind following of one's gut feelings risks making one unable to see the possibil-ity of such arguments. Of course, the paternalistic model could itself be defended on the basis of CARVE principles—giving primacy to the principles of beneficence and nonmaleficence. So having the list of CARVE principles is not going to resolve the question of whether physicians should be paternalistic. But the CARVE principles help articulate the ethical controversy, and they bring one's attention away from the gut feelings inculcated by professional training toward the deeper values at stake.

A Procedure for Moral Reasoning: The AJ Method

The major moral principles are useful tools in moral reflection. The principles help identify the values behind different choices, ensure one has not missed important moral considerations, and provide a common vocabulary for discussions with others. But questions about how to interpret, apply, and weigh the principles are inevitable. As in any case where judgment is involved, there is no substitute for experience and practice in developing good moral reasoning skills: seeing many cases, making tough moral decisions, observing and living with the results. This book provides many cases on which to practice. You may well find that after reading a case, you have a "gut instinct," an intuitive sense of what should or should not be done. The CARVE principles should help you identify the values behind that instinctive position. But after reading some of the commentaries, or discussing the case with others, you will usually find that your intuition needs further support: there are moral arguments and CARVE principles on the other side; and you could imagine an intelligent and decent person having a different "gut instinct" about the case, based on a different understanding of the CARVE principles or their relative importance. Here it would be useful to analyze the case and the moral arguments more carefully, to better understand and possibly reevaluate your initial position.

The procedure for moral reasoning described below involves five simple steps to take when faced with an ethical issue.[7] Going through these steps involves carefully analyzing the ethical issue, and then justifying a position on how to best handle it; we will thus call the method the "Analysis and Justification Method" (or the "AJ Method"). This is not the only possible method of ethical reasoning, and it is not strictly followed by HCPs, ethicists, or other professionals involved in the field of biomedical ethics (lawyers, clergy, etc.). But the AJ Method incorporates most of the elements to be found in any good attempt to analyze and justify a position on a biomedical issue. We thus offer this method as a useful guide. Simply reading through it can help further develop your skills in ethical reasoning, and it can be used more formally to structure group discussions, individual reflection, or essays on ethical issues.

The first four steps in the AJ Method are "neutral" ones, involving a careful analysis of the issue with which all parties should agree; only the last step involves taking a stand on the moral issue, and that step requires explaining and justifying (to oneself or others) why one set of reasons outweighs those on the other side. Going through the procedure does not guarantee avoiding mistakes or coming up with the right view—no procedure can guarantee that everyone thinks clearly and insightfully, and there may even be more than one reasonable stand on a moral question. But the recommended procedure does provide a framework that helps one to minimize mistakes, and to better understand the deeper issues involved. The procedure is thus a way to expand your moral imagination, urging you to take into account more of the moral factors involved in an issue, and making your judgments more subtle, complex, and well-grounded.

Step 1: Information Gathering (IG)

The very first step in tackling an ethical issue is to make sure one fully understands the factual elements of the situation, as well as any background information important to the issue. In bioethics this usually means learning as much as possible about: (1) the *medical circumstances* involved; (2) the *implications* of different decisions for the lives of patients and their families (consequences); (3) the *history* of the situation, especially elements that are important to applying the CARVE principles of rights, virtue, and equality; (4) any relevant *laws or institutional policies*; (5) *economic* considerations; and (6) the *cultural and psychological* dimensions of the situation, especially as they affect the determination of competency and the application of the CARVE principle of autonomy. In hospital bioethics committees, investigating these various kinds of information about a specific case means having extensive discussions with HCPs, families, and patients; in academic contexts, this may mean more scholarly research on factors relevant to the ethical issue under consideration.

As an example, if a family is in disagreement over whether to end life support, we need to be sure we really understand (1) the medical circumstances: What is the medical condition, who made the diagnosis and prognosis, how sure are they, and are there any differing opinions? We also should consider (2) the implications of a decision: What does ending life support really mean for the patient and the family? Does the patient have any prospect of enjoying a sustained life, or would we be causing needless suffering to keep the patient alive (nonmaleficence)? If life support were to continue, would family members be unduly postponing their lives or their grieving (utility)? In addition, we ought to be acquainted with (3) the history: What led to the current disagreement amongst family members? Have they all always felt as they do, or has there been an evolution in their views as the case progressed? How have medical staff dealt with the family over time (virtue, equality)? Of course, we need to also know about (4) law and policy: Who has the *legal* decisional power within the family, as a legal proxy if there is a power of attorney, or as next of kin? What is the policy of the institution about family disagreements: is there a clear directive or informal norm allowing delays until a family works out its disagreements? Is there room under law or policy for questioning decisional power in a case like this one—for example, are there questions about motive or competence which are clearly relevant to applying law or policy (rights)? What are the penalties, if any, for going against the legal or policy mandates? Would jobs be lost, or civil suits likely to succeed against the institution? This raises the matter of (5) economic considerations: What would be the economic burdens of continued treatment, or the risk assessments regarding the likelihood of being sued (utility)? Would continued life support take money from an estate, and are some family members concerned about that? Finally, we should consider (6) the cultural and psychological dimensions of the situation: Are there religious differences between family members leading to their disagreement? Is there evidence of what the patient would have wanted (autonomy)? Do some family members want to avoid the guilt of going along with a decision to end life support? Is there a rift in the family that leads inevitably to fights, no matter the issue at hand? These various questions need to be explored to make progress in figuring out how the situation should be handled.

Step 2: Creative Problem Solving (CPS)

The ideal way of dealing with a tough ethical dilemma is to come up with a creative plan of action that avoids the ethically troubling alternatives, while still solving the problem that created the dilemma. This requires a strategy that cannot be reasonably objected to on moral grounds. In health care contexts, this is often where ethical reflection begins and, with a little good fortune, ends: in a creative strategy which all parties recognize to be consistent with each of the CARVE principles and (thus) ethically untroubling.

For instance, if an expensive, medically recommended procedure is not covered by a patient's insurance, and the patient cannot afford to pay for it, there is an apparent dilemma: forgo the procedure, risking the patient's health, or provide the procedure anyway, billing the patient while knowing payment will never be forthcoming, requiring that others absorb the costs (through higher charges for medical services, government reimbursements, or decreased profits). If we choose to forgo the procedure, we are violating the principles of beneficence and perhaps equality; but if we provide the procedure without expecting the patient to pay, we are arguably violating the rights of those who would have to absorb the costs—perhaps other patients who would be paying higher charges, or taxpayers, or shareholders, depending on how the costs would be absorbed. This is a dilemma about the demands of *justice*, with claims of fairness and rights on both sides. A creative solution would avoid the moral problem—which means finding a way to provide good health care to the patient without requiring that others absorb the costs, thereby not violating any major moral principles. But how?

Here a bit of creative (and optimistic) thinking is in order. Perhaps there is another medical procedure, covered by the patient's insurance, which is a reasonable alternative to the one that is not covered? Or perhaps further negotiations with the insurance agency can convince it to extend the coverage in this instance? Or maybe the funds can be found elsewhere—an organized charity, or a fund-raising campaign by family and friends? If any of these strategies worked, ethical controversy would be avoided; the problem would be solved.

This stage of moral reasoning is perhaps the most important one for the everyday practice of health care. People in the health care professions are very talented at it, and take it to be a major part of their jobs. Psychology and counseling are quite often at the center stage in such creative problem solving, since ethical dilemmas are often raised by conflicts amongst patients, family, medical staff, and insurance companies, and those conflicts may be dissolved through good dialogue, further information, and various other practical strategies (e.g., participation in a support group, viewing of informational videos, etc.). When conflicts between the parties can be resolved, the dilemma goes away; everyone agrees on the proper course of care. But this is not always the case: sometimes HCPs cannot find successful creative solutions, and must face the hard choice between morally troubling options.

Step 3: Listing Pros and Cons (PC)

Faced with the hard choice, one must explore the moral reasons for and against each of the morally troubling choices, the moral "pros and cons." To keep track of the various ethical considerations, one can construct a simple list of the main options, and the reasons for or against each option. As mechanical as such a procedure seems, keeping track of all of the important moral arguments can make a tremendous difference in the quality of moral reasoning. In a group setting, it ensures all participants have their reasons written down and addressed, and in personal decision making it provides a map of the relevant moral reasons for further analysis. In addition, this is the point where the CARVE principles are especially useful. After going through the moral reasons you take to be obvious, go through each CARVE principle and see what it would lead you to consider important about the case. This often brings out moral factors you miss at first glance, given your own initial bias about the case, or your specific moral perspective. Even if a consideration seems trivial, if it is backed by a CARVE principle perhaps it deserves further thought. The resulting list of moral reasons has the following form (with the CARVE principles included in parentheses to identify the general values behind each reason):

	Pros	**Cons**
1st Option	1. Reason for 1st Option (CARVE Principle)	3. Reason against 1st Option (CARVE Principle)
2nd Option	2. Reason for 2nd Option (CARVE Principle)	4. Reason against 2nd Option (CARVE Principle)

The goal at this stage is to provide a map of the moral reasons for further reflection, a map that will be neutral in an important sense: people who disagree about which option is best could still accept the map as identifying the main moral considerations important to the case. Usually it is best not to list trivial reasons, since that can clutter up the chart, and to keep the options to two or three. Note that not every pro/con box needs to be filled: as long as there is a reason or argument listed on each diagonal (in a two-option chart), each option has something in the chart that is in its favor. Also, be prepared for cases where a reason could fit either as a pro for one option or a con against an alternative. For instance, one might argue for providing surgery based on the fact that it could save the patient's life (a pro), or against forgoing surgery because the patient could die (a con). Rather than double-entering this basic idea, it is best to list the reason one place or the other but not both.

Step 4: Analysis (A)

The next step is the most challenging and difficult one, where the *strengths* of the various reasons in the pro/con list are evaluated. The key here is to be thorough, seriously considering whether each reason is a strong one, taken independently or in comparison to other reasons on the pro/con list. One way to do this is to keep in mind the question:

What assumptions are necessary to consider the reason extremely important? Some assumptions will be (1) *factual*, in the sense of not directly involving moral values. They would involve the sort of factual information to be investigated in Step 1, but it may be that there is no good evidence or agreement about the factual issue involved, so that different persons might make different assumptions about it.[8] In bioethics such assumptions are typically about the likelihood of an outcome, the long-term consequences of a decision, or the true motivations or intentions of the parties. In contrast, other assumptions will be (2) about the deeper *values and moral principles* at stake, and their relative importance. For instance, if one is considering a complicated rehabilitative surgery to give a disabled patient full use of his arms, one might be making factual assumptions about the degree of risk or the likelihood of success, or one might be making a value assumption about whether it is worth risking a patient's life to improve its quality in this way. Thus, a reason should be considered a strong one only if it is *quite likely to protect or promote an important value.* These two judgments, of likelihood and importance, rest on factual and value assumptions that need to be examined.

This is especially apparent when people from different religious or cultural backgrounds are involved in a case or its analysis, since such differences often go along with radically different assumptions. For instance, some people from certain religious traditions assume that spiritual strategies of healing have a very good chance of success. So when physicians admit that an illness is not easily treated with a proven cure, some religious people forgo the recommended but uncertain medical strategies in favor of their spiritual approach. Note that this choice is based on a factual assumption by the religious persons that spiritual strategies have good prospects for curing. The assumption is not factual in the sense of provable, but it is factual in the sense that it has to do with the factual outcomes involved, not with the weighting of values. Alternatively, a religious person might place more value on reverence for life itself, apart from the quality of the life. This could lead to avoiding surgical risks, on the basis of a different value assumption than the one made by a person who counts life not to be worth living, once its quality drops sufficiently.

Notice that this analysis step is still "neutral," in the sense that people who disagree about which option is best can agree on the analysis. At this stage one is only further exploring the reasons, considering what might lead a person to view a reason as especially strong (or weak), and raising questions about the factual and value assumptions thus unearthed. This means that even before making up one's mind about a case, or taking a position in a discussion, the proposed method requires one to *imaginatively put oneself in the shoes of those who weigh the reasons in different ways.* Nevertheless, this can bring to light the more vulnerable or unsupported assumptions, thus leading into the next step of taking a position and defending it. For instance, if an assumption that is crucial to considering a reason a strong one is factual, one can ask if there is any good evidence for it, or if one would be making a mere guess. If one would be guessing, is it reasonable to base a morally significant decision on such a guess? Alternatively, if an assumption is evaluative or moral in nature, one can ask if there are any good moral reasons for that assumption: why should we interpret rights or autonomy in the requisite way, and what moral assumptions are built into that way of interpreting the value? This process helps one to see which are the more and less reasonable weightings of the reasons, since some of the assumptions are likely to look more plausible than others.

In addition, looking at the assumptions behind the evaluation of reasons helps identify what really lies at the core of disagreements about which option is best. In this context a useful question is:

*What **difference** in basic assumptions can explain why reasonable people might disagree about the strength of a reason?*

Once again, sometimes the differing assumptions will be about the factual elements of a case—what is the likelihood of a certain outcome, how a patient will accommodate to a certain outcome. At other times the assumptions will be about the values at stake. But it is important to identify the real source of a difference in perspective about the case.

People in health care contexts often focus their discussions and arguments on the strictly factual aspects of bioethics dilemmas: on what the chances are for recovery, on the likely outcome for various parties, on the relevant psychological and legal factors, or on the long-term consequences of a given decision. These are matters about which HCPs can offer their expert judgments, and such matters are reasonably comfortable to discuss. But restricting the conversation to factual matters risks ignoring the underlying value issues at stake, and it is at least equally important to consider those issues. Indeed, there is sometimes little or no good evidence for some of the factual predictions on which people base their arguments, raising the question of whether their positions are really based on something else, specifically on *value as-*

sessments that are more difficult to defend. For instance, one might argue for the rehabilitative surgery mentioned above on the grounds that it is safe and quite likely to succeed, when the real reason is that one doesn't much value a life of disability. So it is important in this analysis step to question any factual assumptions for which there is no real evidence, in case a deeper value commitment is really at work, and then to consider whether that value commitment can be adequately supported.

Step 5: Justification (J)

At this point one has identified the relevant moral reasons, the moral principles on which they depend, and the factual and value assumptions being made by those who take one or another reason to be especially significant. This means one should have a good understanding of the ethical issue, why people might disagree about it, and usually a sense of which option has stronger moral support, in light of the reasons, principles, and assumptions one has determined to be most important or plausible. The next step is to work through a systematic justification of the morally preferable option. The key to a successful justification is this:

> Identify why the reasons for one option are more convincing than the reasons on the other side, based on a reasonable assessment of the factual and value issues important to the case.

Working out a systematic justification can be done in different spirits—simply to test one's initial view, or as a final defense of one's position. It can also be done in different contexts: as a presentation at a meeting, in conversation with friends, as a series of notes on paper for oneself, or in a formal essay for sharing with others. In any of these cases, it is always important to cover all the reasons someone could consider significant—that is, all the reasons listed in the pro/con chart. Here is an outline of this process that can aid in constructing presentations or written work:

I. **Introduction:** Briefly introduce the moral issue, and indicate the option your analysis has shown to be morally preferable.

II. **Support:** For each reason in the pro/con chart that supports the option you prefer, write a paragraph explaining what your analysis has shown about the reason. Identify why it is strong or important (if it is), and discuss and defend any factual or value assumptions behind that judgment. (Note: the reasons that "support" an option include (a) the pros for the option, and (b) the cons against the alternative options, since those provide indirect support by working against the alternatives.)

III. **Defense:** For each reason in the pro/con chart that goes against the option you prefer, write a paragraph detailing what your analysis has shown about the reason. Identify why it is weak or unimportant, and discuss and defend any factual or value assumptions behind that judgment. (Note: the reasons that "go against" an option include (a) the cons directly against it, and (b) the pros that attempt to support the alternative options.)

IV. **Summary:** Summarize the reasoning. Review the most important reason favoring the better option, and remind the reader why the main reason against that option is not as significant.

This format ensures that every reason from the pro/con list is carefully presented and evaluated. All too often presentations and written justifications simply put forward the supporting side, including the reasons against alternative views, without explaining why the reasons on the other side, against one's position, are not just as important. That can lead to parties speaking past one another, or to a kind of tunnel vision when working through moral dilemmas on one's own. A way to avoid this is always to keep in mind a reasonable critic, one who disagrees with your position but is willing to hear your reasons and be convinced if the reasons are good ones. What could sway such a person to weight the reasons as you would? Here the key is to further defend the factual and value assumptions behind your weighting of reasons. What is your evidence for the factual assumption about which someone might initially disagree? What kinds of moral argument can support a value assumption about the importance of one moral principle, as compared to the other principles at issue in the case? Why might someone disagree, and what mistake or misunderstanding lies behind that disagreement?

A Sample Case Study

In the analyses throughout this book you will see commentators use the principles and techniques discussed in this chapter, though not usually in the exact step-by-step manner described here. Before turning to those commentaries, it may be useful to review the framework described in this chapter by considering how the CARVE principles and the AJ Method might be used systematically to tackle a sample case. Here is the case:

> Following an auto accident Ms. A and her four children are admitted to a small rural hospital. Three of the children are doing well, but the fourth, a young girl, was dead on arrival. Ms. A suffers from broken ribs and internal bleeding; she is fully conscious, and deeply distraught over her children. She repeatedly asks how they are doing.
>
> Ms. A's physician, Dr. B, assures her that her children are fine, and writes an order in the chart specifying that Ms. A is not to be told of the child's death until morning, at which time her condition will have stabilized and her husband will have arrived to support her. Ms. A's nurse, Ms. C, understands the physician's concerns but worries that patients have a right to the truth and, in any case, thinks it would be horrible to have to

look her patient in the eye and repeat a lie of such magnitude.[9] *After the physician has gone, Ms. A asks, "Tell me the truth, are my children all OK, and why can't I see them?" Ms. C wonders whether she shouldn't tell this mother what she so clearly wants to know.*

In this case, the right thing to do is not obvious at first glance: if Ms. C tells the truth it might cause Ms. A's condition to worsen, perhaps causing her death; but faced with a direct question the only other option seems to be to tell a lie, one of great magnitude. Telling the truth is responsive to Ms. A's rights and autonomy, but it threatens to violate nonmaleficence, arguably the most important principle governing the care of patients. So this is a genuine moral dilemma, one worth wrestling with.

Step 1: Information Gathering

The most crucial information here concerns the risk to Ms. A: how serious is that risk, and thus what are the chances that we are violating nonmaleficence if we give Ms. A the news of her daughter's death? Investigating this requires more information about Ms. A's *medical condition*, and the potential *implications* of telling her the bad news: how likely is it that being told the bad news would threaten her life or complicate the recovery process? These could be discussed with Dr. B, Ms. C, and other medical experts, if available, and we could do general research on traumatic injury cases, to understand the kinds of injuries involved and the kinds of threats such injuries make to continued survival. We could then look for any studies about the implications of psychological or emotional stress on the relevant physiological conditions involved in traumatic injuries, such as blood pressure and heart rate. Perhaps there is good evidence in the medical or psychological literature that emotional stress or grief has a dramatic effect on such physiological conditions, and thus evidence that there is a substantial risk to Ms. C if she is told the bad news. Or perhaps there is evidence that there are no such dramatic effects (e.g., a study indicating that there are no known cases where emotional trauma was causally important to a patient's death).

We might also investigate the *history* of the persons involved here and their relationships: Does Ms. A have a good and trusting relationship with Dr. B and/or Nurse C? Do Dr. B and Nurse C have high regard amongst other HCPs and patients, or do they have a history of questionable decision making? Was Ms. A promised by medical staff that she would be kept informed about her children—for example, if she protested their absence at some point? These historical factors affect how to apply the principles of rights, virtue, and equality (fairness), and they could substantially shape a decision about what to do.

As for the *law and policy* issues, these are probably quite complex, since the contemplated lie (normally against law and policy) is in defense of a life, which law and policy often explicitly or implicitly allow as an exception. But there might be relevant case law worth exploring, or a history of cases at the specific institution, and these might concern not only the general question of informing at-risk patients, but also the question of the role of nurses in withholding such information on physicians' orders.

It is unlikely that *economic* considerations are crucial here, though it might be worth looking into a risk assessment regarding a potential suit by Ms. A or her survivors should we make one choice or another. But it would clearly be important to know more about Ms. A's *cultural and psychological* situation, if possible: Is she someone prone to extreme emotional reactions, or more even-keeled? Is she from a cultural or religious tradition that might affect her way of seeing the loss of a child, or the event of having been lied to about her child?

Step 2: Creative Problem Solving

The information gathered in Step 1 might resolve the case: perhaps there is clearly no risk to Ms. A's health, and the physician is simply misinformed. But more likely, the information has only enriched our understanding without clearly resolving the issue. So the next strategy is to find a way out of the dilemma of whether to tell such a terrible lie, or risk killing Ms. A with the truth.

A natural thought is for Ms. C to try to avoid doing either, for instance trying to redirect Ms. A's concern by saying "we need to worry about *you* right now." This would not be a lie, and it might avoid causing Ms. A emotional distress. Alternatively, Ms. C could simply pretend ignorance of the children's condition, which would involve a lie, but arguably a less troublesome one than saying that all the children are fine. Notice, however, that these techniques could actually cause Ms. A to become more irritated and anxious about not receiving the answers she is seeking, which may still risk causing her condition to worsen. So the strategies might be worth trying, but if they do lead to psychological frustration and physiological decline, the nurse would still be faced with the question of whether to ease the anxiety by telling the lie.

Another creative strategy would be to find other family or close friends to support Ms. A before telling her the truth. One could even make sure her husband is on the phone, having been informed of the situation—and perhaps he could help assess whether Ms. A would be able to handle the news, with his knowledge of how she deals with emotional difficulties. But notice that these sorts of strategies still involve acting against the physician's orders, a moral concern involving virtue and rights, so they do not completely avoid the dilemma.

Another possibility would be to medicate Ms. A so that she is unable to ask or worry about her children. Of course, this may be an unreasonable option, given Ms. A's condition, but it may be that induced sleep would be medically advantageous, in which case it is a solution that would avoid the dilemma.

Step 3: Listing the Pros and Cons

Let us suppose these creative strategies all fail, or face serious moral objections, so Ms. C faces just two primary options: telling Ms. A about the death of her daughter, or lying and saying her daughter is still alive. Of course, there are lots of different ways of telling the truth—bluntly and insensitively, or with care and compassion. And there are different ways of lying: saying her daughter is perfectly OK, saying you are unsure how she is doing, or saying she is in surgery. The differences are important to consider, but for simplicity, we can speak of two options, telling the truth and lying, keeping in mind that there are various ways of exercising each of the options.

The question then is which of the two options is the better one, and to make progress in answering it we can list the pros and cons, putting down the obvious ones first. In favor of telling the truth is that the mother has a right to know about the condition of her own child, which involves the CARVE principle of rights. But in favor of lying to her, despite her apparent right to know, is the consideration that the physician has instructed the nurse to do so, and ordinarily nurses should follow physicians' orders. This involves the CARVE principle of virtue, since it is appealing to a general trait of character that nurses should have: a tendency to respect and follow the instructions of the physicians in charge of their patients' care. Against that idea is of course the thought that lying is wrong, a violation of the autonomy and rights of patients; but against telling the truth is the thought that doing so could seriously harm the mother, given her vulnerable medical condition. This leaves us with the following chart of basic moral pros and cons, with the related CARVE principles in parentheses:

	Pros	**Cons**
Tell the truth	1. Ms. A has a right to know about her child (Rights)	3. It could cause her condition to worsen (Nonmaleficence)
Lie	2. Dr. B has instructed Ms. C not to tell Ms. A about the daughter's death (Virtue)	4. Lying is wrong (Autonomy, Rights)

To be systematic, let us consider each of the CARVE principles in more detail, to see if we have missed anything. Nonmaleficence is represented by reason #3, the concern not to harm the mother with the news. Beneficence might lead one to try to comfort Ms. A with the lie, but that concern, while morally relevant in most contexts, is trivial in this one, and so it need not be included. Utility requires looking to all those persons affected by one's choices, and that means considering others besides the mother, something not yet incorporated in the pro/con list. Who else might be affected? The other children, of course, if the mother is harmed by hearing the news. There is also a larger concern about the effects of lying on the reputation of health care professionals. If the lie is told, the mother may come to distrust and resent those who lied to her, and that sentiment is one she may share with others. This could harm the reputation of the profession—however important and well-intentioned the lie may have been—leading to future patients not trusting medical professionals, which could mean withholding information or even refraining from seeking medical assistance (at least until it is urgent, and perhaps too late). These are significant concerns overlooked in the first list, and worth adding as a separate reason against lying (see below).

As for the principle of respect for autonomy, it also goes against lying to Ms. A; in misinforming, one would be manipulating Ms. A's view of the world for one's own purposes.[10] This is already reflected in the chart for reason #4. Autonomy might also tell in favor of Ms. C making her own moral decision, rather than just following the physician's directions, which would undercut the importance of reason #2. That is worth noting, but it is something that can be considered later since it concerns an evaluation of the strength of a reason rather than a new reason altogether. Rights are represented—the right to know the truth about your children, and the right not to be lied to. Virtue appears, as the idea that a good nurse should follow a physician's orders. But notice that virtue can also cut the other way: it is not obvious that the virtue of obedience should override virtues of honesty and integrity in the nursing profession. So it would be worth inserting this idea into the chart, especially since Ms. C's own concern, as reflected in the case description, seems to have to do with the matter of her own personal integrity in participating in the lie (see below). Finally, equality (and the related concept of fairness) do not seem directly relevant, unless one speaks of the unfairness of lying to the mother, something better captured by the idea of her rights. The revised pro/con list then reads:

	Pros	Cons
Tell the truth	1. Ms. A has a right to know about her child (Rights)	3. It could cause her condition to worsen (Nonmaleficence)
Lie	2. Dr. B has instructed Ms. C not to tell Ms. A about the daughter's death (Virtue)	4. Lying is wrong (Autonomy, Rights) 5. May contribute to loss of trust in the medical profession (Utility) 6. Violates the nurse's honesty and integrity (Virtue)

Step 4: Analysis

All the reasons listed in the chart are morally relevant, and have some moral force. What assumptions must be made to consider any one reason substantially stronger than another?

The most obvious place to start is with *factual assumptions* about how likely the truth is to cause the mother serious harm. One might assume that there is a significant risk, on the grounds that this must be why the doctor wanted to wait until the morning, or based on general knowledge of the effects of emotional stress on the physiology of those under critical care. But is this sufficient evidence? Alternatively, one could argue that it is just as likely the doctor simply wanted to wait so the husband could deal with the mother and her emotional reaction, rather than having to deal with it himself.

If we are forced to admit uncertainty about the likelihood of harm, it raises the question of what the "default" position should be when one is uncertain about causing harm, which can involve *value assumptions* worth exploring. For instance, one might be assuming that even a slight chance of causing death is a powerful, overwhelming moral consideration, based on the idea that the most significant moral principle for health care is to avoid harm (nonmaleficence). Note that this is an assumption about values, not an assumption about the facts: people who *agree* about the chance of causing death could *disagree* about its moral importance. For why think nonmaleficence should override prohibitions on lying, or considerations of rights and autonomy? In recent years more emphasis has been put on respecting the rights and autonomy of patients, even when doing so means that patients may be harmed by hearing bad news, or be allowed to make poor choices. Why not extend this argument to cases where risk of death is involved? Here it might be useful to consider what led to the increased importance of autonomy and rights in health care, and whether the reasons extend to the current kind of case.

Alternatively, one might assume patient's rights and autonomy are so important that they can only be overridden if there is *clear and convincing evidence* of its necessity to avoid serious harm. What could justify putting the burden of proof on the side of the paternalist here? Is this based on a suspicion of the motives of physicians, or on a prioritization of principles of autonomy and rights? If the former, what is the evidence; if the latter, what considerations (or examples) might be used to show that the patient's welfare should not be the sole or main focus of health care ethics? One way to think about this is to notice that there is a chance the mother will die even if lied to, and then she would die under the false belief that her daughter was fine. Is that a terrible thing, suggesting that there is something important about knowing (and telling) the truth regardless of the consequences? Or is it a mercy that the mother did not have to spend her last hours agonizing over the loss of her child, and perhaps her own responsibility for the death?

Similar factual and value assumptions lie behind assessments of the other reasons in the chart. Why think a nurse should follow a physician's orders (reason #2), even when those conflict with the nurse's own moral judgment? Is that based on a factual assumption about the role of nurses in medical practice, and the worry that if nurses were to second-guess physicians' orders it would undermine that role and thereby cause patients harm? What is the evidence for that? If one assumes nurses should follow their own moral compass, valuing integrity and professional autonomy over obedience to physicians, what justifies that assumption? Again, is it based on assumptions about what would work better for the health care profession, for example that nurses are needed in certain cases to advocate for patients or protect them against mistaken or unethical conduct by physicians? What justifies that assumption? Or perhaps there are value assumptions at the root of this question of virtue: perhaps anyone, in any job, should always consider his or her own own moral compass, at least when asked by superiors to do things which would be a serious violation of one's own moral conscience. Perhaps that is a view based simply on the dignity of human beings, on their ultimate autonomy to live by their own values.

Another reason worth examining is #4, that lying is wrong. Some people assume all lies are serious moral violations, while others take beneficent and "white" lies to be morally legitimate.[11] What is behind these differing assumptions? In the case at hand, all would agree the lie is one of great magnitude or import, so it isn't a trivial or white lie, but arguably it is a beneficent lie, designed to save a life. What assumption must be made to think this beneficence sufficient to justify the lie? Is the assumption that lying is wrong based on the belief that it typically is harmful to persons to lie? Is that the essence of the wrongness of lying? Or is lying an interference with rights not so easily overridden by considerations of utility? What assumption must one make to think lying is wrong independent of such utility considerations? If no one is harmed by a lie—indeed, if people are helped—what is left to make the lie wrong?

Step 5: Justification

At this point, having worked through the analysis, one should be better prepared to determine which option is morally preferable. There may be room for reasonable people to disagree about the current case, but let us consider the position that the nurse should lie to the mother, waiting until the morning and the arrival of her husband to tell her of her loss. A simple justification, fitting the recommended format, and with minimal information gathering involved, could be offered as follows:

I. Introduction

Faced with Ms. A's continual request for information about her children, Ms. C should follow the physician's orders and tell Ms. A her children are fine, seeking to calm the mother and help her make it through the night, when she will be in a more stable and safer condition to receive the news about her loss.

II. Support

The most significant reason for this course of action is the need to protect Ms. A from harm (reason #3). Telling Ms. A of the death of her child could cause her condition to worsen, and increase the risk that she will die. These are reasonably likely consequences, given that she is likely to feel substantial grief and anguish about her involvement, and those emotions are well known to cause physiological stresses that threaten those under critical care. The likelihood is further supported by the physician's order, written in the chart, which indicates the seriousness of the threat in the eyes of the physician. It is not for a nurse to second-guess such a medical judgment. Moreover, it is extremely important that a nurse not cause such harms, or take substantial risk of doing so. That is the primary ethical command in health care, since its purpose is defined by the goal of tending to the well-being of patients.

Another reason for telling this difficult lie is that the nurse is on orders from the doctor to do so (reason #2). This is not a trivial reason, since physicians are in a clear line of command over nurses. It is an important virtue of nurses that they respect and obey the directives of physicians, since that is their nursing role and generally reflects the differences in levels of education, training, and expertise. Nevertheless, it must be admitted that there is also an important role for nursing autonomy, even on medical questions about which the nurse is especially experienced, and certainly on ethical questions, since a physician's medical training is no guarantee of superior ethical instincts. In addition, respect for moral integrity requires that nurses be considered free to consult their own moral conscience. So if a nurse believes that following a physician's orders would involve a serious violation of ethics, it should be open to the nurse to not do so. As a result, this reason is not a strong one in this case: the nurse has serious reservations, and the existence of a physician's orders does not alone settle what to do.

[Notice: each supporting reason listed in the chart above has been considered, although the author says one of the reasons is not a very important one. The goal is to represent one's own genuine views, not to simply use any reason that one can.]

III. Defense

A significant reason against lying is the simple idea that lying is wrong, a violation of patients' rights and their autonomy (reason #4). For this reason to prevail, in the face of the risk to Ms. A's life, we would need to assume that considerations of rights and autonomy are of equal or greater import than ones of welfare in health care contexts. But what could justify such an assumption? The central mission of medicine is by any lights to serve patient well-being, and any rights or other moral rules are themselves best understood in the service of that mission. It is true that in recent years medical paternalism and its prioritization of patient welfare over autonomy has become less accepted, cut back by various rules and laws about informed consent and the rights of patients. But the history of these changes shows that the new rules and laws were developed precisely because they were seen as necessary to protect patients. Thus informed consent rules have their birth in the discovery of the abuse of patients in medical research (most importantly in the case of the Tuskegee Syphilis Study). And many of the other rules are due to the decline of the family doctor and the rise of bureaucratic, specialized medicine, where the familiarity and trust crucial to a paternalistic model are far more rare. So while there are some good utility reasons for taking rights and autonomy seriously, they do not extend to situations where a person's unwanted and preventable death might be the result. In such a context, one should always look to the ultimate mission of medicine, and err on the side of life.

Another argument against lying is that the mother has a right to know information about her own daughter (reason #1). This is true, but there is the question of timing. The mother has the right to know at some point, but not necessarily right away, in a situation where knowing could endanger her health (or that of others). The right to know is like the right to free speech: it generally holds, but not when someone wants to yell "fire" in a crowded theatre. Telling the mother the truth immediately would be like yelling "fire," possibly leading to serious harm or death, and so we need not do so.

There are also concerns about whether lying in this case, or in cases like this one, could lead to a decrease in trust and respect for the medical profession (reason #5). Again, this is an important consideration, but not a crucial one. The mother will learn the truth in the morning, and it can be explained that the delay was to protect her own life given her unstable condition. Some mothers would focus on the loss of their child, and forget, forgive, or even be grateful for the beneficent lie. Others may be indignant and severely upset, but it is doubtful that would last very long. The chance that Ms. A will reject the paternalistic justification, leading to a long-term distrust of the medical profession that leads to her not seeking necessary care, is fairly small—and worth risking in face of the alternative of definitely risking her health and survival this very night.

Finally, the point can be raised that for the nurse to tell a lie goes against the virtues of honesty and integrity—virtues which we would want nurses to cultivate (reason #6). Here the key is to recognize that those virtues, like all virtues, need to be evaluated in context. Honesty is important, as a basic disposition to tell the truth, but there are exceptions where telling the truth can be a vice. That is obvious when it comes to truths which are confidential or inappropriate, but it also means that there are some cases where lying is consistent with virtue, as in the trivial cases of white lies to put people at ease in social situations ("fine, how are you?"). As for integrity, if the nurse thinks through the arguments put forward here, she would recognize the moral legitimacy of the lie, and thus it would not violate her integrity to do so. So the virtues of honesty and integrity are insufficient to undermine the beneficent lie in this case, as important as they are in other contexts.

IV. Summary

As difficult as it may be for Ms. C, she should tell Ms. A that her children are doing well, to help increase Ms. A's chances of getting through the night. The sole reason is to avoid worsening Ms. A's condition with the terrible news of her child's death. Though telling the lie flies in the face of many ordinary moral norms, it is justified by the motive behind it—protecting the well-being of the patient—and the primacy of that motive in the mission of health care.

Further Steps: Moral Theory and Moral Philosophy

This use of the above framework—the CARVE principles, and the five-step AJ Method—may lead different people to different conclusions about the morally best way to handle ethical issues, in health care contexts and elsewhere. The advantage of using the framework is that it helps make each person's reasoning more complete, subtle, and complex, but it does not ensure that all reasonable people will end up agreeing with one another. Perhaps nothing can do that, but some have tried, and in closing let us briefly consider two additional stages in the process of moral reflection.

The first is the realm of *moral theory*, in which we step beyond our judgments about specific ethical issues and develop a more general moral outlook.[12] This is a natural and common theoretical step, as we seek to organize our moral ideas and make them more coherent, usually by basing them on a set of more fundamental moral principles or values. The theoretically simplest way of doing this is to find a *single* moral principle on which all our moral judgments can be based. One example of such an approach is a moral theory called *utilitarianism.* Someone who has committed to a utilitarian moral theory takes the CARVE principle of utility to be the most fundamental principle for moral thinking. This means that a utilitarian takes concern for the welfare of all to be the deepest, most general, and most important moral consideration, lying at the base of all other thoughts about right and wrong, goodness and evil, virtue and vice. For instance, *why* should we respect individual rights, or the choices and autonomy of individuals? The answer, according to a utilitarian, is that doing so generally involves more benefit than it involves harm: people do not like being interfered with, and generally fare better if left to their own devices. Yet in some cases—such as when the rich want to keep all their income despite the health care needs of the poor, or when a sick person is fearful of life-saving surgery—the utilitarian would set aside claims of rights and autonomy to do what would be best for all concerned. So a utilitarian offers a general answer to the question of what is morally right or wrong in any given situation: it is the choice, of the alternatives, that would promote the most general welfare for all who might be affected by one's choice.[13] Sometimes the benefits and harms are difficult to calculate, so there can be moral controversies based on different factual assumptions; but if utilitarianism is right, there is no basis for a dispute over fundamental values: we should all share a fundamental concern for promoting the general welfare, and that value will decide any questions about whether to follow a certain moral rule or value in a given case. John Stuart Mill is the most well-known historical proponent of this moral theory, a theory which has had tremendous influence on moral and political thinking in the Western world.[14]

Of course, there are other influential moral theories, which prioritize different moral principles, and that's the rub: to enter into moral theory is to enter the realm of controversy all over again, though at a more general level. For instance, those following the philosophy of Immanuel Kant prioritize a version of respect for autonomy over utility.[15] On a Kantian view, the most fundamental moral idea is that we should recognize other moral agents as rational beings—as able to think and evaluate and reason for themselves—and we should respect the dignity of all such rational beings. This means putting far less emphasis on how people *feel*, and more on how they *reason*; less emphasis on promoting health or well-being, and more on respecting individuals; less emphasis on good *outcomes*, more on *duties*. Kantians thus embrace the idea of absolute restrictions on how we can treat other persons. As a result, they reject the utilitarian idea that we should treat persons in ways that promote the general welfare, for that may involve an insult to the dignity of an individual we may be using as a means to greater good. Instead, Kantians seek to base all moral reflection on some idea of respect for the autonomy and dignity of rational beings. There are different versions of Kantianism, based on different ways of fleshing out this basic idea of respect for autonomy, and there is controversy over which of the different approaches is best. But like utilitarianism, Kantianism has been quite influential in Western ethical thought, helping create the recent emphasis in health care ethics on informed consent procedures, as well as having an influence on moral and political thought more generally.

There are also moral theories that reject the attempt to base all ethical thought on a single principle, while still seeking to provide a coherent story about what it is to take a moral point of view. One approach, called *pluralism*, insists that none of the major moral principles is fundamental; different principles have more or less importance in different contexts, with only our moral intuition to judge which principle should prevail in a given case.[16] Other theories stress the importance of virtue, and the development of a virtuous character, rather than the application of principles or rules.[17] Traditional virtue theorists have sought to further develop Aristotle's ancient theory of virtue, while some feminists have argued that the virtue of caring for others should be understood as the organizing idea for moral theory.[18]

To enter moral theory is to investigate these various alternative moral theories, and the kinds of arguments that have been offered for thinking one or another provides a better sense of how to organize and improve ethical reflection. The advantage of engaging in moral theory is that the focus can be on the general value dis-agreements, which may lead to progress on the larger questions of how to under-stand and prioritize basic moral principles and values. But a disadvantage is that one may lose a sense of why the value disagreements matter. One may only see what is truly at stake in taking on a general moral outlook if one considers individual deci-sions about cases and specific moral judgments. Those who study and write about moral theory usually handle this quandary by seeking what John Rawls has defined as "reflective equilibrium"—by adjusting their moral theory in light of considered judgments about individual cases, and vice versa, until there is an overall coherence between the moral theory and what the theorist thinks, on reflection, is the morally best approach to individual cases.[19] This reflective equilibrium may not fit perfectly with some intuitions or gut instincts about cases, due to considerations at the more general level introduced by the moral theory; but one is searching for the most co-herent fit one can find between theory and specific moral beliefs. Once again, how-ever, even if you do find a moral theory that is in reflective equilibrium with your various considered judgments about cases, other people may find that a different and competing moral theory is in reflective equilibrium with their own considered judgments. So how can the difference over moral theory be resolved, once the same level of reflective equilibrium has been reached by each party to the dispute?

Moral philosophy is the field of study that seeks to make further progress through the most abstract kinds of questions about the nature of moral thought and discourse.[20] What is the relationship between our different moral concepts of the right, the good, and the virtuous? What would it mean to have a good argu-ment for one moral theory or judgment over another? Is it a matter of finding ab-solute certainty, or is some kind of intuitive probability sufficient? What would be the ultimate grounds of such a judgment? Indeed, what are we even doing when we make an ethical claim? As G. E. Moore put it, how can we know what is good if we do not first figure out what we mean when we talk about good?[21] What kind of judgment is it that something is good, or that an act is morally wrong? Is ethi-cal judgment the ascription of an objective property, like the property of being red or of weighing two pounds?[22] Or are ethical judgments subjective, matters of personal taste or emotion that make no claims to objectivity, as when we judge a fashion or a musical style to be good or desirable?[23] Yet could a mere difference in subjective tastes be the essence of disagreements about whether patients have a right to refuse treatments, or whether the rich and famous should be given pri-ority in organ transplants?

This level of moral reflection, while quite abstract and seemingly detached, can sometimes enter into practical ethical thinking. A common example is when some-one argues against interfering in the affairs of another person or culture, on the grounds that we and they have different ethical judgments, and it is not for us to im-pose our ethical judgments on them, since ethical judgments are merely relative. This line of reasoning argues from a relativist position in moral philosophy to the conclusion that we should respect the moral views of others. Note though the paradox: the ethical conclusion about respecting others is not taken to be a relative one, so there must be at least some ethical norms that are not relative. This provides an example of how reflections at the most general level of moral philosophy sometimes enter into everyday ethical life, for better or for worse.

The upshot is that there is no end to the process of reflecting on moral questions. Which kinds of reflection are most important is itself a matter of controversy, as is even the question of whether reflection is itself a good thing. This essay has offered a fairly uncontroversial approach, emphasizing principles and basic reasoning steps useful in evaluating moral issues and justifying one's position. The CARVE principles and the AJ Method procedure are more than enough for most of us, busy as we are, to make our moral choices and get on with our lives. But for those who seek to go further, moral theory and moral philosophy are ways to deepen and enrich one's understanding of the moral domain.

Notes

1. Kurt Baier, *The Moral Point of View: A Rational Basis of Ethics* (Ithaca, NY: Cornell University Press, 1958).
2. Some writers have made distinctions between "the moral" and "the ethical," with the moral being more closely tied to everyday notions of guilt, punishment, and explicit social rules. We will follow the more common usage and take *moral* and *ethical* to be roughly synonymous.
3. The judgment that moral considerations should prevail is an overall normative assessment, not a narrowly moral one, a sense of what would be best "all things considered."
4. See Tom L. Beauchamp and James F. Childress, *Principles of Biomedical Ethics*, 4th ed. (New York: Oxford University Press, 1994), 28–40.
5. This version of the list of principles, and the acronym, is from Becky Cox White and Eric H. Gampel, "Resolving Moral Dilemmas: A Case-Based Method," *HEC Forum* 8, no. 2 (1996): 89–90.
6. The Principle of Equality does allow unequal treatment if people are different in a way that *is* morally relevant. As an obvious example, emergency room personnel may treat a person with a jammed finger "differently" than one in cardiac arrest, treating the latter more quickly and more intensively than the former, without being in violation of the Principle of Equality.
7. The use of a similar method in teaching is discussed in Eric Gampel, "A Method for Teaching Ethics," *Teaching Philosophy* 19, no. 4 (1996): 371–83.
8. The "facts" in this sense are not known or provable, but we might find that our own views presuppose that the facts are a certain way.
9. This case is adapted from B. Tate, *The Nurse's Dilemma* (Geneva: International Council of Nurses, 1977). The discussion is based on White and Gampel, note 5, above.
10. The principle of autonomy is usually understood to prohibit misinforming while requiring the provision of accurate information. Both involve shaping a person's choices, but misinformation does so in a way that serves one's own purposes—even if one's purpose is beneficence—and thus counts as a kind of manipulation, whereas informing a person as to the facts simply allows the person to make a decision in light of all the relevant information.

11. Sisela Bok, *Lying: Moral Choice in Public and Personal Life* (New York: Vintage Books, 1989).
12. For an accessible overview of moral theory, see James Rachels, *The Elements of Moral Philosophy*, 2nd ed. (New York: McGraw-Hill, 1993).
13. This is a version of utilitarianism called "act utilitarianism," since we are applying the principle of utility to the individual act to see if it is morally best. A different suggestion is that we should follow the rules that would, if generally followed, promote the greatest overall welfare. See Richard B. Brandt, *A Theory of the Right and the Good* (Oxford, England: Oxford University Press, 1979), 271–305.
14. John Stuart Mill, *Utilitarianism* (New York: Bobbs-Merrill, 1957).
15. For a good historical survey of Kantian and other moral theories, see T. C. Denise, S. P. Peterfreund, and N. P. White, eds., *Great Traditions in Ethics*, 9th ed. (Belmont, CA: Wadsworth, 1999).
16. William Ross, *The Right and the Good* (Oxford, England: Oxford University Press, 1932).
17. For an overview of virtue ethics, see Rachels, note 12 above, 159–79.
18. Nel Noddings, *Caring: A Feminine Approach to Ethics and Moral Education* (Berkeley: University of California Press, 1984).
19. John Rawls, *A Theory of Justice* (Cambridge, MA: Harvard University Press, 1971), 20–21, 46–50.
20. For an overview that emphasizes these more abstract questions, see Gilbert Harman, *The Nature of Morality* (New York: Oxford University Press, 1977).
21. G. E. Moore, *Principia Ethica* (Cambridge, England: Cambridge University Press, 1903).
22. Moore defended this sort of objectivity of ethical properties in *Principia Ethica*. For a defense of ethical objectivity in the tradition of virtue ethics and natural law, see John Finnis, *Natural Law and Natural Rights* (Oxford, England: Clarendon Press, 1980). In the Kantian tradition, see Christine Korsgaard, *Sources of Normativity* (Cambridge, England: Cambridge University Press, 1996).
23. For an account that emphasizes ethical attitudes and emotions, see Allan Gibbard, *Wise Choices, Apt Feelings* (Cambridge, MA: Harvard University Press, 1990). Another kind of subjectivism has been developed by Simon Blackburn, who draws an analogy between subjective color judgments and ethical judgments; see "How To Be an Ethical Anti-Realist" in *Essays in Quasi-Realism* (Oxford, England: Oxford University Press, 1993).

Chapter 1

Whose Pain Is It Anyway?

Mr. T, a 58-year-old retired executive, was admitted to the orthopedic unit after an open reduction of a fractured ankle under spinal anesthesia. He is in a short leg cast and Dr. U, the orthopedic surgeon, intends to discharge him in 24 hours. On admission to the unit Mr. T was extremely restless and complaining of pain in his ankle and of a severe headache. His nurse, Mr. V, administered two doses of Tylenol Extra Strength, the only pain medication ordered; but Mr. T received no relief. Using a subjective pain-assessment scale, Mr. T indicated that his pain was a "10" on a 1–10 scale. Mr. V contacted Dr. U, who stated that Mr. T has a history of narcotic abuse. He began taking narcotics for severe headaches several years ago. An extensive diagnostic workup failed to reveal any explanation for the headaches. Attempts to wean Mr. T from the narcotic failed repeatedly. He attended Narcotics Anonymous without success and finally became drug-free only after joining a new church and receiving support from the congregation. Dr. U is reluctant to prescribe any narcotics, fearing read-diction. After further discussion Dr. U orders that 2 cc's of normal saline (salt water) be given by injection every 2 hours for complaints of pain.

Saline does not have any intrinsic pain-relieving qualities. A sub-stance that contains no pharmacologically active ingredients, but which is given to relieve pain, is called a placebo. Research done on the use of placebos for pain shows that about 35 percent of patients receiving place-bos experience relief of even severe pain. This response, known as the placebo effect, *is attributed either to a psychological effect (the patient be-lieves it will work, so it does) or stimulation of the body's production of natural narcotics, known as endorphins and enkephalins. Why either of these effects occurs is unclear.*

Mr. V administered the saline as ordered by Dr. U. When Mr. T asked what drug he was receiving, Mr. V replied "what the doctor ordered." He reasoned, correctly, that a placebo effect would not be achieved if the patient knew he was receiving a placebo. Mr. T received no relief, and became increasingly agitated. He continued to report the severity of his pain as a "10."

Mr. V is ambivalent about accepting Mr. T's assessment, believing that drug users often exaggerate pain reports to get as much pain medication as possible. However, Mr. T is not a current drug user and fractures are quite painful. Further, Mr. T may be suffering from a headache as an effect of the spinal anesthetic, a type of headache which is also quite severe.

Mr. V believes that deceiving Mr. T is wrong. He is convinced that such deception not only violates Mr. T's autonomy, but may result in a loss of trust of present and future health care professionals, should Mr. T discover the deception. He also believes that allowing Mr. T to continue to suffer from pain that can be relieved violates his professional obligation to the patient to relieve suffering. Mr. V appreciates the burdens of narcotic addiction, but wonders if Mr. T would in fact resume his addictive behavior after his pain subsides. Research shows that most patients who use narcotics for pain control, even for long periods of time, are able to discontinue them when the pain is resolved. However Mr V. is uncertain whether the research applies to persons with a history of drug abuse.

Mr. V discusses his concerns and Mr. T's continued pain with Dr. U, who still refuses to change the placebo order. Mr. T is again asking for pain medication.

What is Mr. V's moral obligation at this point?

Introduction

This case raises at least four significant moral questions:

1. When, if ever, is placebo use morally permissible?
2. How stringent is the moral obligation to relieve pain?
3. What is the moral obligation of physicians to continuing education?
4. To whom do health care providers (HCPs) owe (primary) professional allegiance?

The AJ Method

Step 1: Information Gathering   What facts are necessary for resolving this case? Dr. U is *assuming* that prescribing narcotic analgesia for Mr. T would result in readdiction, though some evidence contradicts that claim. (Brody; Brown)* Is Mr. T currently capable of autonomous decision making? Have Mr. T's HCPs failed to maintain currency regarding professional standards of care? (Brody) Dr. U and Nurse V assume that Mr. T is an addict, but is he? (Borneman; Brody) Mr. V believes he is bound to follow Dr. U's orders, but he may be mistaken. (Borneman)

HCPs typically appreciate that, other things being equal, deceiving patients is morally impermissible. Professional codes of ethics promise honest communication with clients, and the American Hospital Association's Bill of Patient's Rights explicitly recognizes a right to information about treatment.[1] So how could HCPs justify patient deception, of which placebos are one instance?

Step 2: Creative Problem Solving   Any creative solution would have to relieve Mr. T's pain without (1) (re)addicting him, and (2) without exposing Mr. V to noxious work environs.

Step 3: Pros and Cons   Survey CARVE principles to identify important moral reasons that support conflicting options for resolving this case.

Consequences   Mr. T appears to be at risk of harm no matter which route is taken. If he is medicated, he is thought to be at risk of readdiction. If he is not medicated, he is at risk of uncontrollable pain and the psychological and physiological harms that attend it. (Borneman; Brody; Brown) Depending on his actions, Mr. V is at risk of being reprimanded or fired; or at risk of moral distress at failing to address the needs of his patient. (Brody; Brown)

Typically, deceit is undertaken when HCPs believe a patient, if given a choice, would choose poorly and as a result be seriously harmed. Interestingly, placebos are effective in roughly one-third of the patients to whom they are administered.[2] Mr. T is in the unlucky two-thirds, but presumably Dr. U believes the burden to Mr. T of readdiction would be greater than a few days of severe pain. But is Dr. U better able than Mr. T to compare these burdens? Experts in pain control argue that only the patient can accurately describe the nature and intensity of his pain(s). If only Mr. T can compare his postoperative pain with the pain of addiction, the choice to risk readdiction should be his (albeit in consultation with his physician), assuming he is capable of autonomous choice.[3]

---

* Names in parentheses in case study introductions refer to commentators on the case study; their analyses follow the introductions.

Autonomy   Deceit is morally problematic because it robs persons of information needed to make autonomous decisions. Because rational choices begin with facts, missing or misrepresented facts (e.g., that one is receiving genuine analgesics) derail rational decision making. (Brody; Brown) Nonetheless, some deceit is thought to be morally permissible if it sacrifices short-term loss of autonomy in favor of preserving long-term autonomy. Is placebo use one such legitimate exception to deception? How stringent is the moral obligation to relieve pain?

HCPs often worry that patients in severe pain are incapable of choosing autonomously, that the pain itself is coercive to the extent that patients will eschew any option that does not promise immediate relief. Such concerns drive policies in academic health care centers that conduct research in which placebos play a part. Consent to placebo use must be obtained *prior to* the need for medication administration (i.e., consenting to the *possibility* of being deceived), thus avoiding coercion and preserving autonomy.[4] Community health care centers, however, are rarely sites of research. Thus nonacademic institutions may be less familiar with the moral issues attached to placebo administration, more likely to erroneously view their use as morally unproblematic, and unlikely to have policies to guide placebo administration (e.g., an option of prior consent to deception).

Rights   Within the context of the patient-professional relationship, Mr. T has a right to be aided. He also has the right of self-determination. But does aid consist in relieving acute pain or preventing (re)addiction? In either case, which right is stronger?

Virtues   If Mr. V is to practice with integrity—that is, with commitment to the values espoused in his code of ethics—to whom does he owe (primary) professional allegiance—his patient or his physician colleague? (Borneman) Is compassion better demonstrated in relieving acute pain or preventing (re)addiction? (Borneman) Does courage require the nurse to stand up to the patient or the physician? (Borneman; Brody) Surely the virtue of honesty is relevant to this case. (Brown) Similarly, if Dr. U is to practice with integrity, what are his moral obligations regarding continuing education? (Brody)

Pain control has over the last decade received increasing attention. Oddly, HCPs rarely take pain as seriously as patients do—"oddly," because pain is experienced by most patients and has a profound impact on the quality of life, negatively affecting physical, psychological, social, and spiritual well-being.[5]

Precisely why HCPs fail to give priority to patients' pain is unclear. Various hypotheses include medicine's preferential attention to objective issues (e.g., discrete pathology with measurable indicators) rather than to "mere" subjective reports (e.g., presence and severity of pain); incomplete continuing education (e.g., inadequate information about the therapeutic need to or *how* to relieve pain); or concern about noxious side effects of medications to pain—to name a few.[6] William Ruddick, in an exceptionally trenchant analysis, argues that HCPs must, as a defense mechanism, psychologically distance themselves from pain and are educated and socialized to do so.[7] Taken to its logical extreme, one might argue that ignoring (at least some) patient suffering is a necessary condition for professionals' psychological stability and practical success.

Whether this is true is not only a compelling consequential issue, but relevant to the virtue of professional integrity. All our commentators report that attitudes regarding the importance of and practices to achieve adequate pain control—including for addicts—are all-too-commonly outdated. Given that HCPs cannot be current in every evolutionary change in therapeutic practice, is continuing education about pain control essential to fidelity to patients? Put differently, is currency with the importance of and the methods for pain control critical to promoting patients' welfare—an obligation admitted as paramount in codes of ethics?[8] If so, what about logistical problems for practitioners who lack easy, convenient access to continuing education?

Next, how do HCPs balance the conflicting obligations to colleagues and patients? The American Nurses Association and the American Medical Association both recognize an obligation to collaborate to achieve patient welfare. And both recognize the potential for disagreement, urging their members to work toward resolution. But what if resolution is not forthcoming? If collegiality and patient welfare fail to coincide, which should integrity privilege?

Equality/Fairness (Justice)   Is Mr. T being treated unequally or unfairly because of his history of (alleged) addiction? (Brody; Brown) Or does his history justify disparate treatment?

The Law   In conclusion, the following legal considerations are relevant to various parties in this case. (1) Are HCPs legally obligated to avoid deceiving presumably competent patients who hold decisional authority? (2) Are HCPs legally obligated to provide the best possible (as that is currently defined) care? (3) Are HCPs legally obligated to continue their education—and to maintain currency in clinical practice—that is more substantial than that recommended by the American Medical Association? (4) Finally, not only professional codes of ethics but state boards of nursing may have practice standards for practitioners; failure to comply with such standards may result in loss of one's license to practice.[9]

The following commentaries examine the application of various moral principles to this dilemma, thereby assisting the reader to undertake *Step 4: Analysis* and *Step 5: Justification.*

Notes

1. American Hospital Association, "A Patient's Bill of Rights," (Chicago: American Hospital Association, 1998), #3, adopted 1973, revised 21 Oct. 1992, http://www.hospitalconnect. com/aha/about/pbillofrights.html (13 Aug. 2003); American Medical Association, "Principles of Medical Ethics," 15 July 2002, http://www.ama-assn.org/ama/pub/category/8292.html (14 Aug. 2003), Principle II; American Nurses Association, *Code of Ethics for Nurses with Interpretive Statements* (Washington, DC: ANA, 2001), 2001, http://nursingworld.org/ethics/code/ethicscode150.htm (12 Aug. 2004), § 1.4.
2. Tamar Nordenberg, "The Healing Power of Placebos," *FDA Consumer Magazine* 34, no. 1: (2000), http://www.fda.gov/fdac/features/2000/100_heal.html (14 Aug. 2003).

3. Fiona A. Stevenson et al., "Doctor-patient Communication about Drugs: The Evidence for Shared Decision Making," *Social Science and Medicine* 50 (2000): 829–40.

4. But consider Karin B. Michels and Kenneth J. Rothman, "Update on Unethical Use of Placebos in Randomised Trials," *Bioethics* 17, no. 2 (2003): 188–204.

5. Betty R. Ferrell, "The Role of Ethics Committees in Responding to the Moral Outrage of Unrelieved Pain," *Bioethics Forum* 13, no. 3: (1997): 11–16.

6. David B. Resnik, "Why Modern Medicine Has a Problem with Pain," *Ethics & Health Care* 5, no. 1 (2002): 1–4.

7. William Ruddick, "Do Doctors Undertreat Pain?" *Bioethics* 36, no. 4 (1997): 246–55.

8. See note 1, above: American Hospital Association, #8; American Medical Association, Principles 1 and 5; American Nurses Association, §§ 1.3, 1.4.

9. Rebecca F. Cady, *The Advanced Practice Nurse's Handbook* (Philadelphia: Lippincott, Williams & Wilkins, 2003), Chapter 6, "Professional Liability Issues," 127–68.

   Legal discussions of informed consent are explored in American Medical Association, Council on Ethical and Judicial Affairs, *Code of Medical Ethics: Current Opinions with Annotations*, 2000–2001 ed. (Chicago: American Medical Association, 2000), §8.08, "Informed Consent," 165–69.

   Compromise of the general obligation of truthtelling under the claim of therapeutic privilege, as well as the principle of informed consent, are explored by Arthur S. Berger, *Dying & Death in Law and Medicine: A Forensic Primer for Health and Legal Professionals* (Westport, CT: Praeger, 1993), 24–28, 95–96.

A Physician Ethicist's Analysis

Howard Brody, MD, PhD

This case raises a set of internested ethical questions, including at least these:

1. When, if ever, should practitioners prescribe placebos?
2. What duties do practitioners owe patients for the adequate treatment of pain?
3. What should nurses do when they disagree with physicians about the care given to patients?

The American Medical Association's (AMA's) compilation of opinions on medical ethics states (§ 8.12): "It is a fundamental ethical requirement that a physician should at all times deal honestly and openly with patients." This advice would immediately preclude the course taken by Dr. U. Technically speaking, one does not lie to Mr. T if one tells him that the injection is "what the doctor ordered," but withholding the name of the drug is not "dealing openly and honestly" with him. If Mr. T continued to ask follow-up questions, one would eventually either have to lie or else refuse to speak to him further. This is why it is almost never ethical to prescribe placebos, unless one can obtain the patient's consent for doing so.[1] Obtaining consent is an option in practice under special circumstances—the option is very commonly employed in research trials—but this is not consistent with the way placebos have traditionally been used in medicine over past decades. The case of Mr. T drives home another empirical fact about placebo use in practice: placebos tend to get used on troublesome or disliked patients.[2]

Why is Mr. T a "troublesome" patient? He presents a problem that Dr. U does not really know how to address, and so he ends up getting blamed for other people's discomfort. Dr. U, like most physicians trained until very recently, received a very poor grounding in the modern principles of pain management, and probably learned a lot of things that aren't really so. Let's assume that Mr. T has a history of narcotic abuse and see where that leads us. The evidence-based clinical guideline on *Acute Pain Management,* compiled by the U.S. Agency for Healthcare Policy and Research in 1992, includes a section on treating acute pain in addicts.[3] The guideline makes clear that many aspects of the care of these patients need special attention, but the bottom line is: first, withholding narcotics from a patient who has a fracture *is not* appropriate pain management in this group; and second, of all former addicts, Mr. T's case is actually relatively easy to treat since he has not used any narcotics recently. Moreover, even if Dr. U is correct in not prescribing narcotics, many nonnarcotic options would make much more sense for Mr. T's specific sort of pain than Extra Strength Tylenol.

If Dr. U was intent on utilizing the strongest possible placebo effect on Mr. T's behalf, while still avoiding the deceptive use of a placebo, he could do so by ordering injections of ketorolac. Double-blind studies have shown that ketorolac given by injection is really no stronger than other nonsteroidal anti-inflammatory drugs given orally.[4] But most emergency room physicians seem to think that injectable ketorolac is a stronger painkiller than oral medications, probably because of the heightened patient expectancy of relief from a shot as opposed to a pill.[5]

But is it really true that Mr. T is a former addict? What is the evidence? He had headaches which got better with narcotics, and a diagnostic workup revealed no explanation for the headaches. The most common types of headaches are vascular (migraine), tension, and mixed tension-vascular. None of these can be "objectively" proven by laboratory tests or imaging studies. Pain is essentially a subjective experience; it is known only to the person who has the pain. For research purposes, the 10-point scale for reporting the level of one's pain is considered as "objective" a yardstick of pain as is available in medical science.[6] Quite possibly Mr. T had severe headaches which got better with narcotics and he kept seeking narcotics because they made his headaches go away. He may have quit using narcotics after joining his present church because he was an addict who reformed, or he may have quit because his congregation shares the dominant view in our society that narcotics and their users are evil, and Mr. T eventually decided to grit his teeth and tolerate his headaches rather than go on battling against the phobias and misinformation that characterize our society's reaction to chronic pain.

If these speculations about Mr. T's previous use of narcotics are plausible, Mr. T may not be an addict at all but rather a pseudoaddict.[7] That is, because our medical system and our society are so fearful of prescribing adequate amounts of strong analgesics for persons with chronic pain from "invisible" sources, patients with inadequately treated pain may become "drug-seekers"—not in the usual sense of addicts looking for a fix, but as people desperate to get adequate pain relief. From a behavioral point of view, however, we cannot usually tell the difference between the "drug-seeking" that accompanies true addiction and the "drug-seeking" that accompanies poor medical treatment. Patients in pain without enough analgesia may go to multiple doctors, visit emergency rooms, lie about their symptoms, and eventually show all the same signs as addicts. The only difference is that people with pseudoaddiction stop "drug-seeking" as soon as they reach a level of analgesic prescribing sufficient to treat their pain and to allow them to function in their jobs or home life, while addicts go on seeking even more drugs and become ever more dysfunctional in the rest of their lives as a result.

The pseudoaddiction scenario suggests the sad possibility that Mr. T has been severely punished by the medical system twice. First he was punished for having hard-to-diagnose headaches and for trying to use the medication that actually gave him some relief. Now he is being punished for being in pain from a fractured ankle and for having the label "addict" stamped on his forehead from his previous punishment.

Dr. U is probably treating Mr. T exactly as he was trained to treat pain, showing that the failure is less Dr. U's personally (although his management falls short of the best current practice guidelines, as noted) than our entire medical system's. It is not merely that Dr. U doesn't know how to treat pain properly; worse, he doesn't know that he doesn't know. Few physicians who have not made a special effort to become informed about the more recent ideas in pain management are aware of the traditional gaps in medical knowledge. Lying to patients by giving them saline injections when they think they are getting pharmacologically active analgesics is, in this case, simply covering up the deeper ethical problem of inadequate management of pain.

What should the nurse, Mr. V, do? Ideally, when a nurse sees a patient receiving inadequate medical care, he or she should act as patient advocate and try to secure an improvement in the care. The usual official channel is to work upward through the nurse supervisor to the director of nursing, who should then take up the matter with the chief of the medical service. The nurse raising the concern should, in a well-functioning hospital, be protected from retribution from the attending physician for raising such complaints as a matter of conscience. If the physician is truly interested in seeing the patient receive the best possible care, he will welcome more active input from nursing rather than feel threatened by it. The problem in this case is that there is every likelihood that the nursing administrator, and the chief of medical staff, are as poorly informed on modern principles of pain management as Dr. U is. In that case Mr. V's concerns will fall on deaf ears.

The AMA code of ethics has no statement on a physician's duty to relieve pain. This reflects the unfortunate lack of attention the issue has received in ethics circles. Numerous studies were published in the 1990s documenting inadequately treated pain in even the best American hospitals and nursing homes—in some cases, affecting as many as one-third to one-half of the patients.[8] Untreated pain is bad for one's health as well as for one's quality of life. Medicine possesses today the technology needed to adequately control pain nearly 100 percent of the time. Our failure to control pain adequately so much of the time signals that we simply have not made this a priority. Our refusal to make this a priority is, I would argue, an ethical as well as a technical failing. Much work needs to be done at all levels, in community facilities as well as in academic centers, before things improve.

Notes

1. Howard Brody, "Placebo," *Encyclopedia of Bioethics,* 3rd ed., ed. S. G. Post (New York: Macmillan, 2003).
2. J. T. Berger, "Placebo Medication Use in Patient Care: A Survey of Medical Interns," *Western Journal of Medicine* 170 (1999): 93–96.
3. Agency for Healthcare Policy and Research, Department of Health and Human Services, *Acute Pain Management: Operative or Medical Procedures and Trauma. Clinical Practice Guideline,* AHCPR Publication No. 92-0032: Feb. 1992, n.d., http://hstat.nlm.nih.gov/hq/Hquest/db/local.arahcpr.arclin.apmc/screen/Browse/xid/74/s/52453/cmd/PD/action/GetText (16 Aug. 2003).
4. M. L. Neighbor and K. A. Puntillo, "Intramuscular Ketorolac vs. Oral Ibuprofen in Emergency Department Patients with Acute Pain," *Academic Emergency Medicine* 5 (1998): 118–22.
5. Howard Brody, "The Placebo Response. Recent Research and Implications for Family Medicine," *Journal of Family Practice* 49 (2000): 649–54.
6. F. Berthier et al., "Comparative Study of Methods of Measuring Acute Pain Intensity in an ED," *The American Journal of Emergency Medicine* 16 (1998): 132–36.
7. D. E. Weissman and J. D. Haddox, "Opiate Pseudoaddiction: An Iatrogenic Syndrome," *Pain* 36 (1989): 363–66.
8. C. S. Cleeland et al., "Pain and its Treatment in Outpatients with Metastatic Cancer," *New England Journal of Medicine* 330 (1994): 592–96.

A Nurse's Analysis

Janet Brown, RN, MSN, CNS

Pain management is a crucial and difficult aspect of nursing practice, but it is especially difficult when the patient has a history of substance abuse. In addition to posing the therapeutic challenge of devising an individual plan of care for Mr. T because of his past problems discontinuing narcotic use, the issue of using placebos presents a major ethical challenge.

The American Nurses Association's Code of Ethics identifies the fundamental moral principle directing professional nursing behavior as respect for the person.[1] This principle encompasses the principles of autonomy, nonmaleficence, beneficence, veracity, and justice. Examining these principles in relation to Mr. T's pain management and placebo use may help Mr. V make morally appropriate choices about Mr. T's care.

The principle of autonomy requires Mr. V, as a professional, to respect Mr. T's ability to decide for himself. One opportunity for respecting autonomy is informed consent. Informed consent promotes and respects a person's autonomy by providing information needed to rationally make health care choices. If Mr. T has the capacity to understand the benefits and risks of treatment options, he is considered competent to make personal decisions about his care. Then, from a moral point of view, he has full authority to decide what happens to him.

A critical component of informed consent is *veracity*, or the duty to tell the truth. The use of placebos requires deceiving Mr. T about what is being done. Deceit circumvents the process of informed consent. Mr. T wrongly assumes he is receiving a medication with active ingredients to relieve his pain. When he asks, he must be given a false or evasive answer. His decision about his care can not be considered an informed or autonomous decision since it is based on inaccurate or incomplete information.

Mr. V also has the duty to avoid deliberate harm, or to adhere to the principle of nonmaleficence. Since the placebos have not eased his pain, Mr. T is harmed by his continued suffering. The primary consideration must not be his history of substance abuse but rather his acute medical problems, including unrelieved pain. Inadequate pain control puts him at risk for a variety of harmful effects. The impact of unrelieved pain on Mr. T's quality of life may include anxiety, fearfulness, and/or hopelessness about his recovery. Continued pain may also decrease his physical activity, which is counterproductive to healing. Pain also triggers a number of physiologic stress responses that can produce harmful effects. The heart, lungs, and gastrointestinal and immune systems do not work as well when the body is stressed by unrelieved pain; this results in decreased oxygen, nutrients, and other tissue-building materials needed for wound healing.

Accepting the placebo as appropriate treatment may further harm Mr. T because it keeps physicians and nurses from looking for more effective methods of managing pain. The American Society of Pain Management Nurses holds that "placebos should not be used by any route of administration in the assessment and management of pain in any patient . . ."[2] And the California Board of Registered Nursing, for example, has stated, "Use of placebos would breach the basic premise of pain management, which is that patients who report pain are entitled to the best possible treatment reflecting current research on methods that are safe and effective."[3] So giving a placebo conflicts with Mr. V's professional code of ethics, professional nursing standards, and, if he is practicing in California, the policy of the state licensing board.

The relationship between Mr. T and his nurse may also be harmed if it is based on deceit. If Mr. T discovers his health care providers have been lying to him, he loses trust in them and their ability to care for him. This can contribute to Mr. T's feeling anxious about his care and may also decrease his willingness to participate in planned treatment, such as following physical activity recommendations of the staff.

Dr. U and Mr. V's concern that giving narcotic medication will contribute to Mr. T's addiction or create an additional addiction is a legitimate moral worry. Aggravating or extending addiction would surely violate the principle of nonmaleficence. But no scientific evidence shows that giving narcotics for pain control to a person who has a history of drug addiction will make the addiction worse, and withholding narcotics does not assist the recovery of a substance abuser.[4] During the acute phase of pain treatment the priority is to treat the pain.

The last ethical principle challenged by Mr. T's care is justice. Justice requires Mr. V to ensure that all of his patients are treated fairly. It is important to examine whether a prejudice about Mr. T's substance abuse is affecting the type or quality of care being provided. A negative attitude about Mr. T's history of substance abuse could result in his physicians or nurses believing he is lying about his pain and/or that he does not have a legitimate need for pain medication. This bias will certainly color the judgment of Mr. T's clinicians as they plan his treatment. But treating Mr. T fairly means his pain must be assessed and treated in the manner employed with a person who does not have a history of substance abuse.

What can Mr. V do to meet his moral obligation to Mr. T? He needs to start by addressing Dr. U directly with his concerns about the moral conflict inherent in this situation. He could suggest nonnarcotic analgesics for Mr. T, but if Dr. U continues to insist on placebo use, Mr. V needs to refuse to participate and must take his concerns up the chain of command in his organization. Because placebo use conflicts with both ethical and professional standards, his superiors in nursing administration should support him. And while working to change the pain management order Mr. V is obligated to use every resource and nonpharmacologic technique available to help relieve Mr. T's pain until an effective analgesic is ordered.

Notes

1. American Nurses Association, *Code of Ethics for Nurses with Interpretive Statements* (Washington, DC: American Nurses Association, 2001), 2001, http://nursingworld.org/ethics/code/ethicscode150.htm (12 Aug. 2003).
2. American Society of Pain Management Nurses, "Position Statement: Use of Placebos for Pain Management" (Pensacola, FL: ASPMN, 1996), 18 Apr. 2000, http://www.edc.org/PainLink/placebo.html (12 Aug. 2003).
3. California Board of Registered Nursing, "Frequently Asked Questions Regarding Pain Management," (File NPR-B-38), Nov. 2001, http://www.rn.ca.gov/ (28 May 2003).
4. P. Compton and M. McCaffery, "Treating Acute Pain in Addicted Patients," *Nursing* 32, no. 9 (2001): 17.

A Nurse's Analysis

Tami Borneman, RN, MSN

Relevant to ethics are doing good and avoiding harm. The Florence Nightingale Pledge emphasizes the consequences of actions and promises: "I will abstain from whatever is deleterious and mischievous . . . and devote myself to the welfare of those committed to my care."[1] The American Nurses Association (ANA) Code for Nurses states that "The nurse's primary commitment is to the patient. . . ."[2] This commentary will focus on the nurse's moral obligation to the patient.

After Nurse V administered the placebo for pain, he realized the deception was wrong. The fact that Nurse V administered the first placebo may indicate the tension he felt between his moral obligation to the patient and his collegial obligation to the physician whose orders he was responsible for carrying out. Choosing between obligations of fidelity to the physician on the one hand and to the patient on the other is a pervasive struggle in nursing. Regardless of the struggle, Nurse V's moral obligation is first and foremost to the patient. The ANA Code for Nurses states "When the patient's wishes are in conflict with others, the nurse seeks to help resolve the conflict. Where conflict persists, the nurse's commitment remains to the identified patient."[3]

The ethical dilemma occurs because the patient is a former drug abuser. The physician's fear of causing readdiction is genuine, but he allows this fear to guide his judgment, leaving the patient in pain. As a result, neither he nor Nurse V is fulfilling the obligations of beneficence and nonmaleficence.

Dr. U and Nurse V, in their effort to avoid the harm of readdiction, actually distort the principle of nonmaleficence. The obligation of nonmaleficence requires neither inflicting nor imposing risks of harm. Harm, defined as "thwarting, defeating, or setting back" a person's interests, may be intentional or unintentional.[4] Nonetheless some harms may be morally justified because they are unavoidable side effects of promoting important benefits. For example, titrating analgesics to diminish the pain might also precipitate a negative effect, such as a relapse into drug addiction. The ethical issue in this case is the undertreatment of pain. Possible readdiction is not the worst outcome of treatment; rather, suffering needlessly may be.[5]

One might analyze this dilemma in terms of the Rule of Double Effect (RDE). The RDE is used to justify actions having two foreseen effects—one good, one harmful. According to the RDE an action is morally permissible if four conditions are met:

1. The act *itself* must be good or morally neutral.
2. The agent only intends good effects (bad effects can be foreseen, but cannot be intended).
3. Bad effects cannot be the means to good effects.
4. Good effects must outweigh bad effects.[6]

Does the RDE justify placebo use? Probably not. The goodness or moral neutrality of the act of administering a placebo becomes morally problematic as soon as Nurse V knows that the placebo does not relieve pain. Thus, condition #1 is not met. If we assume that Nurse V only intended the good effect of avoiding readdiction and not the bad effect of ongoing suffering, condition #2 is met. (One could, however, question whether Dr. U's decision was based *on self-interest*—fear or concern that he would be held responsible for readdiction in Mr. T, should that occur—

or was *genuinely altruistic.*) Condition #3, however, is clearly violated. The bad effect of unrelieved pain is *the means* to avoiding readdiction. That is, the only way to avoid readdiction is to administer placebos that fail to relieve suffering.

Condition #4 is probably violated as well. It is unclear why the physician thought the harm of *potential* readdiction would be greater than the *actual* benefit of pain relief. First, the immediate result is a patient in excruciating pain. The decision to avoid opioids was not based on current facts of drug abuse. In fact, Mr. T is not a current drug user. Second, severe pain isolates a patient. The only thing the patient can think about is relieving the pain and all choices are focused on that end. "In its extreme, pain destroys the soul itself and all will to live."[7] Third, undertreatment of pain may provoke drug abuse in a patient with a history of substance abuse.[8] Fourth, the *immediate* relief from *actual* pain (intended good effect) for Mr. T would appear to outweigh the *possible future* effect of readdiction (unintended bad effect), if only because pain relief is certain and readdiction is only possible. So: appealing to RDE supports replacing placebos with analgesics. (But I'm talking as a health care professional. Certainly I would not push pain management on someone who wouldn't want it.)

The discussion of the RDE may appear to apply more to Dr. U's order than to Nurse V's actions. Does Nurse V have his own moral obligation to Mr. T? Nurse V believes that leaving Mr. T in pain violates his obligation to relieve suffering. On the other hand, he believes he should avoid harming Mr. T through readdiction. How might he compare these two obligations?

Persons have a moral obligation of beneficence—a moral obligation to *act* for the benefit of another—if five conditions are met: (1) One person is at significant risk of harm; (2) Another person's act is necessary to prevent the harm; (3) The act is likely to prevent the harm. (4) The act would not likely risk serious harm to the actor; and (5) Benefits to the needy person will outweigh harms to the actor.[9]

Applying these conditions to the present case, we note: (1) Mr. T is at risk of significant harm—ongoing unrelieved pain; (2) Nurse V's action—getting an order for and administering a genuine analgesic—is needed to prevent this harm; (3) Nurse V's action has a high probability of preventing the harm; (4) Nurse V's action would not significantly harm Mr. T; and (5) the benefit to Mr. T outweighs (nonexistent) harms to Nurse V. Nurse V needs to fulfill his moral obligation of beneficence by taking a more active role to relieve his patient's pain.

The obligation of beneficence requires a commitment to accountability. *Accountability* involves holding oneself responsible for the well-being of patients under one's care, including (as we just saw) the obligation to act for the benefit of another. In order for Nurse V to provide effective nursing care to Mr. T, he needs to start with a good assessment of the physical, psychological, social, and spiritual well-being of the patient. Knowing that the patient is experiencing pain on a level of 10 is not enough. Inquiring about the patient's thoughts on readdiction could provide a basis for collaborative planning regarding his treatment. It would provide an opportunity for Mr. T to make choices about his care, including preparation for readdiction, should that occur.

The bottom line is that Nurse V's moral obligation requires him to provide adequate pain relief to his patient. He is responsible and accountable for his nursing practice, and that includes the undertreatment of pain.[10] He may consider consulting his immediate nursing supervisor to see what could be done to alleviate the patient's pain. And, if appeals to appropriate officials in the hierarchy of authority are unsuccessful, he could, as a final step, present the case to the ethics committee. But even if support from others is not forthcoming, Nurse V has a moral obligation to provide pain relief to Mr. T through standard nursing practices of assessment, intervention, and evaluation.

RECOMMENDED READINGS

American Pain Society, *Principles of Analgesic Use in the Treatment of Acute Pain and Cancer Pain*, 4th ed. (Glenview, IL: American Pain Society, 1999).

Hill, T. Patrick "Freedom from Pain: A Matter of Rights?" *Cancer Investigation* 12, no. 4 (1994): 438–43.

Notes

1. L. Gretter, *Florence Nightingale Pledge* (Detroit, MI: Farrand Training School for Nurses, 1863).
2. American Nurses Association, *Code of Ethics for Nurses with Interpretive Statements* (Washington, DC: American Nurses Association, 2001), 4.
3. Ibid, § 2.1.
4. Tom L. Beauchamp and James F. Childress, *Principles of Biomedical Ethics*, 5th ed. (New York: Oxford University Press, 2001), 116.
5. For nurses, effective pain management is not just an ethical issue; they are also legally liable for the undertreatment of pain. See M. Frank-Stromborg and A. Christiansen, "A Serious Look at the Undertreatment of Pain. Part I," *Clinical Journal of Oncology Nursing* 5, no. 5 (2001): 235–36.
6. See note 4, above, 129.
7. E. Lisson, "Ethical Issues Related to Pain Control," *Nursing Clinics of North America* 22, no. 3 (1987): 654.
8. R. Savage, "Assessment for Addiction in Pain-treatment Settings," *Clinical Journal of Pain* 18, no. 4 (2002): S28–S38.
9. See note 4, above, 171.
10. See note 2, above.

Further Reflections

General

1. What moral principles justify deceit in this case and what principles might argue against lying to this patient? Compare Howard Brody's use of beneficence and Brown's use of the principle of respect for autonomy as the justifications for *not* using placebos. How might Dr. U respond to these arguments?

2. How should one deal with the disagreements between nurses and physicians concerning the care or treatment of patients? All commentators insist that when a patient's interests conflict with the demands of collegiality, the patient's welfare is primary. But what if the HCPs have differing conceptions of what would promote the patient's interests?

Consequences

3. Identify and evaluate the consequences of placebo use in a nonresearch clinical situation.
4. Brown and Brody both urge that HCPs give greater attention to acquiring currency in pain medication and management. What, specifically, are the problems and challenges that result from the inadequate assessment of addiction, poor pain management, the anemic and improper use of pain medication, and the use of placebos? What myths and attitudes about pain, narcotic use, and pain management need to be overcome in our society? Borneman notes that "undertreatment of pain may provoke drug abuse in a patient with a history of substance abuse." If this is true, then what does this suggest about how we ought to think about pain management and medication?

Autonomy

5. Identify the challenges that pain and addiction might present to autonomous decision making. What symptoms or behavior would trigger a suspicion that patients in pain or that addicts are incapable of autonomous choice about analgesics?
6. Is deception necessary to the successful use of placebos? Why or why not? If so, is it legitimate in some settings and not others?
7. Borneman's discussion of the Rule of Double Effect (RDE) raises the possibility that respectful intentions might support deception or placebo use. Review the requirements of RDE and indicate what conditions would have to be present to support deceiving Mr T.

Rights

8. Do patients have a right to pain relief? Justify your answer.

Virtues

9. Under what circumstance would lying be virtuous? vicious?

Equality/Fairness (Justice)

10. Does Mr. T's status and label as a "former addict" justify placebo use for Mr. T? Is it because, as Brody suggests, Mr. T. is a "troublesome or disliked patient" or because of a general negative opinion about drug addicts?

Chapter 2

Mommy Dearest

Mrs. K is an 84-year-old retired librarian who suffered from transient is-chemic attacks (temporary interruptions of blood to her brain) for several years, and then had a stroke last year. The stroke left her with a complete paralysis of her dominant arm and leg. Rehabilitation has had limited suc-cess; her disabilities are considered permanent. As a result, Mrs. K entered a skilled nursing facility (SNF), where she receives assistance with activi-ties of daily living (ambulation, eating, personal hygiene). Because her dis-abilities are significant and persistent Mrs. K is unlikely to be able to move to a step-down facility or return to her own home.

Mrs. K's son and his wife live in the same town. They visit her fre-quently, chatting and dining with her. On occasion Mrs. K has been able to leave the SNF and visit them in their home for Sunday dinner, short family outings, etc. Mrs. K's son has been very supportive during her re-habilitation and long-term care. When the SNF staff have difficulty coax-ing Mrs. K to cooperate with therapy, her son successfully nudges her into accepting their advice. He has been a conscientious and concerned part-ner with the staff in ensuring that his mother receives the best of care.

Throughout her stay Mrs. K has remained alert and competent, though she has become increasingly irritable, demanding, and defiant. She frequently refuses her medications; has torn out an intravenous line inserted to rehydrate her after a bout of diarrhea; refuses to eat on the meal schedule of the SNF; and refuses to get out of bed to use the toilet, brush her teeth, or get dressed (although she is capable of all of these ac-tivities with assistance). At the same time, she complains that the staff "either treat me like an idiot or a baby." She abhors "being told rather than asked what to do." Over the last several weeks Mrs. K has become

44

intractably uncooperative. She rejects all new interventions because "no one asked me about this," " it won't get me home anyway," or, simply, "I don't want to."

Although uncooperative, Mrs. K shows no sign of incompetence. When she chooses to discuss her care, she demonstrates appreciation of the importance of her medications and physical and occupational therapy. But all too frequently her son arrives to discover his mother arguing with or berating the staff. Originally proud of his mother's spunk and independence, her son has begun to realize (as have the SNF staff) that Mrs. K's noncompliance with medications, feeding, and treatment regimens is beginning to affect her health. She is losing weight, experiencing frequent elevations in her blood pressure, and has suffered two urinary tract infections thought to result from dehydration. Her response to these observations is unconcern: "If I die, I die."

Mrs. K's advance directive names her son as her surrogate decision maker; but other than during her hospital stay after her stroke, he has never had to act as her surrogate. However, yesterday as he was leaving, the SNF administrator approached him to discuss his mother's care. The administrator asked him to give permission to insert a feeding tube to enable the staff to provide adequate nutrition and hydration, as well as to administer Mrs. K's medications without having to do battle each time one is due. She also informed him that Mrs. K's doctor would like to begin an antipsychotic, in hopes that this drug would restore Mrs. K's previous enthusiasm for life and eliminate her irritability and other unpleasant, obstructive behaviors. She added that when the doctor mentioned this to Mrs. K, she explicitly refused the drug, indicating "my mind is just fine."

Mrs. K's son agrees that these changes would probably be in Mrs. K's best interest. Nonetheless, he is troubled that he, rather than his mother, is being asked to make these decisions. He protests that his mother is still competent and, when cooperative, is capable of making treatment decisions. The administrator agrees, but observes that "catching" Mrs. K during her episodic cooperative moments is inordinately difficult, while her need for treatment is continuous. In her estimation, having her son make decisions for Mrs. K would be much more efficient and effective in improving her health.

Mrs. K's son does not know what to do. He observes that "My mother is still able to decide these things for herself and she wants to do so; she's made that clear to me over and over. She is especially unhappy with any decision that is made without consulting her. Don't we still need to get her permission for these sorts of serious treatments?"

The administrator agrees that "in principle" Mrs. K should make these choices, but notes that unless someone decides—and soon—to institute these treatments, Mrs. K is likely to be beyond help. She adds that Mrs. K obviously trusts her son's judgment; why else would she designate him as her surrogate? Mrs. K's son replies that, while his mother does trust his judgment, she would be quite dismayed if he assumed formal decisional authority while she was still capable of deciding for herself.

The administrator nods in understanding, but repeats her earlier warning: if Mrs. K does not soon receive adequate nutrition, hydration, and medication, her health will probably deteriorate beyond recovery. She adds that waiting for Mrs. K to deteriorate into incompetence before providing necessary care seems irresponsible. Mrs. K's son agrees, but is still reluctant to usurp his mother's decisional authority.

What should Mrs. K's son do?

Introduction

This dilemma raises the familiar problems of conflicting values and conflicting interests; its resolution requires addressing at least three moral questions:

1. Whose interests should be considered when preserving the interests of some requires sacrificing the interests of others?
2. In health care settings, do patients' preferences automatically "trump" those of families or health care professionals (HCPs)?
3. What role does the virtue of integrity play in managing the care of obstreperous elderly patients?

The AJ Method

Step 1: Information Gathering   What motivates Mrs. K's rejection of medicine and care? (Rysberg) Are her rejections autonomous? What are her actual preferences—a shorter life with more control or something else? Who has *legal* decisional authority about Mrs. K's care? What motivates her son? What motivates the administrator? What are her actual goals regarding Mrs. K? How difficult is giving care to Mrs. K—virtually impossible or just annoying?

Step 2: Creative Problem Solving   A creative solution would have to simultaneously respect Mrs. K's choices while providing the care from which she would benefit.

Step 3: Pros and Cons   Survey CARVE principles to identify important moral reasons that support conflicting options for resolving this case.

Consequences   Will Mrs. K be harmed or benefitted if health care professionals (HCPs) comply with her requests? if they do not? (Hill; Rysberg; Spiegel) Who else will be affected? Will these effects be negative or positive? How likely are they to occur? (Flescher)

From the broadest perspective, the interests of all persons are on a par.* Practically, this implies that the welfare of all who will be affected must be considered before acting. This utilitarian approach does not mean that everyone's interests must be promoted or even protected, only that they must be taken into account. Thus, if the benefits to some are sufficiently great (e.g., Mrs. K), others (e.g., HCPs) may be burdened to produce them. Conversely, if burdens outweigh benefits, the benefits must be forgone. Most important choices generate burdens and benefits; as long as benefits outweigh burdens, the action is morally permissible—and may be morally required. (Think of the rule of the majority while respecting the rights of the minority.)

Here the broad utilitarian perspective requires identifying and evaluating the interests of Mrs. K, her son, and the skilled nursing facility (SNF) and its personnel. Mrs. K has an interest in controlling what happens to her, and in minimizing her pain and suffering (psychological and physical). Her son has an interest—derived from the virtue of filial loyalty—in promoting his mother's interests; but he also has an interest in his own welfare—minimizing his own burdens while meeting his filial responsibilities. Finally, the administrator and SNF employees have interests—grounded in professional integrity—in providing good patient care under good working conditions.

If all affected parties' interests are equal, we might reasonably expect that Mrs. K's interests (or those of any SNF resident) could easily be overridden by the more numerous interests of family members and HCPs. Do good reasons exist to give priority to patients' interests?

Autonomy   Recall that autonomy, most broadly understood, applies to choosing the values in terms of which to live one's life, as well as the means to achieve those values. Whose autonomy will be respected if the HCPs comply with Mrs. K's

---

*Moral theorists have identified many problems with assuming equality—and sometimes even the legitimacy—of all interests. We will ignore these important questions and assume that in health care settings the range of interests may be limited to health care and their sequelae.

requests? if they do not? (Rysberg) Whose autonomy is relevant here? (Flescher; Hill; Spiegel)

Determining which interests are weightier is essential to ranking them. Here, all parties value self-determination, quality of life, and life itself, but prioritize them differently. Mrs. K appears to value autonomy over her health, while the SNF administrator apparently values patient health over patient self-determination. Mrs. K's son's ranking vacillates.

Health care institutions (HCIs) and HCPs exist to serve the interests of patients. This policy is thoroughly rational because patients would be unlikely to turn over their care to persons or facilities that failed to give priority to their interests. This commitment is articulated in HCIs' and HCPs' codes of ethics.[1] These codes speak to the primacy of promoting patients' welfare and protecting patients' dignity and self-determination. Thus the virtue of fidelity binds HCIs and HCPs to preferentially promoting patients' welfare, even when doing so is inconvenient or annoying. Further, patients, if competent, get to call the shots—at least in terms of treatment goals and *effective* means thereto.

Nonetheless, choices that pose *inordinate* hardships on others may sometimes be resisted, even when the choosers are autonomous patients. And we might wonder whether persons, on entering a SNF, relinquish some freedoms in order to contribute to the smooth functioning of the facility. In either case, we must determine if Mrs. K's behavior, which is admittedly annoying and often inconvenient, poses an inordinate hardship or is merely a not uncommon approach to illness or incapacitation.

Further, if some other value "outranks" autonomous choice, that value might justify treating Mrs. K, even over her objections. Such rankings have been notoriously difficult to articulate, typically assuming a religious stance that defines (mere) life as the ultimate value. Those who do not accept the religious foundation do not consider themselves subject to its implications. To treat persons on the basis of a religious belief they do not embrace is to hold them hostage to others' values.

If one accepts the possibility of a life not worth living, one must accept that death can be preferable to a life whose quality is too low. Who decides when the quality of a life is so low that death is preferable? Appeals to autonomy suggest that the person living that life should weigh its quality against its extension. When the stakes of (non)action are so high, those involved must be especially vigilant in assuring the decisions are autonomous. In Mrs. K's case, this mandates careful assessment of her competence.

Competence is the necessary precondition for autonomous choice.[2] Competent patients possess the most complete knowledge of their values and goals and, barring coercion or lack of information, are capable of autonomous choices to promote or preserve those values and goals. A charge of incompetence is often raised when patients reject HCPs' suggestions, the thinking being that no "rational person" would reject sound advice.[3] Rejection of suggestions is common in institutional settings, where patients often resist both therapeutic and scheduling requests.[4] But disagreement is not compelling evidence of incompetence. Patients may be structuring their objections in terms of long-held values and goals that are opaque to their caregivers. If established values or goals, rather than psychopathology or cognitive deterioration, are motivating patients' behavior, then competent patients' rejections of suggestions should be seen as autonomous choices rather than mere recalcitrance.

If Mrs. K has made an autonomous decision that her life is not worth living, or that she prefers a lower quality of life with more control over living it, her resistance must be taken seriously. If her rejections of treatment are respected, her son and HCPs would, sadly, have to witness her decline, knowing they could prevent or forestall it. Would their moral distress be justified?

Rights Mrs. K's right to self-determination is central. (Hill) Rights to not be harmed and to be aided also apply. (Hill) Are the rights to privacy and confidentiality still in force, given Mrs. K's declining health and aggressive rejections of care?

Virtues Does professional fidelity indicate which option is better? Does tolerance? compassion? Does fidelity to family-centered role-related responsibilities give any direction? (Flescher; Spiegel)

The HCPs might worry that, in respecting Mrs. K's rejection of care, they would have to eschew some of the very actions that define their professional practice, thereby threatening their professional integrity. HCPs and HCIs, by their very description, focus on health and—because one cannot be healthy without being alive—on life. They are committed to basic levels of care and modes of treatment, guided by practice standards that indicate required behavior for members of their professions. They are obligated not only to establish beneficial therapeutic relationships with their patients, but also to construct and maintain a positive reputation in their social and professional communities. Thus, Mrs. K's HCPs are rightly concerned with her health and her preventable death. However, professional fidelity requires them to meet not only her needs, but the needs of the community in which she and they participate. They might reasonably see her deterioration as not only failing to meet her own interests, but as shoddy professional practice or a threat to the welfare of the community (e.g., other patients may worry that Mrs. K is being neglected, a state of affairs with potentially fatal consequences—and a fate that may befall them next).

Further, they might feel that failing to meet her needs constitutes abandonment. However, some professional opportunities—minimizing Mrs. K's pain and suffering—remain, even if saving her life or minimizing her disability are no longer possible.[5] Does professional integrity permit such trade-offs?

Further, the appeal to the virtue of family-focused fidelity forces us to consider the effects on Mrs. K's son. The effects on him of watching Mrs. K decline into death are likely to be quite painful. If he believes he could have—and that a good son would have—prevented her death, he may suffer pangs of guilt, regret, or feelings of failure. Typically we think that the avoidable imposition by others of significant burdens can, morally speaking, be resisted. Are families of patients somehow different?[6] Are they, by virtue of some particularly powerful role-related responsibility, required to bear whatever burdens family members' choices impose (recognizing that patients do not have as their goal making their families' lives difficult)? This demand is frequently resisted in other important spheres of life; for example, no one would expect a son to submit to his mother's demand to divorce his wife, or to not have children. So, can even "good sons" insist their parents not behave in certain ways or override their choices when they behave badly?

Justice Is Mrs. K being treated equally with other patients with similar needs? Does the extra time spent trying to gain Mrs. K's cooperation pose an unfair burden on other patients? (Hill)

In summary, resolution of this dilemma requires determining whether patients' desires always outweigh others' interests or if family or professional interests can outrank those of patients. Embedded in evaluating patients' desires is evaluating their autonomy, while a comparative analysis of welfare must also attend to obligations of filial fidelity and the professional integrity of the HCPs.

The Law   The following legal considerations are relevant to this case: (1) Who, legally, has decisional authority for Mrs. K? (2) Does the SNF administrator breach confidentiality by discussing Mrs. K's case with her son? (3) Under what conditions, if any, can Mrs. K's autonomous decisional authority be legally overridden? (4) Would inserting a feeding tube legally constitute a violation of privacy? assault or battery? (5) If Mrs. K is not treated, could the SNF or its HCPs be held legally liable for her medical deterioration or her death (due to negligence)? (6) If she is treated, would SNF staff be guilty of assault and battery?[7]

The following commentaries examine the application of various moral principles to this dilemma, thereby assisting the reader to undertake *Step 4: Analysis* and *Step 5: Justification.*

Notes

1. American College of Healthcare Executives, "Code of Ethics," 25 Mar. 2000, http://www.ache.org/abt_ache/code.cfm (8 Aug. 2003); American Nurses Association, *Code of Ethics for Nurses with Interpretive Statements* (Washington, DC: ANA, 2001); Public Affairs, Parliamentary and Access Branch, Commonwealth Department of Health and Aged Care, Canberra, Australia, "Guide to Ethical Conduct for Providers of Residential Aged Care: Code of Ethics for Residental Aged Care," *Nursing Ethics* 10, no. 1 (2003): 89–94.
2. Ruth R. Faden and Tom L. Beauchamp, *A History and Theory of Informed Consent* (New York: Oxford University Press, 1986), 287–293.
3. Becky Cox White, *Competence to Consent* (Washington, DC: Georgetown University Press, 1994), 7–10; Stephen Wear, *Informed Consent: Patient Autonomy and Clinician Beneficence within Health Care,* 2nd ed. (Washington, DC: Georgetown University Press, 1998), 132–42.
4. For a description of patient demographics in SNFs, see Sheel M. Pandya and the Independent Living/Long-Term Care Team, Public Policy Institute, Public Affairs, American Asso-

ciation of Retired Persons, "Nursing Homes," Feb. 2001, http://research.aarp.org/health/fs10r_nursing.html (9 Aug. 2003).

5. Franklin G. Miller and Howard Brody, "Professional Integrity and Physician-assisted Death," *Hastings Center Report* 25, no. 3 (1995): 8–17. For an extended discussion of the values inherent in medicine as a profession, see eds. Robert M. Veatch and Franklin G. Miller, *The Journal of Medicine and Philosophy* 26, no. 6 (2001): 555–662.

6. John Hardwig, "What About the Family?" *Hastings Center Report* 20, no. 2 (1990): 5–10; James Lindemann Nelson, "Taking Families Seriously," *Hastings Center Report* 22, no. 4 (1992): 6–12; Jeffrey Blustein, "The Family in Medical Decisionmaking," *Hastings Center Report* 23, no. 3 (1993): 6–13. But cf. Insoo Hyun, "Conceptions of Family-Centered Medical Decisionmaking and Their Difficulties," *Cambridge Quarterly of Healthcare Ethics* 12, no. 2 (2003): 196–200.

7. Helpful for providing an overview of the full range of challenges facing nursing home administrators (including issues related to patient care) is James E. Allen, *Nursing Home Administration*, 4th ed. (New York: Springer, 2003). George P. Smith, II, *Legal and Healthcare Ethics for the Elderly* (Washington, DC: Taylor and Francis, 1996), 91–106, provides an overview of the Patient's Bill of Rights, long-term care ombudsman representation, the use of physical and chemical restraints, forced psychotropic medication, and elder abuse issues. Peter J. Buttaro and Emily L. H. Buttaro, *Legal Guide for Long-Term Care Administrators* (Gaithersburg, MD: Aspen, 1999) provides an overview of issues related to torts, negligence, administrative and vicarious liability, corporate negligence, and protective arrangement for person and property. Most concrete in its attention to legal decisions, federal criminal and elder abuse statutes, and a review of residents' rights is California Advocates for Nursing Home Reform (CANHR), *Nursing Home Abuse: District Attorney's Reference Guide* (San Francisco: CANHR, 2000).

An Adult Child's Analysis

Harriet Spiegel, PhD

Mrs. K, the 84-year-old retired librarian, seems justifiably unhappy. The nursing staff, while perhaps well-intentioned and almost assuredly short-staffed and with limited financial resources, is nevertheless not listening to her. They are treating her more like a begonia than a mentally competent human being, worrying about her hydration and nutrition and keeping her alive, but not much more. And, in a way, these are the visible problem areas for Mrs. K: she cannot feed herself, her mobility is restricted, and her health is deteriorating.

I see nothing in this case that suggests a loss of intellectual acuity; indeed Mrs. K's responses seem appropriate to a mentally competent person who is frustrated and discouraged by physical limitations. Her rejection of the doctor's antipsychotic medications also seems appropriate: medication will not make her life a meaningful one. And it does seem that she will need to remain at a care facility.

The main problem I see is that Mrs. K's son, while acknowledging Mrs. K's complaints and conveying them to the nursing staff, seems to feel he needs more to please the administrator than his mother. He worries more about how to get his mother to take her medication than how to make her life meaningful.

My comments come from my upbringing as a Jew in an extended family with four generations in the same town. First I see the centrality of honoring the elderly and honoring one's parents as meaning more than supplying physical maintenance. Honoring means listening to our parents and our elders and learning from them. Mrs. K wants to be treated as the intelligent human being she is, reminding her caretakers, "My mind is just fine." If the son would listen to his mother, he would hear that she is asking her caretakers to treat her as the person she was and is.

In Mrs. K's case, several options exist for providing Mrs. K with experiences that would allow her to value her life, and give her reason to live and to cooperate with the nursing staff. She has been a librarian. Again, my background gives me reason to embrace her profession, for Jewish tradition values books, learning, and their vital connection to our human experience.

I would suggest that both the son and the nursing staff seek ways to engage Mrs. K's mind and professional history. They might solicit a visiting librarian service to supply books and occasional company as a way to engage her mind and expand her current life beyond its limitations. When my grandmother was ill and confined to her bed, she greatly looked forward to her weekly visit from a librarian. Additionally, she should be encouraged—and enabled—to attend reading groups in the community, including those in senior centers.

Locally, our synagogue has a reading group; two elderly community members, one of them blind (he reads using a computer-voice system), come regularly, picked up by other reading group members, and participate enthusiastically. I know they greatly look forward to these gatherings. Bookstores, libraries, schools, and religious institutions often have reading groups. As Mrs. K is able to leave the nursing home for visits with her son, I should think she would welcome outings that would engage her mind.

If the physical acts of holding a book and turning pages present difficulties for Mrs. K, agencies even in our small town can arrange for delivery of books on tape. If Mrs. K has an interest in childrens' books, local schools might be contacted; several schools in our town make regular visits to "adopted grandparents."

The son seems to know his mother well, and his desire to respect her intellectual abilities is to be commended. But he seems to have forgotten the need to foster continued intellectual activity in his attempts to get his mother to acquiesce to the institution's desires. I would suggest that he focus not so much on forcing his mother to cooperate with the institution's current approach, but rather on finding ways to revise their current aims to include intellectual nourishment, helping her keep alive her sense of self and, indeed, thus honoring her as a person, rather than as a plant.

A Psychologist's Analysis

Jane Rysberg, PhD

Mrs. K's son is in an approach-avoidance conflict, as he sees both positive and negative consequences to assuming decision-making power for his mother. In considering the placement of the feeding tube, he weighs physical health benefits against disruption of their relationship. He wonders whether, if he assumes responsibility for this decision, he can sidestep important questions in the future.

What does a person in an approach-avoidance conflict do? Typically, nothing. One way to break this behavioral log jam is to gain more information. Mr. K must try to answer two questions: (1) What is his mother thinking? (2) What is his mother doing?

What is mother thinking?

As a start, Mr. K requests to be present at his mother's next appointment with her physician. He asks pointed questions of the doctor and his mother to ensure that Mrs. K's increasing irritability and negative emotionality are not the result of previously undetected health problems, drug interactions, or poor pain management.[1]

Mrs. K's thoughts are not those of a demented patient, but neither are they the thoughts of her son. He measures his personal time against the date of his birth; at 84, his mother is likely to measure time in her distance from death. She has never been in this situation before and has no mental script for being an institutionalized elder. The "average resident," however, is someone like Mrs. K: female, with few social activities, and unable to perform activities of daily living unassisted.[2] This does not mean that Mrs. K finds her co-residents congenial, as about 60 percent of them suffer from mental as well as physical disabilities.[3]

Mrs. K clearly does not want to be in this situation, nor does her son. Neither is likely to have planned for any other alternatives. Americans, in general, are made anxious by the topics of aging and death; their thinking is likely to center around what they do not want in old age, rather than what they intend to do. Communications between those who might experience the process of aging together, such as parents and adult children, may be scanty, so they may have very different views on how care should be ensured.[4] Not knowing what to do may lead to unasked-for assistance and advice; elders find these advances unwelcome and unpleasant, carrying the message that the elder is incompetent.[5]

The relationship between an adult child and an aged parent is a product of their earlier relationship and present circumstances.[6] It is unlikely that Mrs. K is thinking about the anxiety and discomfort the present situation is creating. She is likely to be focusing upon herself.

What is mother doing?

The best predictor of future behavior is often past behavior. Mr. K reviews his mother's past life. He thinks of her "spunk and independence." Mrs. K worked outside of the home during a time when this was a rarity. She worked in a profession where she was master of all she surveyed. She valued precision and things of the mind. Mrs. K liked being in control. Her personality had suited her well to achievement in the world of work. She was very satisfied by her accomplishments. Though she had colleagues in the work world, she did not have a large social circle. Psychologists would have called her a "happy isolate," content to interact a few times a month with a friend outside of the workplace. Mrs. K had a great deal of practice in taking charge, organizing situations, controlling access, and providing final answers. She is unlikely to be consciously plotting to thwart the good intentions of the staff, but may be using behaviors that have become automatic.[7] It would take a very significant effort for Mrs. K to develop a new repertoire of social responses and attitudes. She might not think that the length of her remaining life span justifies the effort.

What should Mrs. K's son do?

Can Mr. K make it possible for his mother to return to her past lifestyle and habits? Humans tend to select environments that complement heredity ("niche picking").[8] All through adolescence and adulthood, Mrs. K was able to suit herself, picking hobbies, an occupation, and living arrangements that fostered her capacities. Her predispositions to be highly introverted and low in agreeableness made her successful as a research librarian and happy with a small circle of friends. But now Mrs. K has not selected her environment. If economics permit, a move to a first- floor, handicapped-accessible apartment, with full-time professional attendants might provide Mrs. K with the autonomy she craves. She would be able to select furnishings and set standards for dining and recreation.

Can Mr. K lower the perceived cost of change or help his mother to justify the emotional expense? It is unlikely that any skilled nursing facility can perfectly match Mrs. K's temperament and present physical needs, but improvements in the environment are possible. The last room on a corridor with a somewhat taciturn retired school teacher roommate might allow Mrs. K to satisfy her low need for companionship with a person she considers her intellectual equal. Books on tape can bring her back to the literary world without the need to turn a page. Mr. K might write his mother's biography for the staff, including suggestions for styles of social interaction. He might note, for example, that his mother is likely to respond more positively to the question "Would you like to be the first person to be helped to bathe this morning, or the last?" than to the statement "I'm here to get you out of bed for your bath." Finally, he opens negotiations about the feeding tube: "Mom, try it for several months. If you have not gained weight or had fewer infections, you can have it capped off."

Mr. K must decide whether he wishes to be responsible for all aspects of his mother's life. So far, he has been his mother's main contact with the "outside" world. If he does not wish to become solely responsible for his mother's social life, he should investigate other sources of stimulation. If any of his mother's colleagues or friends are able/willing to be available, he might provide them with phone cards and his mother's number to facilitate the continuation of social relationships that were functional in the past. If his mother participated in religious activities in the past, church services, such as Holy Communion or "Friendly Visitors," are possible. Perhaps a paid companion would come to the facility on a schedule set by Mrs. K and perform activities selected by her (e.g., reading *National Geographic* and the *New York Times* out loud, rearranging Mrs. K's belongings, or writing letters on her behalf).

Addendum

Mrs. K was not the client in this dilemma; her son asked for assistance. As a well-educated and alert woman, Mrs. K might benefit from direct professional service. As counseling is under the client's control, Mrs. K might find this alternative more desirable than the medication suggested by the physician.

Prior to old age, Mrs. K might have scored positively on some measures of "well-being." Well-being is a multidimensional concept often referred to as mental health or life satisfaction. One model of well-being applicable to Mrs. K uses six factors: self-acceptance, positive relations with others, autonomy, environmental mastery, personal growth, and purpose in life. Better psychological health is associated with higher scores on the measures of each factor.[9] Presently, Mrs. K seems unwilling to compromise, displays few aims and objectives, and feels unable to change her surroundings. It is unknown whether she now feels positively about herself or sees herself as effective.

The key to success in working with the elderly is building upon past strengths.[10] Mrs. K has been effective and successful. She may find her strengths again through counseling. Cognitive-behavioral approaches assist elders in recognizing and correcting negative thinking. Change can be effected in as few as 20 sessions.[11]

In conclusion, Mr. K has attempted to understand his mother's cognitions and behaviors. Based on his explorations of her past and present, he is trying to help her to restructure her environment so that she can exert as much control as possible, for as long as possible. He is sharing decision-making responsibilities with his mother. He must realize that understanding his mother's cognitions and behaviors will be an ongoing process.

Notes

1. Dorothy Field et al., "The Influence of Health on Family Contacts and Family Functioning in Advanced Old Age: A Longitudinal Study," *Journal of Gerontology: Psychological Sciences* 48 (1993): 18–28.
2. Ulrike Steinbach, "Social Networks, Institutionalization, and Mortality among Elderly People in the United States," *Journal of Gerontology: Social Sciences* 47 (1992): 183–90.
3. Center on Elderly People Living Alone, "Nursing Homes" (Public Policy Institute Fact Sheet FS10R) (Washington, DC: American Association of Retired Persons, 1995).
4. Raeann R. Hamon and Rosemary Blieszner, "Filial Responsibility Expectations among Adult Child-Older Parent Pairs," *Journal of Gerontology: Psychological Sciences* 45 (1990): 110–12.
5. Jacqui Smith and Jacqueline J. Goodnow, "Unasked-for Support and Unsolicited Advice: Age and the Quality of Social Experience," *Psychology and Aging* 14 (1999): 108–21.
6. Alice S. Rossi and Peter H. Rossi, *Of Human Bonding: Parent-child Relations Across the Life Course* (New York: Aldine de Gruyter, 1992).
7. Judith A. Ouellette and Wendy Wood, "Habit and Intention in Everyday Life: The Multiple Processes by Which Past Behavior Predicts Future Behavior," *Psychological Bulletin* 124 (1998): 54–74.
8. Sandra Scarr and Kathleen McCartney, "How People Make Their Own Environments: A Theory of Genotype Environment Effects," *Child Development* 54 (1983): 424–35.
9. Corey L. M. Keyes and Carol D. Ryff, "Psychological Well-being in Midlife," in *Life in the Middle*, eds. Sherry L. Willis and James D. Reid (San Diego: Academic Press, 1999), 161–80.
10. Helen Q. Kivnick, "Everyday Mental Health: A Guide to Assessing Life Strengths," *Generations* 17 (1993): 13–20.
11. Harold G. Koenig and Dan G. Blazer, "Mood Disorders and Suicide," in *Handbook of Mental Health and Aging*, 2nd ed. eds. James E. Birren, Robert Sloane, and Gene D. Cohen (New York: Academic Press, 1992), 379–407.

A Religious Studies Analysis

Andrew Flescher, PhD

In deciding whether to follow the administrator's advice and assume decisional authority in matters pertaining to his mother's care, Mrs. K's son faces the classic dilemma of having to choose between two competing values in tension in end-of-life care. These values are autonomy (respect for one's ability to decide what happens to her) and beneficence (promoting whatever is in the patient's best interests, irrespective of the patient's desires).

Religious and secular traditions alike prize (though weigh differently) these values as instrumental in determining a patient's "quality of life." Western religious traditions such as Judaism, Christianity, and Islam, which often subscribe to a "sanctity of life" doctrine, are likely to maintain that life itself overrides promoting an agent's choices when these values conflict. In this sense, Jewish, Christian, and Muslim ethics tend to prioritize well-being over autonomy. Theologians like the Christian thinker Paul Ramsey, for example, consider all human life to be given by and "on loan" from God. Writes Ramsey: "His essence is his existence before God and to God, as it is from Him. His dignity is 'an *alien* dignity,' an evaluation that is not of him but placed upon him by the divine decree."[1] The traditional theological view, then, is that our life is not our own to terminate under any set of circumstances.

Conversely, most secular traditions (including our legal system) acknowledge a fundamental right for a competent patient to consent to or refuse treatment and, hence, prioritize autonomy over well-being. Since we are given no indication as to the son's own background and, more importantly, that of his mother, we must assume that *both* well-being and autonomy are equally important and thereby direct the son to follow a course of action that preserves each value to the greatest extent possible.

Mrs. K is clearly uncooperative. However she does not yet have dementia or some other condition that would render her incompetent. So we must assume, her stubbornness notwithstanding, that she is capable of understanding the nature of medical decisions that need to be made on her own behalf. At the same time, to the extent that her personality quirks *do* lead her to resist "accepted protocols," she calls into question her competence, and opens the door for her son, who is her designated surrogate, to assume at least some decisional responsibility. We may infer that the situation is fairly urgent, since without basic treatment (e.g., nutrition, hydration, medication), Mrs. K will quickly "deteriorate beyond recovery." In other words, we are given the impression that Mrs. K's well-being cannot be preserved *at all* if the son does not compromise his mother's autonomy *to some degree*. The question then becomes: Is it possible to save Mrs. K's life and still give her some degree of autonomy?

The son is appropriately reluctant to take over his mother's decisional authority. He is in a position to do so because mutual respect and trust led his mother to designate him as her surrogate decision maker. And her son continues to be an active and supportive participant in her care and recovery. Respect and trust demand that before anything is done, he should discuss her health care professionals' (HCPs') concerns with her, taking the time to explain—with all due sensitivity—that they (and he) are beginning to have doubts about her ability to decide in her best interests. Because of the relationship he has with his mother, we might be optimistic that this conversation will be fruitful. In addition, the son should make every attempt to appease his mother whenever her requests do not place her life in further jeopardy. All of this amounts to a "good faith" gesture in the direction of autonomy. Indeed, with this course of action, nothing is done behind Mrs. K's back, and her son may even manage to change his mother's mind in a few key respects, allowing her to maintain a sense that she, and no one else, is in control.

Having said this, Mrs. K's son ought not to allow his mother to refuse treatment altogether, lest he allow her to fall into rapid decline to the point of dying. If the son exhibits good faith by going out of his way to communicate to his mother the administrator's misgivings and fails to cede control to her only when she chooses health- or life-threatening choices, then the son need not feel that he is morally remiss or has let his mother down in some fundamental respect when he opts to follow the administrator's advice. The more his mother acts irrationally and the more he tries to appease her nonetheless, the more his initial reluctance in assuming some decisional authority should give way to a feeling that he is exercising a responsible prudence.

One of the difficulties is that Mrs. K is poised to decline to the point of dying before she deteriorates into incompetence. That is, according to the scenario, the son must choose between sacrificing the mother's will and sacrificing her life too soon. However, this either-or choice, presented as starkly as it is here, is overdrawn and potentially misleading, for there is a *range* of states of mind a patient can exhibit *between* the poles of competence and incompetence.[2] In this case, the mother's conduct seems to indicate that she falls somewhere within this range. On the one hand, Mrs. K can articulate that she understands the purpose and necessity of her medication and therapy, and to this extent she is clearly competent. On the other hand, that she is becoming increasingly uncooperative, which is likely tied to her deteriorating mental state (which we can assume by virtue of the need for an "antipsychotic"), leads us to hold plausibly that Mrs. K is, if not fully incompetent, at least "on the road" to incompetence. But if this is so, then we should conclude that it is possible for her son to assume *some* decisional authority without *fully* depriving her of her autonomy.[3] In support of this qualified assessment, we might observe that nutrition, hydration, and medication, all of which the administrator wants to ensure for Mrs. K, are vital to Mrs. K's maintaining her competence. Thus, in the final analysis, preserving Mrs. K's well-being (and indeed that of patients similarly situated) ironically turns out to be tantamount to providing for her competence, which she must demonstrate in order to be allowed to act against her own well-being in the first place.

Notes

1. Paul Ramsey, "The Morality of Abortion," in *Moral Problems: A Collection of Philosophical Essays*, 3rd ed., ed. James Rachels (New York: Harper and Row, 1979), 45–46.
2. Becky Cox White, *Competence to Consent* (Washington, DC: Georgetown University Press, 1994), 95–106.
3. Ibid., 83–95.

A Medical Director's Analysis

Terry Hill, MD

Although the narrative about Mrs. K ends with a question, it also suggests that her son knows what he should do, at least in regard to having his mother make her own decisions. In discussion with the skilled nursing facility (SNF) administrator, the son "protests that his mother is still competent and, when cooperative, is capable of making treatment decisions." He even seems to have some awareness of legal and regulatory mandates when he asks, "Don't we still need to get her permission for these sorts of serious treatments?" In spite of his knowledge, however, he quickly begins to cede ground to the administrator's arguments, illustrating the vulnerability of emotionally involved family members. Faced with the threat of losing a loved one, we can be swayed even by specious arguments, even by people who hardly trouble to hide their moral deficits.

The question of who should decide about these "serious treatments" is simple. Under the doctrine of informed consent, a person with adequate decision-making capacity has the right to make her own medical decisions. Although Mrs. K can be uncooperative, nothing suggests that she lacks decision-making capacity. Even if her capacity varied from day to day, the clinicians would have an obligation to engage her when she is at her best, when she might be capable of making a fully informed and reasoned decision. If she lacked all capacity and could give no meaningful input, her son as surrogate would have an obligation to use "substituted judgment," to make the decisions consistent with her own prior expressed preferences or her values—in short, to make the decisions he believes she would make, if she could.[1]

The administrator is either ill-informed or manipulative when she argues that these interventions are in Mrs. K's "best interest." Best interest, in the context of medical decision making, is an acceptable fall-back position only when we do not know a person's preferences. Furthermore, best interest should not be narrowly construed as longevity. California law illustrates this point for people near the end of their lives:

> Modern medical technology has made possible the artificial prolongation of human life beyond natural limits. In the interest of protecting individual autonomy, this prolongation of the process of dying for a person for whom continued healthcare does not improve the prognosis for recovery may violate patient dignity and cause unnecessary pain and suffering, while providing nothing medically necessary or beneficial to the person.[2]

It would be hard to argue that stripping Mrs. K of her decision-making authority—her autonomy—would be in her best interest. Her dignity, pain, and suffering also deserve full consideration in decision-making discussions. Efficiency, from the point of view of staff members or the facility, can at times be a legitimate concern in such discussions, supported by theories of justice and equitable distribution of resources. In this case, however, the administrator appears to be disguising her own efficiency interests within her arguments for medical interventions for Mrs. K.

Fortunately the son brings some knowledge about decision making into the situation. He may be able to resist the administrator's pressure. Unfortunately he has no clue that his mother's clinical care is woefully inadequate, at least in two respects. The story provides ample clues that his mother may be depressed, yet she is not being offered appropriate behavioral or pharmacological therapy. Antipsychotics are not appropriate medications for depression. In discussing the antipsy-chotic, both the administrator and the son are victims of bad medical advice. Placing a feeding tube in a cognitively intact person against her will without appropriate assessment is an equally strange and bad idea. Mrs. K may be losing weight because she doesn't like the rigid meal schedule or because she's depressed. The use of feeding tubes in nursing facilities has come under increasing criticism. Even for people with advanced dementia, which Mrs. K does not have, there is no evidence that feeding tubes improve longevity, health, or quality of life, in spite of myths to the contrary.[3]

This nursing facility has not done well by Mrs. K. Her irritability and defiance may have been triggered in part by the staff's lack of respect in treating her "like an idiot or a baby." The administrator and physician have demonstrated a profound lack of respect in discounting her preferences and her right to participate in planning her own medical care. The physician and other members of the care team should have worked with Mrs. K from the beginning to elicit her goals for rehabilitation and to help shape those goals as her rehabilitation potential changed over time.[4] Had they continued to respect her personhood, they might have gained her cooperation. They would also have grounds for asking that she herself be respectful rather than "berating the staff." The facility's failure to do appropriate assessments and its careless handling of the consent issues put it at serious risk of citation by state surveyors.

At this point, Mrs. K's son—and her professional caregivers, if they have a change of heart—should try to turn the situation around on clinical, ethical, and human levels. Mrs. K deserves adequate assessment and a trial of behavioral or pharmacological therapy for depression. Someone needs to engage her as a person and begin to restore her participation in her own care. A nurse, social worker, psychologist, psychiatrist, the medical director, or nursing facility ombudsman might be available and able to help. Communities may have ethics committees or ethics resources available, but trained and conscientious ethics committees are rare in nursing facilities. It may be too late, but honesty and respect are in order. One could start by listening, patiently and persistently, to Mrs. K.

Notes

1. ECHO Long-Term Care Task Force: ECHO Nursing Facility Recommendations, California Coalition for Compassionate Care, 1990, http://www.finalchoices.calhealth.org/pubs_materials.htm#echo (8 Aug. 2003).
2. CA Probate Code § 4650(b).
3. Thomas E. Finucane, Colleen Christmas, and Kathy Travis, "Tube Feeding for Patients with Advanced Dementia: A Review of the Evidence," *JAMA: Journal of the American Medical Association* 282, no. 14 (1999): 1365–70.
4. See note 1, above.

Further Reflections

General

1. How does the concept of quality of life inform discussions of patient interest? Medicine, nursing, and the larger society (often informed by the traditional religious value of the sanctity of life) often talk about the "intrinsic value of life." What characteristics might make life intrinsically valuable? What is the relationship between these characteristics and quality of life?

Consequences

2. Identify the interests of Mrs. K, her son, and the skilled nursing facility (SNF) staff. How are these interests affected if Mrs. K continues to reject treatment? changes her mind and agrees to treatment? is forced to accept treatment? Do patients' self-described interests have any claim to primacy if others construe those interests differently? Why (not)? What sorts of conflicts are possible given the different interests at stake among the various parties in this case?

Autonomy

3. Discuss the relationship of competence to autonomous decision making and to physical deterioration.
4. Can a commitment to personal or professional integrity justify overriding persons' autonomy and acting for their benefit even if against their will?

Rights

5. If competent, Mrs. K has a well-established right to make decisions about her own health care. Yet Flescher suggests that the more consistently Mrs. K resists interventions that compromise her health, the stronger the moral pressure for others to assume decisional authority for her. What moral values does this right protect, and to which moral values does/might Flescher appeal?

Virtues

6. Consider what characteristics are part of a good parent-child relationship. What is required of Mrs. K's son if he is to be a good son and fulfill his obligations to his mother?
7. HCPs are committed to saving life, preserving or restoring health, minimizing disability, and minimizing pain and suffering. When these goals conflict, how might HCPs determine what professional integrity requires? How might this conflict contribute to the many ways in which this SNF has, according to Hill, failed Mrs. K?

Chapter 3

The Not-So-Golden Years

Mrs. O is a 63-year-old Navajo woman who moved with her husband about 20 years ago from an Arizona reservation to a small ranching community (population: 7000) in the northwestern United States. Mrs. O's husband worked for a small company (approximately 30 employees) that sold and transported livestock. She lives in a modest two-bedroom home in which she and her husband raised their three children. Her neighbors are mostly families of employees of this company, as these homes are close to their workplace. When Mr. O died suddenly about five years ago, Mrs. O remained in the house, content to continue working in her garden and tutoring local children in reading and arithmetic. She regrets that she is not closer to a Navajo community or reservation, but she is otherwise content with her circumstances.

Until about four years ago Mrs. O was in good physical condition and continued to drive and keep up her property. But limited exercise tolerance—as a result of chronic obstructive pulmonary disease (COPD), which led to shortness of breath and chronic cough, and severe generalized osteoarthritis, an inflammation of her joints that results in a stiffening and loss of joint use—has made her increasingly sedentary and homebound. She takes Vicodin (a narcotic pain relief and cough-suppressant medicine) every four hours to control her pain and to minimize her nonproductive cough. Two of her children have suggested she move in with them, but both live about 500 miles distant, and Mrs. O is reluctant to leave her home and friends. She has done well with support from her neighbors, who help her with bathing and meal preparation. Because her community is small and remote, she lacks access to home health nurses or physical therapists who might monitor her condition or help her acquire coping mechanisms to compensate for her increasing exercise limitations.

Mrs. O's financial situation has always been precarious. She still makes a mortgage payment of $325/month, something of a struggle, as her sole source of income is social security survivor's benefits of $760/month. When her husband died, she received $50,000 from a life insurance policy carried by his employer. Occasionally she uses the life insurance money to supplement her meager monthly income but is reluctant to do so: this is the only resource upon which she could draw if she needed to move from her home into an assisted living or extended care facility—a very real possibility given her increasing dependence on others to meet her daily needs. She has also entertained the idea of moving back to the Arizona reservation, but—again—prefers to remain with the friends she has made over the last 20 years.

A year ago Mrs. O's youngest son Frank, aged 34, moved in with her. His automotive repair business had failed after he was injured on the job. He was receiving $500 a month in disability payments and his anticipated contribution to the household income made the arrangement attractive. Initially Mrs. O was heartened by his arrival. She welcomed the opportunity to assist in her son's recovery. She assumed he would do the shopping, keep up the property, and drive her to church (she is a converted Catholic) and to her Bible study each week, whereby she could maintain valuable contacts with friends of many years. And in fact Frank performed these tasks conscientiously at first. In addition, he assumed responsibility for managing her financial affairs (difficult for her, given her visual deficits). However, his injuries have healed, his disability payments have been discontinued, and he has made no effort to find gainful employment. Mrs. O's $760 a month must now support two people. This is impossible and Frank indicated he is withdrawing $750 each month from the life insurance money.

Given Mrs. O's long-standing financial difficulties, the neighbors were surprised when Frank purchased a new truck; since then he is gone quite often, sometimes for days at a time. When he is home he drinks to excess.

Recently Mrs. O's neighbors have noticed worrisome changes in Mrs. O. She seems to be coughing more and to be in more pain, and she has begun to lose weight. When her closest neighbor, Mrs. R, asked if anything was bothering her, Mrs. O changed the subject. Mrs. R encouraged her to see her doctor, noting that the increasing distress and unexplained weight loss could portend serious disease. Again, Mrs. O changed the subject, merely commenting in passing that she wishes she could regain her hózhó—or sense of harmony and peace.

One morning Mrs. R discovers Mrs. O crying from pain. When she goes to get some Vicodin to give her, she discovers an empty bottle. She calls the pharmacy to get an immediate refill, only to be told that Mr. O's son had refilled the prescription two days ago. After several failed attempts to make Mrs. O comfortable, Mrs. R calls the ambulance to take Mrs. O to the regional hospital.

When the ambulance arrives, Mrs. R relates Mrs. O's recent history to the paramedic, Ms. M: Mrs. O is eating very little and has suffered serious pain and respiratory distress for several weeks now. Mrs. R speculates that she is eating less, in part because she has difficulty preparing meals (which the neighbors ceased doing when Frank arrived on the scene) and in part to curb expenses. Mrs. R confides her concerns that Frank is pilfering Mrs. O's savings and confiscating her Vicodin (whether for his own use or to sell she is uncertain).

Mrs. R expresses the hope that Ms. M can intervene on Ms. O's behalf. Beyond transporting Mrs. O to the hospital, Ms. M wonders whether she should do anything else.

Introduction

Mrs. O's predicament raises at least three moral concerns:

1. What cues should we take from the traditions (ethnic, religious) and lifestyle enclaves that patients inhabit when deciding on how to treat them medically?
2. What special obligations do friends and family have to the elderly who are infirm?
3. What immediate obligations do first-responders have to patients whose health care needs extend beyond what they are prepared to provide?

The AJ Method

Step 1: Information Gathering   What facts are necessary for resolving this case? What is the actual state of Mrs. O's living conditions? (Douglas) In terms of which community—Navajo or Anglo—does Mrs O define herself, or structure her life? How close are Mrs. O's ties to the Navajo community? (Lustig; Reid) Who does

Mrs. O see as the appropriate decision maker about her care? (Reid) Is Mrs. O capable of autonomous decision making? (Douglas) What form—Navajo or Christian—would appropriate treatment of Mrs. O take? What is the appropriate role of Mrs. O's neighbors in her care? of her son? (Reid) Has Frank been stealing his mother's medications? Is he likely—and, if so, how likely—to continue doing so, given her acute problems? Why does Mrs. O want to protect her son?

Although many Americans imagine that skilled, long-term, or residential care facilities are the inevitable fate of senior citizens, only 1.45 million—just under 4 percent of Americans over age 65—are presently institutionalized. Another 1.4 million seniors depend on formal home health care; but 90 percent of Americans over age 65—about 33 million men and women—are self-sufficient or depend, like Mrs. O, on the informal care of family and friends.[1]

The Navajo culture sees the world as a unified whole, a sacred universe populated by many beings and in which human beings hold no privileged status.[2] Humans are called to live in unity and harmony with this sacred cosmos, and to recognize the importance of the community of people with which one is affiliated and from which one acquires one's true identity. In addition to kinship among humans are important and special connections to animals and sacred places and homelands.[3] When one lives in harmony with the beautiful (achieving *hózhó*)— when one's mind, spirit, and body are compatible with the universe—one is well.[4]

Navajo tradition teaches that persons are responsible for their own wellness, achieved by avoiding forbidden acts and contact with dangerous objects. When a personal error or transgression (whether intentional or accidental, and whether recognized or not) occurs, illness may ensue. In Navajo medicine, the etiology of illness is traced to a variety of factors, including the presence of intrusive objects or spirits (ghosts, witches), bothersome influences, or the corruption or loss of one's soul or life forces.[5] The symptoms of illness are expressed as a range of diseases, personal dispositions, and life disruptions. The goal of treatment—in the context of prayer-centered rituals and ceremonies performed by professional singers or healers—is to banish the cause of the disease and recenter the life of the "one sung over" rather than to simply alleviate the symptoms of a narrowly conceived medical problem or disease.[6] Even traditional Western health care interventions (medications, surgery), when embraced, may need to be undertaken when the timing is "propitious" in the larger cosmic order; such moments are not necessarily defined or determined by medical science, but rather "revealed."

Also critical to health-related issues is the Navajos' belief that thought and language have "the power to shape reality and to control events. . . . In the Navajo view of the world, language is not a mirror of reality, reality is a mirror of language . . . language does not merely describe reality, language shapes reality. . . . For these reasons traditional Navajo patients may regard the discussion of negative information as potentially harmful."[7] To speak of potential events or engage in direct and explicit discussion of negative information or complications is to bring them about.

Thus traditional Navajos typically avoid discussing risks or burdens as part of assuming responsibility for maintaining health; instead they focus on thinking and speaking in a manner that is consistent with the way of harmony and beauty.

These beliefs have profound implications for patient-professional relationships with respect to treatment and decisional authority, including advance care planning. Western medicine and bioethics—which emphasize patient autonomy, self-determination, informed and educated consent, personal decisional authority, the rational balancing of possible responses to various treatment options—may profoundly conflict with traditional Navajo healing ways. These opportunities for misinterpretation and misunderstanding continue to shape the uneasy relationship between Navajo culture and contemporary American society, including its system of health care.[8]

Finally, Navajo tradition locates responsibility for care of the elderly with the family. Family members are critical to providing care, not the least because they accept that aging is a natural stage in the human life cycle.[9]

Mrs. O's life as a practicing Roman Catholic in a small town removed from a Navajo community and culture places her in a world informed by a Western worldview shaped by ancient Judaism, the Greco-Roman and medieval worlds, and some strands of the modern secular Enlightenment. The Roman Catholic community embraces a voluntaristic view of membership in a sacramental community. Participation in the life of the church is open to all, is entered into freely, and confers on its members both the gift of salvation as well as the freedom—and moral obligation—to embrace a life of moral purity in worshipful submission to God.[10] Humans—though part of the created world—possess the *imago dei* (the image of God) at the core of their being.[11] This sets humanity apart from the rest of creation and confers on them a superior status in the cosmos. As a result, the rest of the cosmos (including other living sentient and nonsentient beings, as well as natural resources, science, and technology) are at the service of human beings. And though humanity's moral role is as steward or caretaker of these resources, the sciences and the material wealth of the world are resources for persons and may be employed for the benefit of humanity and its quest to perfect the cosmos consistent with the will of God.

The Catholic worldview, then, gives medicine and health care an important, positive status, and allows—even encourages—the use of the healing arts as a means to maintain and advance humanity.[12] Health care in service to the poor and as a means to empower human beings to creative and productive lives is central to a Catholic theology of health and healing. Because the causes of illness are natural rather than supernatural (Catholic cosmology is for the most part compatible with modern science and scientific understandings of causation and with germ theory, genetics, and modern theories of health and healing), medicine is viewed as the rational and dispassionate mastery of a theoretically finite body of knowledge, applied to humans for the purpose of removing disease and illness, and treating symptoms that might impede or hamper human freedom, development, and performance. While Catholicism certainly is communitarian, in the sense that individuals do not stand separate, apart from, or superior to the integrity of the community, individuals are, for the most part, free to make—and are responsible for—their own medical decisions. On the other hand, there is a strong bias in Catholic health care that interventions that can improve human life and health and should be offered to— and accepted by—those in need of such healing. American Catholicism encourages frank discussions between patients and health care professionals (HCPs) regarding treatment options and their risks and burdens (i.e., negative outcomes). Finally, "propitious timing" of an intervention or treatment is the timing advised by professional physicians and other clinicians.

Roman Catholicism is less settled about caregiving responsibility for those in whom self-sufficiency is no longer possible. Families are usually considered to have the primary obligation, but the mobility of twenty-first-century families often excuses them from or attenuates this obligation. Friends and church members are also expected to help out but are excused if assistance becomes overly burdensome.

Step 2: Creative Problem Solving   Any creative solution would have to promote Mrs. O's welfare and independence without risking harm to the EMT.

Step 3: Pros and Cons   Survey CARVE principles to identify important moral reasons that support conflicting options for resolving this case.

Consequences   Identifying positive and negative effects of actions requires some appreciation of how Mrs. O (and, perhaps, her son) defines "harm" and "benefit," definitions that may be culturally relative. Effects for the EMT can presumably be evaluated from the perspective of the dominant (Anglo) culture. (Douglas; Lustig)

First, we must wonder whether the EMTs (or subsequent HCPs) understand what will count as a "harm" or a "benefit" for Mrs. O, or even whether to explicitly raise the concerns raised by her neighbor. Mrs. O's Navajo heritage and her Catholic tradition offer significantly different approaches to both identifying and resolving medical and social problems.

Autonomy   Which option will best respect Mrs. O's autonomy—including the values and lifestyle she prefers? (Reid) Where does decisional authority lie in this case? (All commentators)

If we hope to provide individuals such as Mrs. O with the treatment, care, and support that they require to flourish, attention to their cultural and community identity is critical. Cultural identity is constructed most basically in terms of how one sees the world (a worldview); how one comes to see the world in this way (the process of acculturation and cultural accommodation); and the place that one occupies in this world (social location).

Mrs. O's cultural identity is complex: she is Navajo by birth and Catholic Christian by choice. Her origins are in the community of the Navajo reservation, but she has made her home in the larger culture and has embraced many of its conventions and values (living alone and in a nuclear family-type setting). If we hope to appreciate Mrs. O's cultural identity, we need to appreciate these—and other—aspects of her life and the choices that she has made.

These competing worldviews have myriad implications for interactions with the health care system. Depending on which worldview Mrs. O embraces (or embraces more strongly), she may not even have defined herself as ill prior to her recent deterioration. She might have seen her pulmonary and joint diseases as discrete pathologies; but she might have believed herself to be in harmony with the universe, in spite of suffering these afflictions. Assume, though, that she did define herself as unwell. What would she consider to be the proper treatment—a Navajo healing ceremony, prayer, Western pharmaceuticals, or some combination of the above? Does she hold herself responsible for her chronic illnesses and believe she must take steps to effect a cure? Are they medical problems that require a physician's intervention? Will she welcome or reject conversations about particular interventions and their potential effects? Finally, who should assist her as her life tasks become increasingly difficult?

An appreciation of Mrs. O's Navajo heritage may provide an important window to better understanding the challenges of her personal situation—but only if Mrs. O continues to embrace that culture. The same claim can be made about her Catholic tradition. Current literature demonstrates much concern for cultural identity, but such attitudes can contribute to pigeonholing patients into one-size-fits-all cultural designations.[13]

Rights Although Mrs. O has a right of self-determination, we might wonder whether she herself embraces—or understands—that right, or if she views herself as a member of a family, neighborhood, or tribe which eschews individual rights-based analyses. Are the rights to privacy and confidentiality relevant here? (Douglas; Lustig)

Virtues Fidelity seems to arise in several versions of role-related responsibilities: Mrs. O's son, her neighbor, and the EMT. Who is responsible for Mrs. O's ongoing welfare? (All commentators)

Who should assume primary responsibility for the welfare of noninstitutionalized seniors: family, friends, communities, the health care system, individual practitioners, others? As Mrs. O's case demonstrates, each of these answers is partially unsatisfactory. Are there moral obligations of intervention or aid that these communities and individuals might have to Mrs. O? Certainly friendship—and familial obligations in the context of Christian and Navajo culture—carry obligations of beneficence and fidelity. But how far and how deep do these obligations extend, particularly as Mrs. O seems to inhabit—at least psychologically—two different communities?

What about the EMT who initially assesses Mrs. O? Her code of ethics commits her to nonmaleficence and beneficence, but Mrs. O's needs exceed the scope of responsibility typically associated with first-responders. If the EMT is culturally sensitive, she must wonder about the questions raised above; if she is culturally unaware, she may intrude in an arena of responsibility Mrs. O is reluctant to concede to others.

Assuming Mrs. O is willing to enter the health care system, meeting her needs may still prove challenging. Providing good care in a less-than-affluent rural community with its sometimes uncoordinated and inadequate health care service requires imaginative problem solving on the part of all local providers. HCPs in small communities necessarily work "outside the box" in providing care. If, for example, the town lacks a social worker, other HCPs will assume the responsibilities that this specialized professional normally assumes. Moreover, rural HCPs are interdependent to an unusual degree, having neither the time nor the resources to see interventions through to a discipline-specific conclusion.

EMTs—as first-responders to medical emergencies—have obligations of beneficence to patients that appear to be narrowly circumscribed by a traditional understanding of their professional responsibilities as limited to acute interventions. EMTs benefit most patients by providing standard care (providing physiological support and stabilizing the patient for transport). But in an environment with limited HCPs, nonemergency HCPs depend on EMTs to assess patients *and* their circumstances, as EMTs' presence on-site may be the only opportunity to acquire this essential information. The concern is that HCPs will exceed both the scope of their education (including cultural and psychosocial training) and their professional standards of practice based on that education—raising concerns about violating the principle of nonmaleficence.

Equality/Fairness (Justice) Does depending on medically naïve friends or family to care for infirm elders constitute an unjust burden? (Reid) Is Frank guilty of elder abuse for which he deserves punishment (Douglas; Lustig)

The Law Which, if any, HCPs have a legal obligation to report Mrs. O's son for possible elder abuse, drug abuse, or theft?[14]

The following commentaries examine the application of various moral principles to this dilemma, thereby assisting the reader to undertake *Step 4: Analysis* and *Step 5: Justification.*

Notes

1. U.S. Centers for Disease Control, National Center for Health Statistics, Table 1: Resident Population, According to Age, Sex, Race, and Hispanic Origin: United States, Selected Years, 1950–2000; Table 87: Home Healthcare Patients, According to Age, Sex, and Diagnosis: United States, Selected Years, 1992–2000; Table 110: Nursing Home Beds, Occupancy, and Residents, According to Geographic Division and State: United States,

1995–2000; Table 97: Nursing Home Residents 65 Years of Age and Over, According to Age, Sex, and Race: United States, 1985, 1995, 1999, 2002, http://www.cdc.gov/nchs/products/pubs/pubd/hus/listables.pdf#Facilities (3 Mar. 2004).

2. For discussions of health and health care in the Navajo tradition, see Stephen J. Kunitz and Jerrold E. Levy, "Navajos," *Ethnicity and Medical Care*, ed. Alan Harwood (Cambridge: Harvard University Press, 1981).

3. Terence Anderson, "The Strangers and the People of the Land: Cross-cultural Implications for Christian Ethics," in *The Annual of the Society of Christian Ethics* (Washington, DC: Georgetown University Press, 1990), 140–75; Åke Hultkrantz, *Native Religions of North America: The Power of Visions and Fertility* (San Francisco: Harper & Row, 1987), 21.

4. Åke Hultkrantz, *Shamanic Healing and Ritual Drama: Health and Medicine in Native North American Religious Traditions* (New York: Crossroads, 1992), 129.

5. See note 2, above, 356–58.

6. Sam D. Gill, *Sacred Words: A Study of Navajo Religion and Prayer* (Westport, CT: Greenwood Press, 1981).

7. Joseph Carrese and Lorna Rhodes, "Western Bioethics on the Navajo Reservation: Benefit or Harm?" *JAMA: The Journal of the American Medical Association* 274, (1995): 826–29; Wade Davies, *Healing Ways: Navajo Healthcare in the Twentieth Century* (Albuquerque: University of New Mexico Press, 2001).

8. Ibid.

9. B. Josea Kramer, "Health and Aging of Urban American Indians," *Western Journal of Medicine* 157 (1992): 281–85.

10. Richard McCormick, SJ, *Health and Medicine in the Catholic Tradition* (New York: Crossroads/Herder & Herder, 1987), 33.

11. Joel Zimbelman, "A Blessing in Disguise: Empowering Catholic Healthcare Institutions in the Current Healthcare Environment," *Christian Bioethics: Non-Ecumenical Studies in Medical Morality* 6, no. 3 (2000): 281–94 .

12. See note 10, above, 39–43.

13. Edmund G. Howe, "Commentary: 'Missing' Patients by Seeing Only Their Cultures," *The Journal of Clinical Ethics* 9, no. 2 (1998): 191–93.

14. Ethical and legal issues differ slightly for home health care professionals and first-responders. See Martha Dale Nathanson, *Home Health Care Law Manual* (Gaithersburg, MD: Aspen Publishers, 1996), Chap. 8, "Fraud and Abuse Issues for the Home Health Provider;" eds., Andrea Walter et al., *First Responder Handbook: Law Enforcement Edition* (Albany, NY: Delmar Learning, 2003), Chap. 4, "Legal and Ethical Considerations," 55–69; and American Medical Association, Council on Ethical and Judicial Affairs, *Code of Medical Ethics: Current Opinions with Annotations,* 2000–2001 Edition (Chicago: American Medical Association, 2000), § 2.02, "Abuse of Spouses, Children, Elderly Persons, and Others at Risk," 4–7.

A Navajo Physician's Analysis

Raymond Reid, MD

A comment frequently heard throughout Indian country is, "Navajos are everywhere." Indeed, according to the 2000 census Navajos were counted in all 50 states. Noted also was that almost 44 percent of the Navajo population lived off the reservation, which is located in the Four Corners area of the states of Arizona, New Mexico, Colorado, and Utah.

The woman described is a 63-year-old Navajo who has lived in a small Northwest community for about 20 years, widowed for about five years, yet choosing to remain among friends. To Navajo on the reservation, this information raises questions regarding Navajo identity, strength of ties to family and clan, and the extent to which commonly taught cultural practices and beliefs are considered relevant when important decisions are made.

The basic Navajo family unit is the extended family. This consists of the maternal grandparents, all grown female siblings, and their husbands and children. Their homes are clustered together. Everyone belongs to the same clan, except the husbands; the husbands' clans become related clans within each single family. All individuals function as a unit with much sharing of basic necessities, money, livestock, chores, and responsibilities. All adults, especially older women, are involved in making important decisions. Help, support, and comfort are given each other in times of hardships and difficulties.

Early in their traditional upbringing Navajos are taught their various individual identities which include name, personal clan, related clans, and the location of residence. One's clan is that of the mother. Related clans include clans of the father, maternal grandfather, and fraternal grandfather. When conveying this information to others, Navajos fulfill their cultural tendency to want to establish relationships with other Navajos, even those with whom there were no previous acquaintances. Many Navajos consider clan relationship as important as or more important than blood relationship. Two Navajo strangers who've never met and who find out that they belong to the same clan can instantly and with cultural legitimacy call each other brother or sister, which is a new relationship that can last a lifetime.

The Navajo concept of "home" goes beyond the location of a dwelling. One's true home on the reservation is the burial place of the stub of one's umbilical cord. The umbilical cord carries the substances of life to the unborn baby and is the spiritual connection between mother, baby, and the outside world. The birthing process and the anatomical structures involved are sacred. Before hospitals were built on the reservation, birth took place inside the traditional Navajo dwelling, the hogan, an octagonal one-room structure made of earth and logs with a door that always faces east, the direction of the rising sun. Entering the hogan is likened to returning to the womb of Mother Earth, a place where protection, nourishment, and a spiritual environment are provided. Ceremonies are performed in the hogan. It's where one returns during times of physical and emotional disorders and to restore harmony, or *hózhó*.

All of the above—the matriarchal Navajo society, clanship descending through women, the role of women within the extended family, giving birth, and the connection between the hogan and Mother Earth—intimately implicate the traditional importance of women.

In the case presented here, the actions taken by the Navajo woman following each unfortunate event are incongruent with Navajo traditional practice. The woman is 63 years old, placing her birth around 1940 or earlier. At that time, most Navajos lived in hogans which had no running water and electricity, herded sheep, spoke only the Navajo language, and had a traditional upbringing. Prior to moving to the Northwest, she had many years' exposure to Navajo lifestyles and culture.

By 63 years of age, most Navajo women would have permanently returned to the reservation because of the strong urge to return to their traditions. Especially after becoming widowed, most women permanently return for emotional support from family, and blood and clan relatives. Because many taboos are associated with death, the urge to be cleansed of evil spirits brings many Navajos back to the reservation where ceremonies can be performed over them. Such a ceremony to restore harmony is done only in a hogan.

Serious illness is also a reason many Navajos return to the reservation, where health care and prescription drugs can be provided free of charge by the Indian Health Service (IHS). The woman in the case should have known this and, considering the seriousness of her illness and the high cost of treatment, the reason for her seeming to have rejected IHS care needs exploration. Returning to the reservation would have placed her near family and relatives from whom she could have received support and care. If she wished, she could have had a healing ceremony performed in an effort to restore *hózhó*.

Considering Navajo traditional practice, most puzzling about this case is the woman's preference to remain "alone" in the Northwest away from the company of her children, and family and relatives on the reservation while burdened by financial, physical, family, mental, and emotional problems. Strong traditional teachings about family, relatives, clans, and the support afforded by this system of relations seemed to have been discarded by the woman. The Navajo concept of "home" and the hogan seem distant if all she did was utter *hózhó* without seriously making plans to return to the reservation. To what degree did she consider her traditional status as a woman to be important? What prevented her from returning to the reservation where so many Navajos return when in a situation such as hers? Does she feel she will be a burden to her family if she went home? Does she think family and relatives feel that she has rejected them by being away from home for a long time? Does she perceive that she has abandoned or rejected family and relatives, and her own children, and to what degree is she guilt-ridden? Finally, if "Navajos are everywhere," which suggests their high mobility, was there at any time any effort by family members on the reservation to travel to the Northwest to check on the welfare of the woman? How frequent have contacts been between the woman and family and relatives?

To help this woman, the strength of her ties to family and relatives on the reservation needs to be assessed. The strength of her ties to home, culture, and tradition also needs to be assessed. These should be compared to the strength of her ties to her friends and to her community. How did she respond to past medical treatment she received in her community? Did she feel adequately supported and comforted by friends in the community when her husband died? Answers to questions asked in the previous paragraph should also be sought. What are her suggestions for treatment? Therapy and assistance might need to be a combination of support and encouragement given by family and local friends and appropriate modern clinical care.

A Religious Ethicist's Analysis

B. Andrew Lustig, PhD

Mrs. O continues to live in the home where she and her husband raised their children. As a widow she has both emotional attachments to memories of her life with her husband and children and ongoing social connections with her neighbors. As a Navajo woman she has, it would appear, some nostalgia for her earlier life on the reservation (feeling some "regrets"), but apparently she has chosen to remain in her current circumstances, preferring the friendships she has formed during the last two decades. (One assumes she has not retained close ties with her earlier reservation life, because no individuals from that life are mentioned as currently in communication with her.) Her Navajo heritage might, in principle, be an important element to consider in analyzing her current circumstances. However, in light of her conversion to Catholicism and her attendance at church and Bible study, whether the Navajo tradition should play any decisive role in interpreting an appropriate course of care is unclear. And although moving back to reservation life might ease her housing and medical costs (hard to assess without more data about the relative costs in each environment), Mrs. O's reasons for remaining in her current community appear to transcend mere financial concerns. Given the significant changes in her health status during the past four years, she has become increasingly reliant on her neighbors for daily assistance. Before Frank's arrival, their regular help had been crucial because of the geographical isolation of her community and her lack of access to home health care.

With the changes from Frank's initially responsible behavior, Mrs. O's physical and financial circumstances have sharply deteriorated. The crisis that prompts Mrs. R to call an ambulance is the culmination of a number of negative changes in Mrs. O's health, including weight loss and increased pain. That pain surely includes both physical and emotional components: the negative sequelae of her chronic obstructive pulmonary disease and osteoarthritis, but also her shame and possible anger at Frank for his failure to seek employment, his drawing down her financial reserves, his neglect of his caretaking commitments and, most recently, his confiscation of her medicine. In addition, Mrs. O's reticence in speaking about the situation with her friends may indicate elements of coercion and emotional abuse by Frank, especially during his bouts of heavy drinking.

In relating Mrs. O's history to the paramedic, Mrs. R requests that the paramedic "intervene" on Mrs. O's behalf. On the one hand, the paramedic, as a matter of course, is required, in consultation with the attending physician, to keep the patient stable during transit. But while that minimal duty may fulfill the letter of the law, a richer understanding of the paramedic's moral obligation is warranted here. The troubling information Mrs. R has shared with the paramedic, while anecdotal, is potentially quite relevant to Mrs. R's treatment and discharge planning. While Mrs. O has been reticent about discussing Frank with her friends, certain facts—especially the missing medication—suggest a pattern of neglect and/or abuse that requires further scrutiny. Whether the paramedic should explore such details with Mrs. O in her current condition is less important than that such concerns be relayed to the attending physician at the time of admission. Moreover, one should not confuse preliminary probing of such areas of personal privacy with a professional breach of confidentiality after a clinical partnership has been established. The determination of Mrs. O's appropriate care requires professionals to make beneficence-based judgments of her condition and circumstances, including the concerns shared with the paramedic by Mrs. R.

A number of alternatives are open to the paramedic. At the very least, on arrival at the hospital the paramedic should contact the attending physician and social services about the need to speak to Mrs. O about her family situation. In addition, social services may wish to contact Mrs. R, who can convey directly the information she is asking the paramedic to relay. In pursuit of the same end the paramedic might also recommend that Mrs. R speak directly to social services on Mrs. O's behalf.

Mrs. R, as Mrs. O's closest neighbor, has been supportive of her friend. At the same time, she has appeared passive at key points in the situation, as have other friends. Given the apparent pattern of Frank's neglect and/or abuse, one might reasonably question Mrs. R's apparent acceptance of Mrs. O's reticence. There may be mitigating circumstances here: a concern to respect Mrs. O's privacy, a small-town respect for keeping family problems private, or perhaps something specific to Mrs. O's Navajo heritage that equates accepting her reticence with maintaining her pride. Nonetheless, in light of Mrs. O's physical deterioration, greater efforts by Mrs. O's friends might have been expected. They might have contacted the other adult children, who earlier suggested that Mrs. O move in with them. If that offer still stands, Mrs. O may wish to reassess her earlier concern with being 500 miles away from her friends. Significant changes in health status often lead persons to make different decisions because of changing priorities. If Mrs. O does desire to stay in her current community, her other adult children may become significant sources of emotional and financial support.

One other important resource should also be emphasized. In light of Mrs. O's interest, until recently, in church attendance, the local pastor should be contacted as a source of spiritual and social support for Mrs. O. The broader church congregation may also be an ongoing source of spiritual, physical, and even financial support. For many homebound religious patients, regular visitation by clergy and fellow parishioners is an import dimension of their coping with chronically debilitating conditions. Moreover, in this case recurring visits from Mrs. O's local pastor might reasonably be expected to serve as a potential check on Frank's abuses.

RECOMMENDED READINGS

Brody, Baruch A., *Life and Death Decision Making* (New York: Oxford University Press, 1988).

A Paramedic's Analysis

Laura Douglas, EMT-P

Should Ms. M, as an ethical paramedic, do anything beyond treating and transporting Mrs. O to the hospital? The Emergency Medical Technician's Code of Ethics states the paramedic is obligated " . . . to conserve life, to alleviate suffering, to promote health, to do no harm, and to encourage the quality . . . of emergency medical care."[1]

To help Mrs. O our paramedic needs to go beyond the normal professional boundaries involved in patient treatment and transport. Paramedics have to be advocates for their patients—defending them, protecting them, and acting in their best interests.[2] The line between emergency and ongoing care may need to be crossed to meet these obligations. How Ms. M handles this ethical dilemma will help to determine the quality of Mrs. O's future years. Her life will differ, depending on how Ms. M intervenes, and she has some conflicting moral issues to consider.

Confidentiality The paramedic's Code of Ethics states, "The Emergency Medical Technician respects and holds in confidence all information of a confidential nature obtained in the course of professional work unless required by law to divulge such information."[3] In a small rural community, discussing the details of this case with coworkers without violating confidentiality will be difficult. Ms. M needs to be discrete about with whom she discusses Mrs. O and what information she shares. Small details may give away the patient's identity, especially if her coworkers have responded to the home in the past. Discussing Mrs. O's situation with the other children or neighbors would violate her confidentiality.

Autonomy Is Mrs. O able to make her own informed decisions without controlling influences? She may not have all the information about her resources and options. Is she misinformed, believing (for example) that she cannot resume control of her finances? What is the source of this misinformation? Is Mrs. O coerced by feelings of dependence, hopelessness, shame, or guilt regarding her inability to manage her own son, or fear of losing her home and independence? Is she under the control or influence of her son and unable to report him? Is she being coerced by her son's explicit or implied threats? Mrs. O may have slipped into this abusive situation without realizing it. She may fear reprisal. Mrs. O may be embarrassed or in denial about what is happening to her. She may believe that everything will be better as soon as her son recovers, stops drinking, gets a job, pays for his car, or whatever excuse he is giving her. Abusers can be very manipulative. Mothers can be very hopeful regarding their children.

Beneficence   Our paramedic's first priority should be alleviating Mrs. O's suffering to improve the quality of her life. In addition to stabilizing and transporting Mrs. O, this obligation may require Ms. M to look closely around the house. Often the paramedic is the only professional to see the patient's living conditions. Is the home safe? Is it clean? Does she have use of the entire house or is she confined to one room? Is there enough food? Are there expensive purchases in the home that are not hers? Are her medications missing? Are things broken or are there signs of violence in the house? Is she getting the personal hygiene care she needs? The paramedic needs to quickly assess the entire scene.

Mrs. O's home reveals some signs of possible elder abuse: Mrs. O's weight loss, her missing medications, the neighbor's expressed concern. If Ms. M does not intervene, no one else may see what is happening inside the home until it is too late. To not intervene would break one of the paramedic's primary professional promises and the moral obligation of the principle of beneficence (in this case, alleviate present and prevent future suffering). No elderly person should be uncared for, lonely, or abused. But what is going to be the most effective way to help Mrs. O and still respect her autonomy and confidentiality? How will our paramedic weigh Mrs. O's interests, which seem to be in conflict with the interests of her son?

Ms. M must determine whether Mrs. O wants help, what fears she may have, the benefits and burdens of her help, and further assistive resources in this rural community. To achieve her objective, Ms. M may have to consider the law in her jurisdiction. Most states have laws requiring paramedics to contact authorities in instances of suspected abuse of the elderly.[4] We recall that "The Emergency Medical Technician respects and holds in confidence all information of a confidential nature obtained in the course of professional work unless required by law to divulge such information." But in addition "The Emergency Medical Technician as a citizen, understands and upholds the law. . . ." Reporting abuse justifies breaching confidentiality because the benefit to one who is being harmed outweighs the right to confidentiality.[5] But does upholding the law extend to the point of risking further harm to Mrs. O by her son, thereby violating the moral principle of nonmaleficence?

Nonmaleficence Mrs. O may be harmed if her son's abusive behavior is exposed, but he is not removed from Mrs. O's home. Ms. M needs to realize that Mrs. O may lie about the nature or source of her problem to protect herself from further harm (e.g., placement in a skilled nursing facility, physical abuse by her son) or to protect her son from harm (e.g., criminal prosecution or homelessness). The son is dependent on Mrs. O's income—a situation that can cause resentment, anger, or even violence. Caregivers with personal problems of their own are more likely to abuse elders. Mrs. O may mistakenly blame herself for her son's situation. She may feel that she failed as a mother.

Ms. M lacks the information she needs to answer these questions. Further, she is unlikely to be able to acquire the relevant facts. Paramedics generally meet patients, survey their environment, perform a physical exam, and question them about their most intimate personal, demographic, social, and psychological history—things they may have never discussed with their families. The patient is evaluated, treated, and transported in a time frame of about 25 minutes, often never seeing the paramedic again.

Ms. M's best option for not contributing to the harm Mrs. O has already suffered is to contact the patient's primary physician when she gets to the hospital. Physicians often develop close, personal relationships with patients and their families, especially in rural communities. Ms. M can inform Mrs. O's physician of the physical findings at the house, the neighbor's concern, and the fact that the prescription filled two days ago is gone. Mrs. O's physician can assess the situation. He can contact her other children. With community resources, a care plan can be worked out. Ms. M also needs to contact her community's law enforcement agency and file a report of potential elder abuse.

Paramedics should always defend, protect, and act in the best interest of their patients. Patients call paramedics for pain relief, reassurance, and rapid, safe transport to rescue them from harmful situations of many kinds. Ms. M has a duty and obligation to initiate changes to prevent further harm to and promote the welfare of Mrs. O, but it is up to the system to follow through. The paramedic should always err on the side of the patient when the best interest of the patient or the right thing to do exceeds normal practice.

Notes

1. Charles Gillespie, MD, "EMT Code of Ethics" (adopted by The National Association of Emergency Medical Technicians, 1978), http://www.naemt.org/about/ethics.htm (9 July 2003).
2. Bryan Bledsoe, DO, FACEP, Robert Porter, MA, NREMT-P, and Richard Cherry, MS, NREMT-P, *Paramedic Care: Principles & Practice: Vol. 4: Trauma Emergencies* (Upper Saddle River, NJ: Prentice-Hall, Inc., 2000).
3. See note 1, above, #4.
4. See note 2, above.
5. See note 1, above.

Further Reflections

General

1. Mrs. O's situation clearly requires more than intervention for an acute problem. Her challenges are more systemic and concern her living situation, financial state, and the type of support she needs to maximize her independence. Are these issues the moral responsibility of the health care community? If not, who has the responsibility to address them? (All commentators)
2. What should be done about Mrs. O's son? Who should do it?
3. Part of the meaning of *community* is that its members are interdependent. Which of Mrs. O's communities—her Navajo clan, the Catholic church, her nuclear family—have moral obligations to Mrs. O? What moral principles serve as the foundation for such obligations? (Lustig; Reid)

Consequences

4. Which cultural systems of benefits and harms are relevant to assessing Mrs. O's needs? (Lustig; Reid)
5. Reid and Lustig both suggest a series of steps that might be taken and resources that might be explored in resolving Mrs. O's situation. Which of these are most likely to result in a good outcome?

Autonomy

6. What would autonomous choice look like to Mrs. O? Is she capable of autonomous choice? (Douglas)

Rights

7. What rights (if any) are relevant to this dilemma? Is the concept of a right relevant to Mrs. O's life?

Virtues

8. Does the fact that Mrs. O has chosen to live independently of her family and Navajo clan release them from any or some of their usual role-related moral obligations?
9. Beyond immediate treatment and transportation (the typical role-related responsibilities of EMTs), Douglas and Lustig argue for a broader moral obligation of the EMT in this case. What are the foundations for such an obligation, and what, concretely, might it require of the paramedic? How should first-responders decide the limits of their obligations to patients with such complex needs? Are some interventions unethical or improper for an EMT or paramedic to pursue because they are beyond the scope of

professional training? Does the small community setting of this case give Ms. M greater latitude—and responsibility—in what she can and should do for Mrs. O? (Douglas)

10. Who should take the lead in following up on Mrs. R's case and making sure that things are taken care of? (Lustig; Reid)

Equality/Fairness (Justice)

11. Does justice require establishing more extensive health care facilities and professionals to meet the needs of (partially) dependent elders? (Reid)

Chapter 4

Patients We Love to Hate: The Noncompliant

Ms. C is a 45-year-old with adult-onset diabetes (AOD). She has a good understanding of the disease and its complications, gained from watching her mother, aunt, and sister manage their AOD and its complications, and from having attended several diabetes education courses. When diagnosed five years ago, Ms. C was 20 percent over her ideal body weight. She was advised to lose weight, exercise at least twenty minutes three times a week, follow a 1500-calorie American Diabetic Association diet, and take an oral medication (Diabeta) twice daily to control blood sugar levels.

Ms. C has complied poorly with this regimen. As sales director for a major corporation, she travels frequently. Her job requires that she wine and dine clients. When traveling, she often skips lunch, drinks more wine than is advisable, and exceeds 1500 calories a day. She reports, with a grin, "Wine and desserts! Those are the things I really enjoy! You could call them my hobbies." She rarely exercises because she "hates to sweat" and occasionally misses one of her daily doses of Diabeta because she is "rushed." She has steadily gained weight and is now 40 percent over her ideal body weight. Her self-monitored daily blood sugar levels reflect huge swings between striking elevations (when she overeats or forgets her medicine) and life-threatening hypoglycemia (when she remembers her drug but fails to eat at regularly scheduled intervals).

As a result of her poorly managed diabetes, Ms. C is a regular visitor at various emergency rooms (ERs). In the last six months she has been admitted seven times with depressed or elevated blood sugars. On three oc-

casions the police brought her in because she was driving erratically. She has begun to experience visual blurring and numbness in her feet.

Ms. C claims to understand both the short- and long-term risks of her disease, but has no apparent interest in altering her behavior to avoid complications. Her physician, Dr. Z, one of only three internists in her hometown of 12,000, has repeatedly spent lengthy sessions counseling Ms. C in an attempt to motivate changes in her behavior. He has also referred her to a diabetic nurse educator to identify techniques to control her diabetes, techniques Ms. C might find more "user-friendly"; to a dietician to educate her about dietary control when she is working; and to a psychologist to help her understand her (in his opinion) obstructive behavior—all to no avail. Ms. C has refused to see any of these providers more than once or twice. She reported that the nurse specialist was "so thin he couldn't appreciate what I go through"; that the dietician "needed to lose 20 pounds herself, so how much could she know?" and that the psychologist's staff rudely refused to accommodate her schedule. Most recently Dr. Z recommended that she begin insulin injections to better manage her blood sugar levels. Ms. C refused, stating that she fears her hypoglycemic episodes would be even worse with insulin. When Dr. Z insisted that her health requires behavior modification and change in medication, Ms. C yelled, "How many times do I have to tell you I am not interested in giving up the few things I enjoy? It's your job to get rid of these problems, not mine!"

Dr. Z finally reached his limit. Six weeks ago he told Ms. C that he could no longer care for her, that she should find another doctor because, two months hence, he would refuse to see her. Today Ms. C showed up at his office and reported that none of the other internists or primary care physicians (most of whom have cared for her during one or more of her ER visits) would agree to take her as a patient. Dr. Z replies that he will only continue as her physician if she agrees to the previous behavioral changes they have discussed. Ms. C insists her life will be devoid of any pleasure if she follows Dr. Z's instructions, adding, "Look, I just want to minimize my symptoms. My mother took drugs to improve her circulation. Why can't you just give me those and quit trying to make me someone I'm not? If I am willing to put up with the aggravation, why aren't you?"

Dr. Z really does not want to care for Ms. C. He is tired of arguing with her and believes he is fighting a losing battle in terms of managing her disease. Still, since none of his colleagues will assume medical responsibility *for her, his termination of their relationship will mean her only care will be through the ER. This will mean that no single physician is coordinating her care, that her "normal" status is never checked, and that no proactive approach is taken. Still, he is not convinced she will be worse off; after all, his coordinated care and proactive approach have not made any apparent difference in her health status.*

Is Dr. Z morally obligated to continue to care for Ms. C?

Introduction

This case raises three important moral issues:

1. What is the relationship of the moral principle of autonomy to rejecting therapeutic advice? Are noncompliant patients *morally* responsible for adverse outcomes?
2. Do the professional virtues of fidelity, tolerance, compassion, or courage give any direction to Dr. Z?
3. Can the health care interests of other individuals or communities ever make utilitarian or justice-based claims on noncompliant patients?

The AJ Method

Step 1:Information Gathering   What facts are necessary for resolving this case? All commentators *assume* Ms. C will continue to be noncompliant, even if Dr. Z agrees to her terms, and that noncompliance will cause harm to Ms. C. Are these assumptions founded on facts or the product of biases? Other salient facts include why Ms. C is so aggressively noncompliant (Rechtin and Mirvish; Swanson); what broader social effects might accrue, should Dr. Z discontinue this patient-professional relationship (Lincourt); whether Dr. Z will himself be harmed by continuing to see Ms. C; and whether Dr. Z is legally obligated to continue to care for Ms. C.

Ms. C is not unique. Nearly 100 percent of diabetics fail to strictly follow dietary recommendations, and 98 percent of obese dieters gain back lost weight within two years.[1] Up to 50 percent of medications prescribed for chronic conditions are never taken; 14 percent–21 percent of patients never even fill their prescriptions.[2]

Step 2: Creative Problem Solving   A creative solution would have to minimize Ms. C's physical and psychological risks without harming Dr. Z or compromising his integrity.

Step 3: Pros and Cons   Survey CARVE principles to identify important moral reasons that support conflicting options for resolving this case.

Consequences   What does a realistic assessment suggest regarding Ms. C's future health status if Dr. Z "fires" Ms. C? if he continues to care for her? In either case, who will be harmed? benefitted? In what ways? (Lincourt; Rechtin and Mirvish)

The consequences of patient noncompliance are severe. Not only do individual patients experience increased morbidity and mortality as a result of no or inadequate treatment; but health care costs—and, thus, insurance premiums, government budgets, and taxes—rise, reducing health care availability for low-income citizens. Further, limited health care resources are overburdened.

Autonomy   What is the relationship of the moral principle of autonomy to rejecting therapeutic advice? Are noncompliant patients *morally* responsible for adverse outcomes? (All commentators) Whose autonomy is (more) relevant here?

Is noncompliance a moral issue, or merely an interesting observation about human behavior? Freely chosen noncompliance seems morally permissible, even if imprudent. Patients who consult health care professionals (HCPs) are presumably acting freely to advance their own interests. This line of thinking suggests that physician consultations are analogous to other professional consultations: a client solicits advice which she is then free to accept or reject.

In health care settings, respecting patients' choices about whether to embrace care plans reflects the moral commitment to respect for autonomy. The principle of autonomy and the right to self-determination protect the freedom of persons to structure their lives as they wish. This freedom, in its most expansive sense, protects the liberty to choose one's own values and pursue them as one sees fit. Respecting autonomy requires that others not obstruct such pursuit (assuming harm to others is not intended)—even if they personally abhor the ends or the means.[3]

Note, however, that the right of self-determination carries an often overlooked correlative responsibility. Persons are responsible for the effects—bad as well as good—of their autonomous choices. If HCPs repeatedly rescue noncompliant patients from their own health-risking choices, they treat patients paternalistically, *not* autonomously, and, in so doing, fail to respect patients as responsible decision makers.[4] Established, ongoing clinical relationships place rights *and* responsibilities on both parties. If the patient-professional relation is collaborative (as autonomy requires), responsibility for negative outcomes, including the unraveling of the therapeutic relationship, must fall, at least in part, on the noncompliant patient.[5]

The situation is complicated in cases where a patient is unable, for whatever reason, to adhere to the prescribed regimen. In such cases one must question to what extent the patient is, causally or morally, responsible for adverse results.[6] When an apparently competent, informed patient rejects reasonable treatment, HCPs need to give significant attention to ascertaining the reasons for noncompliance. The first question is whether the patient's choice actually *is* autonomous (since nonautonomous choices do not command the same degree of respect). A choice is autonomous *if and only if* it meets certain criteria: it is made by a *competent chooser who possesses and understands relevant information and is not coerced.*[7] A noncompliant patient may fail to meet some less obvious criterion of competence[8] or may be nonobviously coerced (e.g., psychologically or circumstantially).[9] When, however, choices are autonomous, HCPs must determine how extensive noncompliance must be for a patient to violate the (admittedly, unwritten and probably differently understood) "contract" that structures the relationship. Physicians should no more be held captive to their patients' unreasonable demands than patients should be held captive to their physicians' unreasonable pronouncements.[10]

Rights   Ms. C has a right of self-determination (Rechtin and Mirvish); but so does Dr. Z. Which has greater moral force in a patient-professional relationship? (Lincourt; Swanson) Within the context of the patient-professional relationship, Ms. C has a right to be aided—a right she clearly has not waived. Has she, in virtue of her noncompliance, forfeited this right?

Virtues   Do the professional virtues of integrity, fidelity, tolerance, compassion, or curiosity give any direction to Dr. Z? (All commentators)

Most physicians and patients believe that the professional promise to promote the patient's welfare and the virtues of integrity and fidelity strongly bind physicians to patients with whom they have an established relationship. After all, nothing in their code of ethics indicates that troublesome patients can be abandoned. Physicians should expect patients to be unpleasant, at least intermittently, as a result of the physical and psychological suffering that attend their illnesses, injuries, or disabilities. Such unpleasantness constitutes a common working condition of HCPs rather than license to abandon patients. The appropriate response is compassion for the patient's suffering, toleration for the patient's ungraciousness, and courage and determination in shepherding the patient through rugged terrain.[11]

Still, virtues need not be exercised each and every time their expression is possible. The virtuous physician need not enslave himself to his patients. Not all suffering demands a compassionate response and not all ungraciousness should be greeted tolerantly. Sometimes one must draw a line; the problem is determining when and where to do so. When can a physician "fire" a patient without incurring a moral (as opposed to legal) charge of abandonment?

Though nearly all patients demonstrate some degree of noncompliance with HCPs' recommendations, most do not believe their noncompliance undercuts the integrity of the therapeutic relationship or the right to the time, advice, or treatment by HCPs. It is worth noting that HCPs often deride patients for demanding perfection in their HCPs. Are HCPs being equally unreasonable in requiring patients to be perfectly compliant? Do physicians have—as some would argue nurses do—an obligation to care for patients in spite of their inability (for whatever reason) to maximally ("perfectly") benefit patients? In the face of noncompliance, what is the proper response—and responsibility—of the HCP? (Swanson)

Equality/Fairness (Justice) Can health care interests of other individuals or of institutions or communities ever make consequence- or justice-based claims on noncompliant patients? (Lincourt; Rechtin and Mirvish)

Can the health care needs of other parties place moral claims on Ms. C and/or her physician to pursue a particular resolution to this problem? The present health care system is overburdened in many respects, most generally by an inability to provide good quality care to all persons at an affordable price. State and local governments and private third-party payers establish reimbursement rates for health care practitioners and institutions on the basis of cost analyses and treatment efficacy (anticipated health outcomes of patients). A patient's decision to eschew treatment that carries with it the prospect of deteriorating health that will require more extensive and more expensive future care will have ripple effects on access to health care for others.

These effects may be especially burdensome in the face of limited resources (physicians' time). Although resource allocation may not strictly be a zero-sum game (that is, resources are finite, and use of a resource by one person means the resource will no longer be available for others), the time a doctor spends either in his office or the emergency room with one patient is time that cannot be spent with another. If Dr. Z washes his hands of Ms. C, she will ever more frequently resort to expensive ER care to manage her AOD. Further, if Ms. C fails to comply with an aggressive weight loss, exercise, and management plan, her deteriorating health will put significant pressures on the health care system for more expensive, more extensive future care. Thus, present and future patients, health care institutions, insurance companies, employers, and state and federal agencies all appear to have a stake in Ms. C's compliance. What claims—if any—can justice make regarding choices to ignore sound medical advice? Put another way, does justice require Dr. Z to tough it out with Ms. C?

Allocation concerns require some assessment regarding to whom the physician is primarily responsible—the patient or society. Historically, the physician has promised to work primarily for the welfare of the individual patient and only secondarily for greater social welfare.[12] Can such singleness of purpose be morally justified in a world of limited resources for which competition is increasingly stiff? Or does justice require limiting individual freedom for the greater good? And, if so, how might such limitations be defined and enforced? If Dr. Z terminates his relationship with Ms. C, she will have to use the ER even more frequently than she does currently. This additional expense will take resources away from others who could profit from their availability.

The Law Finally, a partial list of relevant legal considerations includes: (1) Does a patient-professional relationship constitute a legal contract; and if so, under what conditions may it be legally breached or rendered void? (2) Who is legally responsible for any degenerative changes in the noncompliant patient? (3) Given legal protections of patients' decisional authority, are HCPs legally required to follow a patient's "sensible" requests, even when they view such requests as undermining patient well-being, or as neglect?[13]

The following commentaries examine the application of various moral principles to this dilemma, thereby assisting the reader to undertake *Step 4: Analysis* and *Step 5: Justification*.

Notes

1. Norman B. Levy, MD, "A Psychiatrist Answers Questions About Noncompliance," *E-NEPH Archive: Dialysis & Transplantation* 24 (April 1995), http://www.eneph.com/feature_archive/Compliance/v24n4p187.html (24 Mar. 2004).
2. Christine Wiebe, "Following Orders: New Solutions to the Age-old Problem of Patient Noncompliance with Prescription Drug Orders," 20 Dec. 1999, http://www.ama-assn.org/amednews/1999/pick_99/hlta1220.htm (24 Mar. 2004).
3. H. Tristram Engelhardt, Jr., *The Foundation of Bioethics*, 2nd ed. (New York: Oxford University Press, 1996), 288–330.
4. Heather Draper and Tom Sorell, "Patients' Responsibilities in Medical Ethics," *Bioethics* 16 (2002): 335–52.
5. Franziska Trede and Joy Higgs, "The Clinician's Role in Collaborative Clinical Decision Making: Re-thinking Practice Knowledge and the Notion of Clinician-patient Relationships," *Learning in Health and Social Care* 2, no. 2 (2003): 66–73.
6. Alister Browne, Brent Dickson, and Rena van der Wal, "The Ethical Management of the Noncompliant Patient," *Cambridge Quarterly of Healthcare Ethics* 12, no. 3 (2003): 289–99; Scot D. Yoder, "Individual Responsibility for Health: Decision, not Discovery," *Hastings Center Report* 32, no. 2 (2002): 22–31.
7. Ruth R. Faden and Tom L. Beauchamp, *A Theory of Informed Consent* (New York: Oxford University Press, 1987), chap. 8.
8. For a discussion of the characteristics persons must demonstrate to be competent, see Becky Cox White, *Competence to Consent* (Washington, DC: Georgetown University Press, 1994).
9. See note 6, above.
10. See note 4, above.
11. K. Allen Greiner, "Patient-Provider Relations—Understanding the Social and Cultural Circumstances of Difficult Patients," *Bioethics Forum* 16, no. 3 (2000): 7–12.
12. American Medical Association, Council on Ethical and Judicial Affairs, *Code of Medical Ethics: Current Opinions with Annotations* (Chicago: AMA, 2001), Principles VII and VIII.
13. Legal consideration of patient neglect, patient dumping, and moral and legal obligations of nonabandonment are explored in American Medical Association, Council on Ethical and Judicial Affairs, *Code of Medical Ethics: Current Opinions with Annotations*, 2000–2001 Edition (Chicago: American Medical Association, 2000), § 8.11, "Neglect of Patient" and § 8.115, "Termination of Physician-Patient Relationship"; and Jerry Menikoff, *Law and Bioethics* (Washington, DC: Georgetown University Press, 2001), chap. 7, "The Doctor-Patient Relationship," 151–84.

An Ethicist's Analysis

John M. Lincourt, PhD

No, Dr. Z is not morally obliged to continue to oversee Ms. C's medical care. This position is supported by the belief that Ms. C relinquished her role as a responsible partner in the patient-physician relationship when she chose to direct her health care in irrational ways. Competent patients who know the health risks associated with their diseases and who voluntarily choose to adopt them are responsible for negative outcomes. This includes dismissal from a medical practice.

Abandonment is not at issue here because Ms. C has access to medical care through the emergency room (ER) and the possibility exists to retain her current physician if she becomes compliant. Granted, ER care is not the best option for long-term diabetes management, since it is generally reactive and episodic. But Ms. C cannot force the issue by claiming her physician is obliged to treat her regardless of her lifestyle choices. Noncompliance abrogates such rights. In addition, physicians have an established right to choose whom they will accept as patients.[1]

However, Dr. Z may wish to consider an additional step before discharging Ms. C from the practice. It involves her corporate employer. The corporate Employee Assistance Program (EAP) officer should be informed of the situation and a plan set in motion to triangulate the management of Ms. C's care between the physician, patient, and EAP office. Though Ms. C should be informed of the strategy and Dr. Z should seek her consent, consent is not a requirement for the EAP consultation. This strategy goes well beyond the scope of the traditional patient-physician dyad with its emphasis upon the Hippocratic values of confidentiality and compassion. Traditional modes of care founder where noncompliance prevails. Also, noncompliance has serious organizational implications for employers, and the major corporation for which Ms. C is the sales director is no exception. Ideally, the company has a written policy covering disclosure of such information to the EAP.[2]

From the perspective of organizational ethics, Ms. C's noncompliance creates problems for two constituencies in companies with health care benefits: the main arbiter of services and the payer of services. In this case, the corporation is the primary arbiter and payer. As the main broker for employee medical coverage, the corporation—not Ms. C—negotiates and arranges for Ms. C's medical coverage. In terms of medical economics, the corporate employer is the principal customer. In this corporate view, employee noncompliance increases cost, reduces coverage, and erodes corporate leverage with third-party insurers at contract-renewal time. Moreover, it is axiomatic that noncompliance is a variance from payer expectations. Surely, compliance with generally accepted practices of diabetes treatment is expected of Ms. C by her corporate managers. To knowingly and willfully disregard such practices while accepting corporate medical coverage constitutes abuse. The corporation may choose to give Ms. C a choice: comply, assume full financial responsibility for her health insurance costs, or face the possibility of dismissal from the company.

Caring for noncompliant patients is a high calling requiring discernment, compassion, and grit. A common, though false, assumption is that all persons seeking medical assistance will freely comply as best they can with directions and advice offered by medical professionals. In this view, patients and health care professionals share the same goal: medical care of high quality at the lowest cost and with results that can be measured against expectations. Patient noncompliance perverts this view, turning this model on its head because disease conditions tend to worsen, costs over time increase, and expectations and outcomes conflict. In the case of diabetes, harms become serious and irreversible. For example, insufficient insulin for diabetics inevitably leads to serious complications, including high blood pressure, kidney failure, retinal hemorrhages, gangrene, coma, and death.

Ms. C's behavior makes her a medical saboteur. Her omissions and commissions are instances of subversion and are very likely to defeat the efforts of the most dedicated health care professional. Case-hardened veterans would point out that to date Ms. C has not experienced any serious loss, pain, or debilitation from her diabetes. They reason the "obstructive behavior" displayed here needs to play itself out. On the other hand, Ms. C views regimens associated with sound diabetes management as inconvenient, displeasing, and out of sync with her preferred lifestyle. With unyielding noncompliant persons like Ms. C, only pain is obeyed. Extreme measures may be called for when a misguided sense of autonomy holds sway and the risks to patient well-being run high.

The first step might be for Dr. Z to retain Ms. C as a patient with a contingency: expose Ms. C regularly to patients who live with the dark side of diabetes. This includes persons with reduced life expectancy, multiple amputations, early blindness, unsightly gangrene, and deep-seated kidney pain associated with diabetic nephropathy. These harsh and seemingly heartless measures may be in order for the short term to avoid a long-term health calamity for this patient. The next step would be to identify clear and compelling evidence of the existence and progress of these dark side symptoms in Ms. C. If this fails, Ms. C should be discharged from the practice and left in the care of the ER physicians.

Finally, one caveat deserves mention. Ms. C should not be punished by poisoning the well. Dr. Z should not pass on to others his own negative feelings generated by her unwillingness to abide by a sound care plan. This point is especially important for physicians who set up practice in small towns or rural areas where medical providers are scarce. Ms. C is no medical pariah; she is a person who rejects the role of "medical patient" at this time. Also, health workers must avoid the use of belittling, debasing, and fault-finding labels. This includes such designations as "Rooter," "Troll," "Crock," "GOMER," "SPOS," "Turkey," "Dirtball," and other less printable names. This habit of stereotyping difficult patients is demeaning, unnecessary, and wrong.

Notes

1. American Medical Association, Council on Ethical and Judicial Affairs, *Code of Ethics: Current Opinions with Annotations* (Chicago: AMA, 1997), xiv.
2. EAP programs vary between states and institutions. As an example of an EAP Code of Ethics position on confidentiality see United States Office of Personnel Management, "Confidentiality and the Employee Assistance Program: A Question and Answer Guide for Federal Employees," n.d., http://www.opm.gov/ehs/Confibro.asp (24 Mar. 2004) which indicates conditions under which confidentiality can be breached *within the institution:*

   Under 42 CFR Part 2, . . . when a client commits, or threatens to commit, a crime that would harm someone else or cause substantial property damage, law enforcement personnel must be informed.

A Health Educator's Analysis

David Swanson, PhD

Who is responsible for Ms. C's noncompliant behavior? Ms. C? Dr. Z? Do both patient and physician share responsibility for Ms. C's wellness-related behavior?[1] Consider the meaning of the word *responsibility:* it can be thought of as "response-ability." We can now ask, "Who has the ability to respond?" Further, we can ask what mutual response is appropriate for Ms. C and Dr. Z. Finally, we should consider potential barriers to an appropriate response.[2]

First, Dr. Z probably has traditional training in Western medicine. He is well-trained in the scientific aspects of Adult Onset Diabetes (AOD) and his recommendations for modification of Ms. C's behavior are appropriate under that model. However, the Western scientific medical model promotes a posture of objectivity, separateness, and isolation on the part of the physician. This posture gives the physician a position of strength and power with respect to the patient. Although this can be helpful at times, in this case it may be harmful. The patient may feel diminished and disempowered. Western medicine often emphasizes outcome whereas in this case the emphasis should be on process. Western medicine focuses on mastery whereas in this case the focus may need to be on the mystery as to why Ms. C is not complying.

What might explain Ms. C's noncompliance? Consider the following plausible hypothetical explanation.

Ms. C grew up with a diabetic mother. As a child, Ms. C did not understand the disease or its consequences for her mother's behavior. Ms. C experienced a dysfunctional mother. Ms. C's mother became dogmatic about eating habits in the family. Ms. C was not allowed to have candy like the other kids on her block. Whenever Ms. C was caught eating a piece of candy, her mother inflicted harsh punishment which caused Ms. C to feel guilty and unloved. These conditions were such that Ms. C developed an inappropriate relationship to all food.

Ms. C is aware that she is in denial about the implications of her behavior with respect to diabetes. In fact, when she experiences blurry vision and peripheral circulation problems, she dismisses them as not being life-threatening. Furthermore, she is vaguely aware that she is fearful and/or angry about her own diabetic condition and this unexpressed fear and/or anger has led to a chronic state of depression. Sometimes this depression lifts and during moments of clarity she sees her life more realistically. But the discrepancy between the reality of her life's condition and where she would like her life to be is so painful that Ms. C immediately self-medicates through wine and food in an attempt to dull the pain. Furthermore, Ms. C may feel that the stress of her job and her erratic schedule contribute to her non-compliance.

Ms. C states, "My mother took drugs to improve her circulation. Why can't you just give me those and quit trying to make me someone I'm not?" Perhaps this is the treatment of choice. A multifactorial intervention is now recommended for treating AOD, including diet modification and exercise. However, for patients who are not compliant with diet and exercise recommendations, drug therapy can be at least 80 percent effective for restoring normal physiology.

Now let us explore the issue of Dr. Z's obligation to his patient. Dr. Z does not want to put up with Ms. C any longer, but he wonders if he has an ethical obligation to continue caring for her. Dr. Z had given Ms. C two months to find another doctor, but she continued to request that Dr. Z be her physician.

The question is, how aware is Dr. Z of the barriers he and his style of medical practice present to Ms. C? Furthermore, how aware is he of other barriers that Ms. C must overcome? In other words, who has response-ability given the barriers that are evident, as well as those that are not? Can Dr. Z respond appropriately? Can Ms. C respond appropriately?

It seems to me Dr. Z has three options: (1) He can refuse to be Ms. C's primary care physician; (2) He can locate an alternative primary care physician, perhaps a woman, for Ms. C;[3] or (3) He can look differently at his relationship with Ms. C and continue as her primary care physician.

I would argue that Dr. Z's first option is unethical because it would bring harm to Ms. C, especially if he were aware of (but chose to ignore) the potentially surmountable barriers that she must overcome. Option 2 would be ethical, provided that Dr. Z can locate for Ms. C an alternative primary care physician who can more effectively deal with the barriers involved in her case. (This option is less likely in small-town settings with few practitioners.) However, option 3 may be the most appropriate. Given the small-town nature of Dr. Z's practice, he may be the only specialist who can aggressively treat Ms C. The current treatment standards suggest a multidrug regimen as well as lifestyle modification. A family practice doctor may not be able to manage the patient appropriately. Can Dr. Z inspire a transpersonal attitudinal healing,[4] such as often occurs in 12-step programs? Alternatively, could Dr. Z modify his treatment to be more compatible with Ms. C's response-ability?

Notes

1. Barbara Dossey et al., *Holistic Health Promotion: A Guide for Practice* (Rockville, MD: Aspen Publishers, 1989), 3–99.
2. Stephen Covey, *The Seven Habits of Highly Effective People* (New York: Simon and Schuster, 1989).
3. Karen Allen and Janice Phillips, *Women's Health Across the Lifespan* (Philadelphia: Lippincott, 1997), 3–102.
4. David Swanson, "The Wilson Effect: A Case for Transpersonal Healing Properties of Placebo," *International Journal of Healing and Caring* 2, no. 3 (2002).

A Current and Future Psychiatrist's Analysis

Lissa Rechtin, MD, PhD, and Ezra Mirvish

This case raises two ethical issues: patient abandonment and the requirement that a doctor respect a patient's rights of autonomy and self-determination.

The issue of patient abandonment is of special importance for a small town with few alternatives for medical care. All of Dr. Z's colleagues in the town share his experience of Ms. C and so refuse to treat her. He argues that having her receive care only through the emergency room (ER) would be sufficient, but this hardly seems true. It is not clear, for example, how the patient would get her oral hypoglycemics through ER treatment alone. In general, prescribing a long-term medicine without patient follow-up—care which would not be feasible in an ER setting—is considered improper. One could argue that as a frequent traveler, Ms. C could be referred for regular treatment to a doctor in a city where her work often brings her. In this case, one might feel that an equivalent to Dr. Z's care could be obtained by combining periodic checkups in an out-of-town clinic with emergency care in her hometown. This raises the question, though, as to whether the patient's behavior toward Dr. Z is enough of a provocation to allow him to abrogate his responsibility to care for patients in a small town. A threatening patient might certainly merit denial of services in his or her own hometown and referral to an inconveniently located clinic. The question remains whether the more obdurately vexing qualities of Ms. C would be sufficient grounds for such an inconvenient treatment plan. To answer this question, we need to look in detail at their interrelationship.

One can easily see why Dr. Z and his colleagues have such a negative reaction to Ms C. She can be presumptuous, demanding, and disrespectful. In addition, she denies her own responsibility in the matter of her health, stating that "it's your [Dr. Z's] job to get rid of these problems, not mine!" Ms. C's profligate approach to medical care monopolizes resources that could be better used to treat more acute, emergency cases. From a rule utilitarian point of view, if everybody with chronic illness took her approach to their diseases, it would have a highly deleterious affect on the ability to deliver emergency care.

Still, a discussion of the interplay between this doctor and patient would not be complete without turning a critical eye to Dr. Z's behavior. By threatening to refuse routine care if the patient does not comply with the prescribed regimen, Dr. Z flagrantly disregards the patient's rights of autonomy and self-determination. In general, we consider it a coercive act to try to get patients to comply with therapy by threatening to withdraw treatment. Imagine, for example, an internist who refused to follow a patient for medical management of back pain after the patient refused a recommended surgery. One might think that refusing back surgery is more reasonable than ignoring Dr. Z's medical recommendations, and that is probably the case. Certainly, surgical treatment of back pain is more controversial than Dr. Z's recommendations for Ms. C. However, patients have the right to be less than reasonable with regard to their choices regarding their own bodies. They have, for example, the right to continue smoking despite its being the cause of their emphysema. From an ethical standpoint, therefore, people have as much right to refuse as to follow specific medical/behavioral orders; that is to say, patients have a right to be noncompliant.

Moreover, given how widespread noncompliance is,[1] any physician needs to have some sense of how to understand and deal with the noncompliant patient without resorting to coercive ultimatums about withdrawing care. Noncompliance can be rooted in a variety of factors. It could be due to (1) deficient coping mechanisms, as in the extensive denial of a patient who ignores swollen lymph nodes that are a clear sign of recurrence of a cancer; (2) a psychiatric disorder such as depression, as in the case of a cardiac patient who neglects to take his medicine or undergo required blood tests; (3) a patient's high impulsivity and low frustration tolerance (e.g., failing to pick up his or her high blood pressure medication because the line at the pharmacy is too long). Whatever the root causes of noncompliance, working to circumvent this problem can involve skills that lie at the heart of psychiatry and behavioral medicine. For example, a behavioral specialist must avoid arguing with patients, or "reaching one's limit with them," by mastering the skill of handling his or her own emotional responses to frustrating work. Ms. C certainly seems to be particularly irritating, but this still does not mean that she should lack care. Dr. Z was correct in trying to refer his patient to specialists, including dieticians and behavioral professionals; perhaps his greatest mistake was only doing so after "lengthy counseling sessions."

An important part of any specialty in medicine is knowing how and when to make referrals to other subspecialties. Dr. Z should get better at involving other subspecialists early on to avoid "arguing" with patients about compliance. Moreover, he should have behavioral specialists available for consultation with him when he feels himself becoming embroiled in conflicts. Such consultations would be particularly helpful concerning Ms. C, allowing Dr. Z to develop a treatment plan for her. Among other things, such a plan would avoid coercive ultimatums, while still protecting Dr. Z from Ms. C's more provocative behavior. For example, such a specialist would provide advice on how to put issues of her treatment back in Ms. C's lap when she asserts that it is the doctor's job to "get rid" of her medical problems. This approach would ultimately be much more efficacious and satisfying for Dr. Z. Certainly, this would be more in line with the spirit of a physician's work than trying to find a way to get rid of Ms. C without inviting an accusation of abandoning her or violating her autonomy. It may concomitantly help Dr. Z to do his part, as a physician, to limit wasteful use of medical services.

Notes

1. For a good review of the literature on compliance, see E. Vermeire et al., "Patient Adherence to Treatment: Three Decades of Research. A Comprehensive Review," *Journal of Clinical Pharmacy & Therapeutics* 26, no. 5 (2001): 331–42, 12 Jan 2002, http://www.blackwell-synergy.com (7 Aug. 2003).

Further Reflections

General

1. This case takes place in a small community where experienced physicians are in short supply. What role should this fact play in determining the physician's duty to preserve his relationship with Ms. C? Would the morally appropriate response differ in an urban center with easier access to other qualified physicians?
2. Why might Ms. C's noncompliance with her treatment regimen generate such strong feelings among the health care professionals (HCPs)—including Dr. Z—associated with her care? Why might they consider her behavior immoral (rather than merely annoying)?
3. Why is patient abandonment considered problematic by nearly all health care professional associations?

Consequences

4. What consequences to Ms. C, Dr. Z, other patients and HCPs, health care institutions, and insurance companies might result if Dr. Z terminates the patient-professional relationship with Ms. C? If Dr. Z continues the relationship? (Lincourt; Rechtin and Mirvish)

Autonomy

5. What does respect for autonomy require of HCPs who disagree with their patients' choices? How might an argument from autonomy suggest that

noncompliance does (not) justify Dr. Z's termination of his relationship with Ms. C? (All commentators)

6. The commentators arrive at different conclusions concerning what Dr. Z is morally permitted to do. How do their interpretations of the principle of respect for autonomy inform their conclusions?

Rights

7. Lincourt claims that Ms. C has no right to treatment from Dr. Z, though she retains a right to treatment from an emergency room. Why would she retain a right to ER treatment if noncompliance destroys her right to treatment from her established physician?

8. Does entering a profession, with promises espoused in a professional code of ethics, limit one's right of dissent? (Lincourt)

Virtues

9. The commentators variously refer to "the spirit of a physician's work," "a high calling," and "compassion" as character traits, motivations, and visions of the profession that ought to inspire right attitudes and action on the part of Dr. Z toward Ms. C. What professional virtues or character traits are most important for physicians who must deal with noncompliant patients with chronic health care needs?

10. Do the moral virtues of compassion, tolerance, and courage (specified in the Hippocratic Oath and thought to apply to physicians) apply to Ms. C as well? (All commentators)

11. Swanson suggests that the conflict between Dr. Z and Ms. C arises in part as a result of Dr. Z's Western medical training, a particularly narrow medical outlook, the normative relationship with patients that this view engenders, and a lack of holistic and process-oriented clinical care. Do the virtues of integrity, fidelity, or curiosity require Dr. Z to revise the way he practices medicine? What virtues might support Lincourt's opposing conclusion?

Equality/Fairness (Justice)

12. Lincourt suggests that the concerns of fairness and social utility, which include efficient use of medical resources, can sometimes justify leaving noncompliant patients to fend for themselves in the ER. Rechtin and Mirvish suggest that efficient use of medical resources counsels continuing the private patient-professional relationship. Compare their arguments and indicate which is more compelling, and why.

Chapter 5

I'm Doing the Best I Can

Mr. I is a family nurse practitioner in a frontier town of 2000 in a western state. He is in practice with Dr. R, a general practitioner who has been a physician in town for 35 years and will be retiring soon. After seven years in his position, Mr. I is liked and respected by the population. He, his wife, and their two young sons are immersed in and enjoy their life in this community.

Mrs. M, a 26-year-old wife of a local rancher, has been Mr. I's patient since he began his practice. She has been in excellent health, requiring only routine care (e.g., pap smears, flu shots). When Mrs. M arrived for her annual pelvic exam and pap smear, Mr. I was shocked to see that this normally vivacious, energetic, petite woman had lost nearly 20 pounds and looked as if she had aged as many years. With compassionate encouragement from Mr. I, Mrs. M tells the following story:

> *Three months ago her car broke down several miles from town as she was returning home from Wednesday night choir practice. She began to walk the several miles to the family ranch and counted herself fortunate when her pastor came along and picked her up. To her horror, the pastor drove to a deserted area and raped her. She still has trouble believing the rape actually took place, and keeps hoping this is a bad dream from which she will awaken. Since the rape Mrs. M has had difficulty sleeping, eating, concentrating, and completing her normal tasks (common experiences for rape victims). Her husband, whom she loves dearly, is deeply concerned about her and repeatedly asks if anything is wrong. Nonetheless, she has been unable to bring herself to tell her husband—or anyone else—about the rape. The pastor and her*

husband are lifelong friends, hunting and fishing buddies, and confidants. She fears her husband will not believe her or, if he does, will take some violent revenge on his friend. She worries, too, that he will ultimately come to resent her for the loss of the friendship. She also worries that she may now be pregnant.

Mr. I performs a pelvic exam and is relieved to note the absence of any sign of trauma or pregnancy. Nonetheless, he advises that Mrs. M be tested for pregnancy and for several sexually transmitted diseases. Mrs. M absolutely refuses. She indicates that she would never have told anyone about the rape had her husband not been so worried about her health. She certainly is not about to have Mr. I's office assistant fill out forms requesting these tests. ("God knows who she would tell!") When Mr. I assures her that he will fill out the forms himself, Mrs. M still refuses, crying that she doesn't even want the test results in her medical record. And what if the office assistant opened the mail when the results returned?

Mr. I's more pressing concern is how to manage Mrs. M's profound depression. He advises an antidepressant which she rejects, fearing that the local pharmacy could not guarantee confidentiality or that her husband would discover the pills and insist on an explanation. Mr. I suggests counseling, but the nearest family counselor and nearest psychiatrist are about three hours away. Mrs. M insists that she could not travel so far on a regular basis without raising suspicions. She pleads with Mr. I to serve as her counselor.

Mr. I reluctantly begins to see Mrs. M twice weekly. He believes he is her only option, though is keenly aware that his counseling skills are meager. Telephone consultations with colleagues specializing in psychotherapy and rape counseling provide minimal guidance. Mr. I asks Mrs. M at each visit to reconsider seeing a qualified counselor, but she is steadfast in her refusal.

Six weeks later Mrs. M has made no apparent progress; she is still depressed and has lost seven more pounds. Mr. M has called several times, frantic about his wife's condition and asking if he can or should do anything to help her.

Further, Mr. I is himself becoming depressed. He has stopped going to church, long his most important source of psychological support, because he and Mrs. M attend the same church and, thus, have the same pastor. Mr. I cannot bear to listen to the sermons or interact with the man he knows has committed a deep moral evil.

What is Mr. I's moral obligation to Mrs. M now?

Introduction

Three important moral questions are raised by this case:

1. How should the nurse practitioner's (NP's) moral obligation to promote positive or minimize negative outcomes to this patient be balanced against confidentiality concerns?
2. Are Mrs. M's decisions about her care autonomous?
3. How should health care professionals (HCPs) address the larger issue of sexual assault and rape in society?

The AJ Method

Step 1: Information Gathering   What facts are necessary for resolving this case? Mr. I is *assuming* that Mrs. M has been raped, though no direct evidence supports that claim. (Francis and Buccafurni) Other facts that warrant investigation include whether Mrs. M is pregnant, suicidal, autonomous, or has an STD; whether Mr. I has legal obligations in this case; how Mr. M would respond to learning of his wife's situation; and what broader social effects might result from different actions. Finally, is consultative assistance really unavailable? (Eskelson)

According to the U.S. Department of Justice, 140,990 women on average are raped each year; 63 percent do not report the rape to the police.[1] Most authorities estimate that rape is drastically underreported; that for every reported rape, one to ten rapes go unreported. The Centers for Disease Control (CDC) data from a national telephone survey show that 683,000 women are forcibly raped each year; only 16 percent of rape victims (109,280) report the rape to the police.[2] The most common reasons cited for not reporting rapes are that the victim considered the assault to be a personal matter, feared reprisal, or believed the police would be biased against her. (Eskelson) The closer the relationship of victim and rapist, the less likely the victim is to report the rape.[3]

Although rape is a type of sexual assault and involves the act of having sex, it is typically understood to have nothing to do with sex and everything to do with power.[4] That is, rape is a crime in which men demonstrate and perpetuate their power to harm women and to restrict women's freedom and self-determination. These restrictions take many forms: not walking (or jogging) alone after dark, not challenging men who aggressively place demands on women, not asserting themselves in debates with men, generally doing what men want, etc. Women who fear rape are less likely to assert their independence and, thus, are less likely to challenge the constraints of a patriarchal society in which women have limited opportunities to structure their own personal or professional lives. Restrictions and fears are aggravated after rape by a tendency to blame the victim ("she brought it on herself") and to treat her badly (skepticism or harassment by legal or health care professionals, public shunning or denunciation).[5]

Step 2: Creative Problem Solving   Any creative solution would have to improve Mrs. M's health outcomes without exposing her to greater negative effects.

Step 3: Pros and Cons   Survey CARVE principles to identify important moral reasons that support conflicting approaches to this case.

Consequences   What action would best promote positive and minimize negative outcomes to Mrs. M? To Mr. I? To the larger community? (All commentators) What action would benefit Mrs. M (most)? What actions would harm Mrs. M (most)? (Francis and Buccafurni; Eskelson) Mr. I? (Nathaniel; Eskelson)

The effects of actions may be more profound in small-town settings. The anonymity of larger cities permits victims some measure of privacy: as personal, health care, and professional communities are less likely to intersect, a victim need not worry that her assault will become widely known. In small towns, victims rightly fear—a fear affirmed by Mrs. M herself—a breach of confidentiality. Where one's HCPs are also one's friends (or at least acquaintances), and where medical information is easily accessible to a small and socially integrated professional population, secrets may not be well protected and anonymity may be practically nonexistent. Thus, Mrs. M's concerns about protecting her reputation are not unrealistic, and Mr. I faces a significant challenge in preserving secrecy. He must attempt a consequential calculation in which he weighs the burdens of present physical (ongoing loss of weight) and psychological (worsening depression) harms and benefits (protection of her reputation) against future burdens (marital discord, retaliation by the pastor) and benefits (willingness to seek counseling from a distant therapist), should her rape become publicly known.

The dearth of easily accessible referral resources for psychological support raises concerns of nonmaleficence: will Mr. I's well-intentioned but admittedly inadequate counseling efforts cause more harm than good?[26] One justification for consultation is that exceeding one's education puts the patient (and oneself) at risk for further harm. How should these obligations be compared?

Autonomy   Are Mrs. M's decisions about her care autonomous? (Francis and Buccafurni; Nathaniel) What act would best preserve/restore her autonomy?

Perhaps the first order of business is to determine if Mrs. M's rejections of diagnostic tests and psychological referral are autonomous decisions. Mr. I has a moral duty to respect every patient's self-determination.[7] However, respecting nonautonomous choices is not morally required (though the predicted negative outcomes from ignoring Mrs. M's decision might argue for respecting her choice, even if it is nonautonomous). Thus, Mr. I must determine if Mrs. M is informed about and understands the burdens and benefits of forgoing qualified psychological counseling. He must assess whether her decision is uncoerced or driven by fears (e.g., rejection by her husband, loss of her reputation, ruined marriage).

Approximately 4.7 percent of adult rapes result in pregnancy—perhaps sufficiently low to support Mrs. M's refusal of a pregnancy test. But estimates of sexually transmitted disease following rape are as high as 30 percent. In addition to these injuries, rape victims often suffer from chronic recurring headaches, fatigue, sleep disturbance, nausea, loss of appetite, eating disorders, menstrual pain, sexual dysfunction, suicide attempts, and substance abuse[8]—an impressive list of risks that must reasonably be considered in planning therapy.

A second reason for challenging Mrs. M's choice is that moral obligation to respect autonomous choices is weakened when they put others at risk of harm. Exposing her husband to sexually transmitted diseases (STDs) surely puts him at risk of harm (the extent of which cannot be determined without testing Mrs. M for STDs). Asking a HCP to work outside his area of specialty may harm the practitioner (as well as the patient). At the very least, Mr. I is frustrated and worried by his inability to ameliorate Mrs. M's suffering. Confounding this question are the relevant criteria for rape counseling. Is it just "talk therapy" (for which any intelligent, compassionate HCP is capable) or does this intervention require advanced professional expertise, based on specialized training? If the latter, Mr. I violates his professional code of ethics and breaches accepted standards of practice; both could threaten his license to practice.

The autonomy issue is further complicated by enormous unclarity about Mrs. M's goals, broadly considered. We know what she doesn't want, but have no clear indication of any therapeutic aims. Autonomy is typically respected as a means of protecting a patient's self-specified conception of a good life and means thereto. The case study suggests that positive goals and concern with progress have been ignored.

Rights What is the relative force of Mrs. M's rights to confidentiality, decisional authority, and to not be harmed? (Francis and Buccafurni; Nathaniel)

Virtues What is the relative force of Mr. I's professional integrity—e.g., to put Mrs. M's health concerns first (Francis and Buccafurni; Nathaniel) or to not exceed his abilities? (Nathaniel)—of his compassion? (Francis and Buccafurni) of Mrs. M's courage?

Against Mr. I's professional obligation to respect Mrs. M's autonomy[9] is the virtue of integrity. His professional commitment requires that he not practice outside the limits of his professional training.[10] The American Nurses Association Code of Ethics specifically indicates: "When the needs of the patient are beyond the qualifications and competencies of the nurse, consultation and collaboration *must be sought* from qualified nurses, other health professionals, or other appropriate sources."[11] Further the Code indicates a professional responsibility to contribute to the welfare of one's community, broadly construed. Does integrity confer a duty to warn others of the minister's (alleged) threat to other women?

Equality/Fairness (Justice) Assuming the minister did rape Mrs. M, is Mr. I morally complicit in protecting the minister from *deserved* punishment? (Eskelson) How should HCPs address the larger issue of sexual assault and rape in society? (Eskelson)

Specific laws regarding the reporting and investigation of rape differ between states; however states typically allow the victim to determine whether to report the rape (as long as the victim is an adult). As a result, HCPs may have no legal obligation to report rape of an *adult* victim. One may, however, have a moral obligation to report a rape if, for example, one deems the victim to be at further risk from the assailant.[12] Can Mrs. M's continuing physical and psychological deterioration be seen as further risk *from her assailant*? Probably not in any pure sense, but if Mr. I has reason to believe her health would improve by taking the crime public, his professional obligation may require this move.

Each year, tens of thousands of women are raped. Because most rapes are not reported, the perpetrators are not brought to justice. Women suffer; rapists do not. Justice requires raising the question of what can be done to prevent (and punish) rape. Silencing survivors through truncated reporting; failing to empower victims to bring charges against rapists; culturally conditioned avoidance and denial of violence against women; punishments perpetrated on victims rather than on perpetrators; failure to fund adequately support systems for victims and families—all these contribute to a general passivity that ensures the problem will persist. Should HCPs—who often are the only persons to see the victims and hear their accounts of rape—play a more active role in instigating changes in reporting laws and in education of society beyond victims seen in the clinic? If rape is an assault on one's self-determination, do HCPs have a moral obligation to empower victims as a means of reducing rape?

The Law   What role does the law play in determining obligations (e.g., reporting rape) in the context of professional practice? (Francis and Buccafurni) A partial list of relevant legal considerations includes: (1) Does the nurse practitioner (NP) have an obligation to report this rape to law enforcement under a statutorily mandated reporting law? (2) Would a legal obligation to report override the legal obligation to protect patient confidentiality and patient decisional authority? (3) Short of a statute mandating reporting, is there a legal obligation to warn other women in the community that they might be at risk from this alleged rapist? (4) Would the NP's willingness to exceed his professional training in the provision of counseling services be illegal?[13]

The following commentaries examine the application of various moral principles to this dilemma, thereby assisting the reader to undertake *Step 4: Analysis* and *Step 5: Justification.*

Notes

1. Callie Marie Rennison, U.S. Department of Justice, Bureau of Justice Statistics, "Rape and Sexual Assault: Reporting to the Police and Medical Attention, 1992–2000," Aug. 2002, http://www.ojp.usdoj.gov/bjs/abstract/rsarp00.htm (25 Mar. 2004).

2. National Center for Injury Prevention and Control, Centers for Disease Control [CDC], "Sexual Violence," 13 Jan. 2004, http://www.cdc.gov/ncipc/factsheets/svfacts.htm (24 Mar. 2004).

3. See note 1, above.

4. Susan Brownmiller, *Against Our Will: Men, Women, and Rape* (New York: Bantam Books, 1976); Susan Griffin, *Rape: The Power of Consciousness* (New York: Harper & Row, 1979).

5. Lois Pineau, "Date Rape: A Feminist Analysis," *Law and Philosophy* 8 (1989): 217–43.

6. Nelda S. Godfrey and Katharine V. Smith, "Moral Distress and the Nurse Practitioner," *The Journal of Clinical Ethics* 13, no. 4 (2002): 330–35; Lorri N. Turner, Kathy Marquis, and Mary E. Burman, "Rural Nurse Practitioners: Perceptions of Ethical Dilemmas," *Journal of the American Academy of Nurse Practitioners* 8, no. 6 (1996): 269–74.

7. American Nurses Association [ANA], *Code of Ethics for Nurses with Interpretive Statements* (Washington, DC: American Nurses Association, 2001), §1.4.

8. See note 2, above.

9. See note 7, above, §§1.3 and 3.2.

10. Ibid, § 4.3.

11. Ibid., 17, emphasis added.

12. See Turner, Marquis, and Burman, note 6, above.

13. Rebecca F. Cady, "Scope of Practice and Standard of Care," in *The Advanced Practice Nurse's Handbook* (Philadelphia: Lippincott, Williams & Wilkins, 2003), 49–84; and "Professional Liability Issues," 127–68; and Patricia Younger et al, *Physician Assistant Legal Handbook* (Gaithersburg, MD: Aspen Publishing, 1997).

   Legal concerns of mandated reporting and confidentiality for physicians are ably addressed in American Medical Association, Council on Ethical and Judicial Affairs, *Code of Medical Ethics: Current Opinions with Annotations,* 2000–2001 ed. (Chicago: American Medical Association, 2000), § 2.02, "Abuse of Spouses, Children, Elderly Persons, and Others at Risk," 4–7; and "Confidentiality," § 5.05, 105–17. See also Tarasoff v. Regents of the University of California, Supreme Court of California 551 P.2d 334 (Cal. 1076).

A Legal and Philosophical Analysis

Leslie Francis, PhD, JD, and Diana Buccafurni, PhD(c)

This case raises far too many issues for a single comment. But cases in real life often raise multiple issues, particularly in a small community where the practitioner plays many roles and faces difficult ethical issues regarding the boundaries of professional and personal relationships.

This is a case of alleged rape. We say "alleged" advisedly, because no matter how clear the case seems, the alleged perpetrator has not been convicted of the offense and will be entitled to all due process protections. We also say "rape" advisedly, because the case describes what happened as "rape." Rape, however, is a notoriously difficult offense to prove. Under a typical statute the prosecution would need to prove beyond a reasonable doubt that the defendant had sexual intercourse with the victim against the victim's will. With the time that has passed, there is no physical evidence of the alleged intercourse. Moreover, in some states proof that the intercourse was against the victim's will requires evidence of violence or other duress. In addition to the personal pain and perhaps shame that victims may experience in reporting an alleged rape, these difficulties in prosecution must always remain in the background.[1]

In this case, the nurse practitioner, Mr. I, sees Mrs. M for a regular visit. Her appearance is disturbing and, on inquiry, he is told that she was raped three months ago. Mrs. M requests Mr. I to keep the rape confidential and refuses to allow Mr. I to perform procedures that are standard to protect the health of rape victims (a pregnancy test and tests for sexually transmitted diseases [STDs]). Mr. I acquiesces and agrees to try to help Mrs. M deal with the rape through counseling, although Mr. I has no special training in psychiatric nurse practice.[2] At the time of these decisions, Mr. I fails to serve Mrs. M's health-related interests. He does not determine whether she is pregnant, which might affect medical management. Indeed, he offers antidepressants without knowing whether she is pregnant. He does not determine whether she has contracted a STD, which again might affect medical management. Furthermore, this failure risks Mrs. M's husband if she is an unwitting vector of disease transmission. Finally, he agrees to counsel Mrs. M, possibly outside the scope of his practice. He makes each judgment in response to Mrs. M's earnest requests, perhaps reasoning that Mrs. M's autonomous choices should outweigh her health-related interests. There are of course deep ethical conflicts about whether and why patient autonomy should outweigh patient interests, and when health care providers should act in accord with patient choice.

In this case, however, criticism of Mr. I's actions can avoid these deep conflicts and provide direction for future action. First, Mr. I acquiesced in Mrs. M's choices hastily at best. No evidence from the case suggests he took care to explain to Mrs. M the significant risks of her decisions or to ensure that she understood them rather than reacting from distress. Did Mr. I explore risks to her and to a fetus if she were pregnant and did not receive adequate prenatal care or indicated treatment for any STD? Did he discuss health risks to her husband? Did he explain his own lack of counseling expertise? When patients make decisions against their health-related interests, they should do so with clear understanding; Mrs. M's refusals here were not appropriately informed. Second, no evidence indicates that Mr. I ascertained his legal obligations or explained them to Mrs. M. Depending on the law of his state, Mr. I might be required to report evidence of a crime. Third, Mr. I might have sought the advice of other practitioners in this difficult situation. The case is silent about any practice agreement between Mr. I and Dr. R, another alternative left unexplored.

What should Mr. I do now, when counseling has not helped Mrs. M and when the situation has burdened Mr. I as well? Difficult as it may seem, he should do what he should have done in the first place. He should work with Mrs. M to be sure she understands all the risks of her current choices, including their effects on her own health, on that of her husband, and on her marriage. He should explain why, as a responsible practitioner, he can no longer counsel her. He should explore with her possible alternatives, their risks and benefits, including telling her husband and seeking alternative sources of care. He should be prepared with a referral. He should consult his lawyer, to understand his legal obligations, within the practice and with respect to state reporting requirements. Throughout, he should offer to support her in these choices and to continue to provide her with health care within his scope of practice. The most difficult situation for him would arise if she refuses to take any action. She is depressed and he may not be trained to recognize whether she presents a risk to herself of suicide. Under such circumstances, he should tell her that it is his professional obligation to take steps to protect her, including violating her confidentiality, unless she takes steps to protect herself through a referral. Psychologists and psychiatrists have a professional duty to maintain patient confidentiality, unless certain circumstances obtain, including, though not limited to, the patient's being a threat to self or others.[3] Although he is a nurse practitioner (NP), he is acting as a mental health professional; these would be his obligations as a mental health care provider, acting in Mrs. M's interests and attempting to further her well-reasoned choices.

In sum, this is a case in which Mr. I has confused being nice and trying to help with principled practice. He has done so because Mrs. M is deeply upset and because he wants to try to help her. But the result, unfortunately and all too predictably, is not a success. Moreover, helping Mrs. M take steps now is also likely to be beneficial to the community as a whole; if the pastor really is a rapist, Mrs. M is all too likely not to be his only victim.

Notes

1. For the classic account of these difficulties by a legal scholar, see Susan Estrich, *Real Rape* (Cambridge: Harvard University Press, 1987). For a rape victim's personal story of the difficulties of a prosecution, see Alice Sebold, *Lucky* (Boston: Back Bay Books, 2002).

2. For an account of the specialty of psychiatric nurse practice, see the Web site of the American Psychiatric Nurses Association, http://www.apna.org (15 July 2003). Mr. I apparently is not trained or licensed to practice in the specialty of mental health nursing.

3. Ethical Principles of Psychologists and Code of Conduct 4.05 (2002), http://www.apa.org/ethics/code2002.html#4_05, (15 July 2003).

   The American Medical Association (AMA) also endorses the violation of patient confidentiality privilege in cases where the patient is a threat to self or others, though the AMA does not describe such action as a professional obligation: "Psychiatrists at times may find it necessary, in order to protect the patient or community from imminent danger, to reveal confidential information disclosed by the patient" (American Psychiatric Association, "Code of Ethics with Annotations Especially Applicable to Psychiatry" [1998 ed.]: § 4, no. 8). See also American Psychiatric Association, "Opinions of the Ethics Committee on the

Principles of Medical Ethics with Annotations Especially Applicable to Psychiatry: Opinion 4E," 2001 Ed.

These materials can be found on the Web site of the American Psychiatric Association, http://www.psych.org (15 July 2003).

A Nurse Ethicist's Analysis

Alvita Nathaniel, DSN, APRN, BC

The nurse practitioner (NP) is in the type of impossible situation common to nurses. What Mr. I ought to do in this particular situation is unclear. His actions are constrained by competing moral claims, social and professional role expectations, and binding ethical guidelines.[1] For the most part, nursing codes of ethics are based on deontic ethical theories. These theories determine the rightness or wrongness of an act in terms of the nature of the act and an imperative of duty. Within this tradition, nurses are expected to fulfill duties and uphold inflexible principles.

As Mr. I weighs good and harm, he considers the following moral principles.

Autonomy   Western health care ethics presupposes a strong commitment to patient autonomy. If Mrs. M has decision-making capacity, the principle of autonomy leads Mr. I to respect her wishes, even if they cause her harm.

Beneficence   This principle requires one to "do good" and prevent harm, insofar as it is reasonable. The NP must determine what is "good" (not an easy task) and follow through. In this case, he decides that beneficent actions should include reporting the crime, doing further tests, prescribing antidepressants, and referring Mrs. M. for counseling.

Nonmaleficence   This principle requires Mr. I to avoid actively harming Mrs. M. Unavoidable harm that occurs during a beneficent act must be weighed against the benefit.

Confidentiality   Professional codes of ethics require absolute confidentiality for autonomous patients.[2] Mr. I. is compelled to maintain confidentiality, even if a crime was committed and Mrs. M's husband is frantic about her deteriorating condition.

Fidelity   The principle of fidelity is related to faithfulness and promise keeping. Society grants NPs the right to practice nursing through the processes of licensure and certification. Fidelity, in turn, requires that nurses uphold professional codes of ethics, practice within the established scope of practice, remain competent, and keep promises to patients.[3] Mr. I balances the concern that he exceeds his scope of practice against the prospect of abandoning Mrs. M.

Mr. I valiantly attempts to uphold the traditional ethical principles while simultaneously recognizing the professional and legal implications of his actions. Unfortunately certain moral claims in this case are mutually exclusive and are complicated by social and professional role expectations. For example, Mrs. M rejects antidepressant medications, testing for sexually transmitted diseases (STDs), and professional counseling that the NP recommends. Mr. I feels compelled to follow Mrs. M's autonomous wishes. Even though he lacks the requisite skills, he caves in to Mrs. M's insistence that he counsel her—after all, he reasons, some "good" is better than none. He may worry that she will become suicidal if he abandons her. Although Mr. I is uncomfortable in the role of counselor, some forms of counseling are not entirely outside the domain of primary care NP practice (especially in a frontier clinic).

As Mrs. M's condition deteriorates and she continues to refuse professional counseling, Mr. I questions the moral valence of his actions. Gender and social expectations aside, he tries to do what is "right" in a case in which there are no easy answers. Experiencing both physical and emotional problems, Mr. I begins to suffer from moral distress.

Moral distress is defined as the pain or anguish affecting the mind, body, or relationships resulting from a patient care situation in which the nurse is aware of a moral problem, acknowledges moral responsibility, and makes a moral judgment about the correct action—yet, as a result of real or perceived constraints, participates, either by act or omission, in a manner perceived by the nurse to be morally wrong.[4] Moral distress results from a dynamic interplay of the nurse's moral outlook, commitment to moral principles that may be either intrinsically incompatible or incompatible in specific situations, relationships with patients, role identification, and perception of power imbalances or other institutional constraints. Moral distress is a pervasive problem in nursing, contributing to loss of nurses' ethical integrity and dissatisfaction with the work of nursing. Moral distress is a major contributor to nurses leaving their work settings and even the profession.[5]

Familiarity with nurses' codes of ethics will help Mr. I make decisions, though there are no easy and valid "cookbook" solutions. Nursing codes of ethics sometimes fail to provide solutions to moral problems in complex situations such as this, in which there are divergent ethical perspectives, imbalance of power, competing needs, and privacy concerns within a small-town milieu. In the end, there is no *absolute* morally correct path for Mr. I. If he continues to care for Mrs. M, he is morally obligated to respect her, avoid harming her, maintain expertise in practice, remain faithful to promises, and, insofar as it is possible, adhere to other professionally sanctioned ethical principles.

Since moral claims compete in this case, Mr. I can make a valid decision by using one of two methods: lexical ordering or reliance on conscience. Lexical ordering provides a noncapricious means to prioritize competing moral principles.[6] For example, the traditional adage, "first, do no harm" assigns nonmaleficence greater weight than other principles. But Mr. I defaulted to the contemporary Western health care tradition of giving predominant weight to the principle of autonomy. Using lexical ordering, Mr. I can devise a cogent and consistent prioritized list of principles. Once the principles are ordered, Mr. I may conclude that it is more important to benefit Mrs. M and prevent her harm than to support her autonomous decision. Or, he could make the opposite judgment. Either would be valid.

The second option (the one that I would choose) is to view nursing codes of ethics as moral norms while accepting conscience as the ultimate guide for behavior.[7] Conscience serves as an internal alarm when there are threats to core beliefs. If Mr. I believes it is morally wrong to exceed his scope of practice and risk harming Mrs. M, he should refuse to counsel her. By following his conscience, Mr. I preserves his moral integrity.

One final caveat: Both ethics and law treat the suicidal patient as a special case. If Mrs. M is suicidal, she lacks decision-making capacity and therefore is not autonomous. The nurse practitioner is obligated to protect her from harm by making sure she has immediate mental health care.

Notes

1. American Nurses Association, *Code of Ethics for Nurses with Interpretive Statements* (Washington, DC: Author, 2001), http://www.nursingworld.org/ethics/ecode.htm (25 Mar. 2004); International Council of Nurses, *The ICN Code of Ethics for Nurses* (Geneva: International Council of Nurses, 2000), http://icn.ch/ethics.htm (24 Mar. 2004).
2. See ANA, note 1, above; M. A. Burkhardt and Alvita K. Nathaniel, *Ethics & Issues in Contemporary Nursing*, 2nd ed. (New York: Delmar, 2002).
3. See note 2, above.
4. Andrew Jameton, *Nursing Practice: The Ethical Issues* (Englewood Cliffs, NJ: Prentice-Hall, 1984); Alvita K. Nathaniel, *Toward an Understanding of Moral Distress*, unpublished manuscript, 2003; J. M. Wilkinson, "Moral Distress in Nursing Practice: Experience and Effect," *Nursing Forum* 23, no. 1 (1987–1988): 16–29.
5. See Nathaniel, note 4, above.
6. Robert M. Veatch, *The Basics of Bioethics* (Upper Saddle River, NJ: Prentice-Hall, 2000).
7. Tom L. Beauchamp and James F. Childress, *Principles of Biomedical Ethics*, 5th ed. (New York: Oxford University Press, 2001), 18–21.

A Rape Counselor's Analysis

Tiffany Eskelson

An individual's personal setting influences her response to all situations in which she finds herself; for example, being the survivor of a sexual assault. Individuals belong to a number of cultural systems in which beliefs are created and behaviors are supported. In contemporary American society these structures include positive social attitudes toward the clergy; negative social attitudes toward women who "cry rape"; a social perception that rape is the victim's fault and, hence, pressure on rape victims to keep silent and a demand that *they*, rather than law enforcement, produce evidence and witnesses to prove they aren't "crying rape."

When sexual assault occurs, social structures reinforce the survivor's keeping the trauma, the crime, and the whole of the experience contained within her inner world. Without intentionally minimizing the trauma of a sexual assault in an urban setting, we note that a small, rural community can enhance the pressures that keep survivors quiet. In this setting, Mrs. M has a number of things working against her that make her situation more difficult to resolve: confidentiality is not guaranteed; her assailant is not only an acquaintance, but also a respected person with authority in her community; her health care professional (HCP) has experienced a significant change in his world and support system that may set up a conflict between his own interests and those of Mrs. M; and the community as a whole may be threatened by public knowledge of the sexual assault.

One can presume, in part, that the pastor was able to commit the crime as a result of his social status—one that confers distinct advantages. He has an established level of trust, respect, and authority. He is a "lifelong" friend of Mrs. M's husband. Both these factors reinforce Mrs. M's reluctance to make the rape public. Doing so would disturb numerous personal and social relationships in her town. As a result, Mrs. M will quite likely be seen as a trouble maker if she makes his behavior known.

Nonetheless, the pastor's advantages, if protected by secrecy, will allow him to continue his life—at great expense to Mrs. M—as it was before the sexual assault. At the very least, secrecy deprives Mrs. M of access to local resources that may help her to cope with and recover from this assault on her physical and emotional well-being.

We must also wonder if the community contains other victims. How many other times has the pastor sexually assaulted members of this rural community? We are assuming that Mrs. M is the only victim, but the social pressure to silence survivors may have hidden a serious and ongoing threat to the town. Secrecy gives a perpetrator numerous advantages, including the opportunity to continue illegal and immoral actions. Unless communities force perpetrators to stop, they will continue to rape. The community, and its individual citizens, must dissolve the conditions of secrecy that protect the perpetrator.

One cannot blame Mrs. M for not wanting to report the sexual assault. Sometimes keeping the assault secret is safer for the victim, especially in small communities. But to address the problem of sexual assault, communities must educate their members on the topic. It is also critical to go beyond education to intervention and prevention. A national survey studied sexual assault and domestic violence programs in rural areas.[1] The survey, which both documented the problem of sexual assault in rural areas and posited useful responses, found that "43% [of the towns] . . . have Community Awareness programs," and that "78% also provided training for other community or criminal justice agencies." One way in which Mr. I might reduce the threat to his community would be to initiate a program to bring this information to the community. Ongoing commitment to prevention and intervention can decrease the occurrence of sexual assault, as well as increase survivor safety, reporting, and treatment—all of which make the community safer.

In addition to concerns about Mrs. M's welfare, the community's welfare is threatened because Mr. I's professional, emotional, and spiritual welfare are at risk. Are there moral obligations to take care of the caregiver? Mr. I's knowledge of this crime and his efforts to care for Mrs. M may have serious negative effects on him. These effects, if not addressed, can have an adverse effect on his ability to practice. If he cannot survive in this environment, he may be forced to relocate, depriving this small town of access to qualified health care. Although the moral obligation of beneficence may suggest that Mr. I continue his support of Mrs. M, this can have devastating effects for both individuals if he is not aware of his own boundaries. Mrs. M is experiencing long-term effects, the treatment of which is beyond his capabilities. He can continue to be a support system for her short-term effects—being scared, feeling anxious, withdrawing/isolating herself, self-blame, etc. But more intensive therapy is also warranted. Referral to a specialist will be better for both Mrs. M and Mr. I.

Mrs. M is justifiably concerned about the distress she will cause on an interpersonal level. Her relationship to the pastor/perpetrator has been damaged, and there are several ways she may internalize this. She may also have concerns that her marriage will be destroyed. Her husband's obvious and ongoing concern suggest that he cares deeply about her; however, one cannot necessarily predict how family members will react to a sexual assault.

Finally, on a purely personal level, Mrs. M may have concerns about being believed; however the mere fact that Mr. I believes her creates some assurance in this regard. Also, her previous trusting relationship with her pastor, both in his role as spiritual advisor and as a friend, should lend credence to her charge and suggest that it is not one she would make lightly. Finally, Mrs. M is also justifiably concerned about her emotional, intellectual, physical, and spiritual safety. However her safety seems to be endangered rather than protected by her insistence on secrecy—especially since secrecy obstructs her opportunities for identifying or establishing local support systems and for healing.

Although the case suggests few resources are available to Mrs. M and Mr. I, the survey cited earlier demonstrated that: (1) 50 percent of the programs provided outreach services to victims living in isolated jurisdictions; (2) 53 percent had satellite offices open at least on a part-time basis; and (3) 63 percent had interagency task forces in their community.[2] This information dispels the myth that adequate resources do not exist in rural communities. Accessing these services may sometimes require travel; however, most programs have a 24-hour hotline number. National hotlines can also be utilized as an outreach and support system. The Internet is also becoming a widely used resource by survivors; Web sites that offer education, general information, and support are frequently available in libraries, churches, and schools. Mr. I, like other HCPs, could install Internet access in his office.

In conclusion, the largest problem for all involved in the sexual assault is that the perpetrator's actions create secrecy, which has devastating and immediate effects of this secrecy on individuals. Seeking out resources and implementing change are critical for all concerned. If necessary resources truly do not exist within the immediate area, they must be brought in. Like anyone who offers support to a survivor, Mr. I has a moral obligation to not only support the survivor but to also improve the community in which the rape occurred.

RECOMMENDED READINGS

Kilpatrick, D. G., Edmonds, C. N., and Seymour, A., *Rape in America: A Report to the Nation* (Arlington, VA: National Victim Center & Medical University of South Carolina, 1992).

Men Can Stop Rape, n.d., http://www.mencanstoprape.org/index.htm (25 Mar. 2004).

National Sexual Violence Resource Center, 11 July 2003, www.nsvrc.org (25 Mar. 2004).

National Victim Assistance Academy, http://www.nvaa.org/ (25 Mar. 2004).

Violence Against Women Online Resources, 5 Mar. 2003, http://www.vaw.umn.edu/ (25 Mar. 2004).

Notes

1. Steven D. Walker, Christine Edmunds, and Harvey Wallace, "Addressing America's Forgotten Victimization: Model Strategies and Practices for Rural Victim Assistance," Office for Victims of Crime Grant, California State University, Fresno, 2000, n.d., http://www.washburn.edu/ce/jcvvs/research/rural_crime_victimization (25 Mar. 2004).
2. Ibid.

Further Reflections

General

1. This case takes place in a small community where opportunities for referral to and consultation with specialists are virtually nonexistent. What role should this fact play in determining Mr. I's moral obligation to Mrs. M? Would the morally appropriate response differ in an urban center with easier access to qualified personnel?
2. Eskelson suggests that the rural setting of this case increases the difficulty of resolving the situation. What is it about this setting that does this?
3. What crucial facts are missing in this dilemma?

Consequences

4. Identify the consequences to all affected parties if Mr. I violates Mrs. M's confidentiality *and* if he does not. Which set of consequences is morally preferable?

Autonomy

5. An autonomous choice is made by a competent person who is informed and understands her therapeutic options, and who is not coerced to choose a particular course of action. Francis and Buccafurni suggest Mrs. M's choice is not autonomous. If so, how should Mr. I proceed? If not?

Rights

6. Discuss the moral importance of Mrs. M's rights to confidentiality and decisional authority, giving particular attention to the fact that rights can be overridden if respecting them *causes* harm to others.

Virtues

7. Discuss Mr. I's competing professional obligations and specify what actions these obligations require of Mr. I. Do you agree with Nathaniel that the ultimate source of resolution should be Mr. I's conscience? Why (not)?
8. Francis and Buccafurni suggest that the demands on Mr. I are quite clear; that there may be less of a moral dilemma facing him than might at first be apparent. Nathaniel believes the dilemma is quite complex. Examine the reasons given in each commentary and determine which position is more compelling.

Equality/Fairness (Justice)

9. What role, if any, does justice play in this dilemma?

Chapter 6

Must Health Care Professionals Always Tell the Truth?

Marjorie P is a 7-month-old baby who was born with Tetralogy of Fallot, a serious heart defect that can be corrected with surgery. Marjorie had her first surgery—a shunt between the aorta and pulmonary artery to provide adequate blood flow to her lungs—when she was 2 months old. The complete repair of her heart will be performed when she is strong enough and her condition is stable enough to tolerate the stress of a longer, more complicated operation. When these conditions are met, Marjorie's surgical repair will be done at a regional academic medical center. Her local physician and the pediatric cardiovascular surgeon at the medical center estimate that Marjorie will not be ready for surgery for several months, perhaps a year.

In spite of the earlier surgery, Marjorie's heart functions inefficiently. As a result, her lungs frequently fill with fluid and she turns blue and becomes extremely short of breath. When this happens, her parents must rush her from their farm to the nearest hospital in a small town about 15 minutes away. In the emergency room (ER) she is usually given oxygen and medicines to help her breathe more easily and remove the extra fluid from her lungs. Treatment decreases the strain on her heart and eases her breathing. Mr. and Mrs. P have had to rush Marjorie to the ER approximately once a week since she was born.

Mr. P is 18 years old; Mrs. P is 17 years old. Neither has finished high school. They live with Mr. P's father on his farm. In addition to helping his father on the farm, to secure much-needed health insurance for his family, Mr. P works from midnight to 6 A.M. at a local grocery store. He is chronically sleep-deprived and exhausted. Mrs. P is also chronically fatigued, as Marjorie's care makes demands on her day and night. Both parents are terribly frightened by Marjorie's crises and quite fearful that one day they may not make it to the ER in time. They have become very close to the nurses and doctors in the ER and depend on them for psychological as well as medical support.

One night Marjorie arrives in the ER in more distress than usual. The ER staff are working as fast as they can to give the drugs needed to save her life. One of the nurses caring for Marjorie is inexperienced; she rarely works in the ER and has never worked with critically ill children. In the press of the crisis, she grabs the adult rather than the pediatric vial of morphine (the narcotic given to help ease Marjorie's breathing) and inadvertently gives Marjorie an adult dose rather than the pediatric dose. As a result Marjorie receives ten times the recommended dosage. Because morphine is a powerful respiratory suppressant, Marjorie suffers a respiratory arrest and stops breathing completely.

The ER staff is present when Marjorie experiences her respiratory arrest and immediately begin resuscitation. Within a few minutes they discover the cause of the arrest and promptly give Marjorie a narcotic antagonist—a drug to reverse the effects of the morphine. The narcotic antagonist works quickly, and in less than a minute Marjorie is breathing again. In the interim the oxygen and medicines have had a positive effect, and Marjorie's breathing, heart function, and general condition are much improved.

The ER physician, Dr. D, steps out to speak to Marjorie's parents, who were asked to leave the room when Marjorie stopped breathing. As Dr. D approaches, Mrs. P begins to cry. Through her tears she sobs, "This is just what we were scared would happen. She's getting worse, isn't she? That's why she stopped breathing, isn't it? I don't know what we would do if we couldn't count on you."

Dr. D had intended to tell Mr. and Mrs. P the true cause of Marjorie's respiratory arrest, but now she hesitates. She recognizes that, as Marjorie's parents, Mr. and Mrs. P have both the right and the responsibility to make health care decisions about their daughter's care. To decide effectively, they need full and accurate information. However, Dr. D knows these parents well; she has personally resuscitated Marjorie sev-

eral times and has seen firsthand the parents' stress and the difficulty they usually experience coping with the all-too-frequent crises her illness generates. Further, they lack family members to help them make difficult choices. Mr. P's father, the only close relative, is completely terrified by Marjorie's medical condition. He routinely defers to his young son and daughter-in-law when decisions must be made about Marjorie's therapeutic regimens.

Dr. D worries that if she admits the medication error, the parents might choose to take their daughter to a different emergency room. The next closest ER is an additional 30 minutes away, and on more than one occasion Marjorie has barely arrived at this—the closest—ER in time. Had resuscitation been delayed, Marjorie would probably have died or suffered irreversible brain damage. Dr. D suspects that with different parents she would probably tell the truth; but she worries that these parents—young, inexperienced, habitually stressed, exhausted, and frightened—might choose unwisely and act against Marjorie's best interests. Nor does Dr. D wish to destroy either the Ps' trust in the ER staff or their hope that Marjorie will survive long enough to have surgery. And, to be fully honest, Dr. D worries that telling the truth might expose the hospital, the nurse, or even herself to a lawsuit. Mr. and Mrs. P do not seem litigious, but they would probably be shocked, disappointed, and even further frightened to discover their health care professionals are fallible. They might want to "get even" with the HCPs for making Marjorie worse, even if only temporarily.

What should Dr. D tell Mr. and Mrs. P about the cause of Marjorie's respiratory arrest?

Introduction

Four moral issues arise in this case:

1. Do health care professionals (HCPs) have a duty to tell the truth to their patients and their families? If so, is lying (or omitting information) ever morally justifiable? If so, when?
2. Can professional virtues provide useful guidance to Dr. D?
3. Does the principle of justice require truth telling?
4. Do HCPs have a moral obligation to educate the public about medical fallibility?

The AJ Method

Step 1: Information Gathering   What facts are relevant to this dilemma? Has Marjorie been harmed by her respiratory arrest? Would the parents be able to "handle" the truth just now? Do the parents assume their HCPs are infallible? What is the likelihood that Marjorie's parents would fail to return to the emergency room where the HCPs are familiar with her needs? What would be the implications of this choice for Marjorie's future health? Who is responsible for the medication error—the nurse? the physician? the hospital? Will the parents sue?

How to define a medical mistake is the subject of much discussion.[1] Most basically a mistake is "unintentional; partially preventable; and harmful or potentially harmful."[2] Although patients overwhelmingly indicate a desire to be fully informed about *all* mistakes, HCPs share this information infrequently and, when they do, only infrequently tell the "whole truth."[3] For example, a HCP may acknowledge an adverse event or outcome without disclosing the error that caused it. HCPs are reluctant to disclose errors—even when no negative effects result—for many reasons: shame, worries that the patient-professional relationship will be damaged, fear of lawsuits, etc. What role should such concerns play in disclosing errors to patients?

Step 2: Creative Problem Solving   Any creative solution would have to tell the truth to Marjorie's parents without jeopardizing her future health.

Step 3: Pros and Cons   Survey CARVE principles to identify important moral reasons that support conflicting options for resolving this case.

Consequences   What would be the effects on Marjorie, her parents, the HCPs, and the hospital if Dr. D tells the truth? if she lies? (Banja; Douglas; Smith)

Is lying ever morally permissible? Competing obligations to different persons might justify lying (e.g., lying to protect the confidence of a colleague or another patient). In health care contexts HCPs often justify lying if they believe a lie would be *best for the patient* to whom one is lying.[4] Therapeutic privilege—withholding information as a means to promoting patient welfare—can sometimes be morally appropriate in medical contexts, but all too frequently is invoked to avoid difficult conversations with patients or families. Whether lying to Marjorie's parents would be *best for her* hinges on several issues: her parents' mental state; their desire for the truth; the actions they might undertake, should they discover the truth about their daughter's (mis)treatment; and their capability of making autonomous choices for their child. Will their youth, lack of family support, exhaustion, or fear lead them to irrational conclusions about what options are best for their daughter, or to rash actions that might harm or be fatal to her? Might the truth undercut trust or lead to even greater psychological stress for these overburdened parents?

Autonomy   Are the parents capable of autonomous decision making at this time? If not does, their incapacity justify withholding the truth? (Banja; Lindberg and Iserson; Smith)

Medicine's historic code of ethics, the Hippocratic Oath, placed nonmaleficence and beneficence at its moral center, understanding other moral obligations (e.g., honesty) to follow from those two principles.[5] The Oath neither affirmed an independent duty of truthfulness toward nor prohibited lying to or withholding the truth from patients. The ancient medical community presumed deceit was justified if it was necessary to secure patient well-being.

In contrast, the last several decades have seen health care codes of ethics evolve from a preferential commitment to beneficence/nonmaleficence to one of affirming patient autonomy and self-determination. As a result, codes of ethics now speak to the *primary* moral importance of respecting patients' decisional authority and of veracity as a necessary means to demonstrating that respect. But, as in the Hippocratic Oath, no contemporary professional code of ethics frames the obligation of veracity as an absolute moral commitment.[6]

So, contemporary American health care culture embraces a duty to tell the truth to patients. Still, as this case makes clear, HCPs frequently second-guess this obligation as they try to decide whether—in particular cases—other moral values override the commitment to veracity.

Nonetheless, lying to patients is morally wrong for three reasons.[7] First, not being truthful abrogates a fundamental moral obligation to persons. This duty, which has antecedents in the Judeo-Christian concept of neighbor-love, contends that duplicity ignores the moral force of respecting persons as beings to whom the truth is owed *in principle.* Second, trust in relationships characterized by power inequities (e.g., vulnerable patients who depend on HCPs to protect and promote their interests) cannot be realized or sustained without truthfulness. Trusting a liar upon whom one is dependent is not only difficult, but foolish; one always wonders if things are as they seem and worries about being able to protect oneself from unknown threats.[8] Third, in modern secular culture veracity is grounded in respect for autonomy. Deceit both disrespects persons as decision makers and obstructs their right and freedom to make and act on choices about how to live their own lives. Respect for autonomy requires honesty, for without accurate information persons' actions may be misguided and their goals may be thwarted. In health care settings, veracity underpins a commitment to and is a necessary condition of informed consent.

Rights   Within the patient-professional context, Marjorie has a right to be aided and a right to not be harmed. The parents, on Marjorie's behalf, have a right to self-determination (decisional authority). (Smith) The parents also have a right to not be harmed and, perhaps, a right to be aided.

Virtues   The virtue of honesty is relevant here, as is the virtue of compassion. (Banja; Lindberg and Iserson; Smith) How should Dr. D demonstrate these virtues in regard to Marjorie and her parents? (Douglas) What does the virtue of fidelity, which requires putting the patient's interests first *and* fully informing appropriate decision makers, demand? Finally, is truth-telling an opportunity for Dr. D to demonstrate courage? (Banja)

Inappropriate appeals to therapeutic privilege raise questions of virtue. Virtues are personality characteristics and virtue terms typically describe persons who are predisposed to morally admirable behavior. So, for example, a person demonstrates the virtue of honesty if she is predisposed to tell the truth. She need not always tell the truth, the whole truth, or nothing but the truth; but her initial response will be to tell the truth and she will do so unless presented with properly serious and compelling reasons to conceal the facts. Similarly with fidelity: HCPs need not always honor the professional commitment to patient nonmaleficence, beneficence, and autonomy; but they must have very serious reasons to break faith with these professional promises.

One often-overlooked professional promise is the commitment of HCPs to public education. Perhaps one such opportunity is to educate the public about a commonly unappreciated risk: the fallibility of medical professionals. Though HCPs—like all humans—make mistakes, many persons, like Marjorie's parents, fail to consider the possibility that their HCPs will make life- or health-threatening errors. Given this widespread naïveté, if HCPs lie or (more frequently) withhold the truth, subsequent health care decisions are based on inaccurate or incomplete information, particularly appreciation of risks. Deceit also perpetuates unrealistic and inflated expectations of the very human practice of healing and care. The ubiquitous nature of fallibility raises the question of whether HCPs are morally obligated—either under an appeal to consequences or to professional integrity—to educate consumers about the possibility of mistakes. This same question may be asked about health care institutions.[9]

Justice   Are the parents being evaluated unfairly because of their youth? Who can fairly be considered responsible for the error? (Banja; Lindberg and Iserson; Smith)

Discriminating against Marjorie's parents in virtue of their youth surely treats them unequally, when compared to more mature family members; but does it treat them unfairly? Treatment is unfair if it is based on morally irrelevant characteristics (e.g., race or gender). Frequently, HCPs are tempted to withhold information to patients who are young, old, uneducated, or disabled. Other vulnerable groups include those without emotional support or who are simply not assertive. *If* these characteristics are *morally relevant*, persons may *justly* take them into account; but HCPs must first demonstrate *why* these traits justify unequal treatment. Such cases are difficult to make.

The Law   In conclusion, several legal issues are important to this case: (1) Are HCPs legally obligated to avoid deceiving (presumably) competent patients (here, the parents) who hold legal decisional authority; and under what conditions may

HCPs legally override decisional authority of a (presumably) competent patient? (2) Who is legally liable in a case such as this: the nurse who administered the drug; the supervising physician or other medical staff members; or the health care institution (for assigning an inexperienced nurse to the ER)? (3) Are HCPs legally obligated not to exceed their professional training? (4) What standards of professional training ought to govern HCPs who rotate through various specialized services in a modern hospital, that they may be held *legally* liable for errors they make?[10]

The following commentaries examine the application of various moral principles to this dilemma, thereby assisting the reader to undertake *Step 4: Analysis* and *Step 5: Justification.*

Notes

1. See, for example, Martin L. Smith and Heidi P. Forster, "Morally Managing Medical Mistakes," *Cambridge Quarterly of Healthcare Ethics* 9 (2000): 38–40; Thomas H. Gallagher et al., "Patients' and Physicians' Attitudes Regarding the Disclosure of Medical Errors," *JAMA: Journal of the American Medical Association* 289, no. 8 (2003): 1002.

2. Landis Downing and Robert L. Potter, "Heartland Regional Medical Center Makes A 'Fitting Response' to Medical Mistakes," *Bioethics Forum* 17, no. 2 (2001): 13.

3. See note 1, above; and Amy B. Witman, Deric M. Park, and Steven B. Hardin, "How Do Patients Want Physicians to Handle Mistakes?: A Survey of Internal Medicine Patients in an Academic Setting," *Archives of Internal Medicine* 156 (1996): 2565–69.

4. Edmund G. Howe, "Deceiving Patients for Their Own Good," *The Journal of Clinical Ethics* 8, no. 3 (1997): 211–16.

5. "Hippocratic Oath—Classical Version," trans. Ludwig Edelstein, in Ludwig Edelstein, *The Hippocratic Oath: Text, Translation, and Interpretation* (Baltimore: Johns Hopkins University Press, 1943), http://www.pbs.org/wgbh/nova/doctors/oath_classical.html (25 Mar. 2004).

6. See, for example, American Medical Association, *Code of Medical Ethics: Current Opinions of The Council on Ethical and Judicial Affairs* (Chicago: AMA, 1992), 18 July 2003, http://www.ama-assn.org/ama/pub/category/2416.html (25 Mar. 2004); American Nurses Association, *Code of Ethics for Nurses with Interpretative Statements* (Washington, DC.: ANA, 2001), http://nursingworld.org/ethics/code/ethicscode150.htm (25 Mar. 2004); American Pharmaceutical Association, "Code of Ethics for Pharmacists," 27 Oct. 1994, http://www.aphanet.org/pharmcare/ethics.html (25 Mar. 2004); Emergency Nurses Association, "Code of Ethics," 19 Sept. 2000, http://www.ena.org (25 Mar. 2004).

7. Sissela Bok, *Lying: Moral Choices in Public and Private Life* (New York: Vintage Books, 1989), especially chaps. 2, 3, and 14.

8. Jennifer Jackson, *Truth, Trust and Medicine* (London: Routledge, 2001).

9. Donald M. Berwick, "Errors Today and Errors Tomorrow," *New England Journal of Medicine* 348, no. 25 (2003): 2570–72; Andrew E. Thurman, "Institutional Responses to Medical Mistakes: Ethical and Legal Perspectives," *Kennedy Institute of Ethics Journal* 11, no. 2 (2001): 147–56.

10. The best discussion of conceptual, ethical, and legal issues on this topic is Alan Merry and Alistair McCall Smith, *Errors, Medicine, and the Law* (Cambridge: Cambridge University Press, 2001). Issues relevant to nursing practice are discussed in Rebecca F. Cady, *The Advanced Practice Nurse's Handbook* (Philadelphia: Lippincott, Williams & Wilkins, 2003), esp. chap. 5, "Standardized Procedures, Protocols, and Guidelines," 113–26. See also Amer-

ican Medical Association, Council on Ethical and Judicial Affairs, *Code of Medical Ethics: Current Opinions with Annotations*, 2000–2001 ed. (Chicago: American Medical Association, 2000), § 9.032, "Reporting Adverse Drug or Device Events," 202–3; and § 8.12, "Patient Information," 174–75.

A Parent's Analysis

Laura Douglas

Our little girl is really sick this time. She was so blue and having so much trouble catching her breath. These spells are getting worse and worse. She has never stopped breathing like that before. She looked so lifeless. We cannot bear to lose our only child.

The doctor and nurses have never asked us to leave the room before. They took us away so quickly. We did not even have time to give her a good-bye kiss. The room they put us in is so very quiet and small. It does not have much furniture—a few chairs, a little table, a phone, and a box of Kleenex. The door is closed, but we hear all the commotion in the hall and a bit of frantic yelling. We are so worried. We can only imagine the worst. What have we done to our poor little girl? She just has to make it. . . .

The Truth

The doctor just came in and told us the truth why our baby almost died. She said the nurse made an honest mistake. It could have happened to anyone. The doctor does not think the mistake will cause any lasting harm to Marjorie.

The doctor apologized. The nurse also said, "I'm so sorry." The doctor asked if we would be considerate of the nurse's feelings and not tell everyone in the community her name. She is very ashamed.

The doctor said that from now on she would personally double-check all medicine before it was given to Marjorie so this would not happen again. She also said they were making a special "dosage chart" just for Marjorie because she comes in so often. She also asked us to forgive them.

Dr. D asked us if we had any questions or concerns, but we were too numb to speak. We are so confused. Hospitals are supposed to be perfect and not make mistakes. We are so glad it was not our fault.

The doctors and nurses have all been like family to us. It seems we are always crying on their shoulders. There are so many important decisions to make. We just do not understand all this medical stuff. They have really been wonderful. At times, we feel like we live at this hospital more than at home. The nurses bring us dinner.

They give us warm blankets and pillows so we can rest while they get Marjorie well enough to go back home. They have organized the community in a fund-raiser to help pay for Marjorie's big surgery when she is old enough. One of the nurses even crocheted a blanket for Marjorie at Christmas to keep her warm on her long trips to and from the hospital. Of course, we would forgive a family member. Who would not? Still, it is hard to forget. Should we go to another hospital? The next hospital is much farther away, but it is much bigger. They do not know Marjorie at that hospital. They do not know how very precious she is to us. Who is to say they would not make the same mistake too? We still cannot believe that a hospital made a mistake. What if they make a mistake during her big surgery?

We have spoken with the nurse and the doctor again. The poor nurse, she is so upset and feels so guilty. The doctor promises us they will do everything to make sure another mistake does not happen. They do not think Marjorie would make the long drive to the bigger hospital. The doctor and nurses have been truthful and good to us. We trust and respect them and know they want to do what is best for Marjorie. We will still bring her here, but we are a little more nervous now knowing that hospitals do make mistakes. We cannot help but watch their every move a little closer and have asked them not to take us away from her side again. They promised they wouldn't.

The Lie Undiscovered

The doctor told us that Marjorie responded poorly to the medication. She said they almost lost her, but she turned around and is doing fine for now. We are so relieved.

We are very nervous taking her home this time. We have never come so close to losing her. They encouraged us to care for her at home as we always have. We will stay up and watch her closer than ever, we only wish that we did not live so far away.

We should have brought her in sooner. What if we hurt our baby girl? Maybe we are not good enough to be her parents. The drive is getting longer and longer. If only our farm was closer to town. Maybe we should give her to someone in town who is better able to care for her. . . .

The Lie Discovered

We considered staying home from church today because we are exhausted and worried about Marjorie, but we went. We really wanted to give thanks for saving our little girl and ask forgiveness for not being able to take better care of her.

At church, one of our friends came up and told us what really happened in the hospital that night. We are so mad. Why did they lie to us? We trusted and respected them. They were like family to us. Family would not lie. How can we ever trust them again? What else have they covered up? Everyone in town probably knows by now. What will they think if we take her back to that hospital again? What are we going to do now? We do not want to take her back there ever again! But the other hospital is so far away. Can we make it in time? What if we don't make it?

RECOMMENDED READINGS

Back, Tony. "Breaking Bad News." 1998. http://eduserv.hscer.washington.edu/bioethics/topics/badnws.html (25 Mar. 2004).

Braddock III, Clarence. "Truth Telling and Withholding Information." 1998, http://eduserv.hscer.washington.edu/bioethics/topics/truth.html (25 Mar. 2004).

Brazeau, Chantal. "Disclosing the Truth About a Medical Error." *American Family Physician* 60, no. 3 (1999): 1013–16.

Diekema, Douglas. "Mistakes." 1998. http://eduserv.hscer.washington.edu/bioethics/topics/mistks.html (25 Mar. 2004).

Hebert, Philip, Alex Levin and Gerald Robertson. "Bioethics for Clinicians: 23. Disclosure of Medical Error," *Canadian Medical Association Journal (CMAJ)* 164, no. 4 (2001): 509–13.

Prager, Linda. "New laws let doctors say 'I'm sorry' for medical mistakes," 21 Aug. 2000, http://www.mercola.com/2000/sept/3/forgiveness.htm (25 Mar. 2004).

Rubin, Susan and Laurie Zoloth. *Margin of Error,* (Hagerstown, MD: University Publishing Group, 2000).

"Telling Patients about Mistakes Made in Their Care Is the Right Thing to Do and May Reduce Lawsuits," July 2002, http://www.ahcpr.gov/research/jul02/0702RA11.htm (25 Mar. 2004).

Wu, A. W. et al., "To Tell the Truth: Ethical and Practical Issues in Disclosing Medical Mistakes to Patients." *Journal of General Internal Medicine* 12, no. 12 (1997): 770–75.

Wusthoff, Courtney J., "Medical Mistakes and Disclosure: The Role of the Medical Student," *JAMA: Journal of the American Medical Association* 286, no. 9 (2001): 1080–81.

An Emergency Physician's Analysis

Elizabeth Ann Lindberg, MD,
and Kenneth V. Iserson, MD, MBA

What should Dr. D tell Mr. and Mrs. P about the cause of Marjorie's respiratory arrest? This question raises issues of varying standards of care, medical care protocols, and truth-telling.

Standards of Care

Not all hospitals are major medical centers. Small hospitals have varying staffing, professional abilities, and equipment. With much smaller patient volumes than larger institutions, these mostly rural hospitals will have less experience caring for critical patients. This may increase the likelihood that errors will occur.

Nursing may be a particular issue, since a shortage of experienced nurses for all the hospital's units may require them to "float" to units where they are not familiar with equipment, medications and dosages, protocols, and staff. In any hospital, that is a recipe for disaster. The quality of physician staffing may also vary greatly, from highly competent (especially in certain areas) to those using the rural hospital as a place to "hide out" after failing elsewhere. Even physicians who once had the skills needed to attempt pediatric resuscitations will have few opportunities to use these skills, and even the most competent physicians will lose some of their knowledge and skills with lack of use over time.

Standards of care vary with circumstances. Smaller hospitals and those not routinely treating very ill children will not be held to the same standards as those with larger pediatric patient populations. However, pediatric resuscitation standards exist, such as those in the Pediatric Advanced Life Support program.[1] Where these skills are rarely used—but are expected by those in need—it is incumbent upon medical personnel to get periodic updates and to have written protocols readily available.

Medical Care Protocols

In small institutions where not all appropriate personnel and equipment may be readily available, pediatric resuscitation requires that a mechanism be available to rapidly assemble the required materials and expertise. Often, this involves "calling a code," although something more specific may be needed, such as assembling nurses skilled in starting pediatric IVs and managing children's airways and ventilators, and pharmacists with the ability to quickly calculate pediatric dosages. This became easier with the widespread adoption of Braslow tapes, which provide clinicians with information about the appropriate medication doses and equipment sizes based on the child's size.[2]

The question must be asked: why were the parents asked to leave the room during the resuscitation? Although that was once standard practice, we now know that, especially in pediatric cases, having the family observe the resuscitation, when accompanied by a knowledgeable staff member, may actually lessen stress, increase trust in the medical team, and decrease families' anxiety, guilt, and flashbacks if the outcome is not successful. The bottom line is that relatives who are not present for the resuscitative attempt always imagine worse things than if they are allowed to remain in the room.[3]

Truth-Telling

One thing that gives emergency clinicians the confidence to perform with speed and assurance in critical situations is assurance that they know that they will do the right thing. When they err, they may have as much difficulty admitting it to themselves as to the patient or family. Nevertheless, both admissions must occur. People like to think their doctors and nurses are infallible, but they nonetheless appreciate knowing they are honest and human.

Telling patients or family of a medical error is never easy. Whether there are potential legal repercussions, a sense of personal failure, or possible outrage from the recipients, the clinician must "bite the bullet" and deliver this painful message. The key is to deliver the facts honestly and not (as is too frequently the case) blame one individual more than is justified.[4] As the American Medical Association's Code of Medical Ethics says, "A physician shall deal honestly with patients and with colleagues."[5] This obligation derives from, among other sources, basic respect for patients that governs (in the guise of autonomy and informed consent) much of modern medicine.

In this case, the young parents were very concerned that they may have done something to worsen the baby's condition. While one could argue that telling the parents of the error might actually harm Marjorie by having them go to another, more distant, facility in the future, this smacks of the now discredited reason for withholding bad news from patients—"therapeutic privilege." So-called therapeutic privilege allows physicians to withhold vital information on the typically erroneous assumption that the truth will harm the patient (or family). But this "privilege" deprives patients of information they need to make fully informed decisions, essentially depriving them of their autonomy. Indeed, these parents may feel better knowing that a reversible medical error, rather than their own actions, caused the problem.

In addition, this incident occurred in a small town, where everybody knows everybody and there are no secrets—good or bad. If the parents later heard about the medication error from another source, the beneficial trusting relationship would likely be shattered. Most lawyers agree that telling the truth in an open, honest, and timely manner results in the clinician's best chance of maintaining the parents' trusting relationship with the medical profession.

In conclusion, professional standards of care and the moral principles of beneficence, trust, and truth-telling require admitting the error to Marjorie's parents, and supporting them as they come to grips with this mistake.

Notes

1. American Academy of Pediatrics, "Pediatric Advanced Life Support Course" (Dallas: American Heart Association, and Elk Grove Village, IL: American Academy of Pediatrics, 1985 and updated).

2. A. Braslow et al., "CPR Training Without an Instructor: Development and Evaluation of a Video Self-instructional System for Effective Performance of Cardiopulmonary Resuscitation," *Resuscitation* 34, no. 3 (1997): 207–20.

3. Kenneth V. Iserson, *Grave Words: Notifying Survivors About Sudden, Unexpected Deaths* (Tucson, AZ: Galen Press, 1999).

4. James Rachels, "Responsibility to Monitor and Remedy Quality-of-care Mistakes," *Ethics in Emergency Medicine*, 2nd ed., ed. Kenneth V. Iserson et al. (Tucson, AZ: Galen Press, 1995), 346–50.

5. American Medical Association, "Principles of Medical Ethics" (also adopted by the American College of Emergency Physicians), *Code of Medical Ethics: Current Opinions of The Council on Ethical and Judicial Affairs* (Chicago: American Medical Association, 1992), § 8.12: 125.

A Clinical Ethicist's Analysis

Martin L. Smith, STD

A mistake in Marjorie's medical management has occurred: she experienced a preventable adverse event.[1] This "near miss" could have resulted in her disability or death had the resuscitation not been so successful. Dr. D now faces an ethical dilemma: how honest should she be with these young and frightened parents who are worried that their daughter's condition is worsening?

Significant ethical and legal emphasis on patient autonomy and informed consent presume that health care professionals (HCPs) will be honest with patients or their surrogates. In order to make informed choices, decision makers (usually patients themselves, but in this instance, Marjorie's parents) need accurate and adequate information about diagnosis, prognosis, and risks/benefits/alternatives/ possible outcomes of recommended interventions, procedures, and tests. This principle-based "standard of care" for truth-telling and the educative process of informed consent probably propel Dr. D to disclose to the parents what happened to their daughter. Dr. D's ethical intuition to be honest is supported by the American Medical Association's Council on Ethical and Judicial Affairs:

> *It is a fundamental ethical requirement that a physician should at all times deal honestly and openly with patients. Patients have the right to know their past and present medical status and to be free of any mistaken beliefs concerning their conditions. Situations occasionally occur in which a patient suffers significant medical complications that may have resulted from the physician's mistake or judgment. In these situations, the physician is ethically required to inform the patient of all the facts necessary to ensure understanding of what has occurred. Only through full disclosure is a patient able to make informed decisions regarding future medical care. . . .*

Concern regarding legal liability which might result following truthful dis-
closure should not affect the physician's honesty with the patient.[2]

The Ethics Manual of the American College of Physicians offers a similar appeal: "Physicians should disclose to patients information about procedural or judgment errors made in the course of care if such information is material to the patient's well-being. Errors do not necessarily constitute improper, negligent, or un-ethical behavior, but failure to disclose them may."[3]

Although Dr. D is initially inclined to meet these expressed ethical duties, she engages in some consequentialist and paternalistic thinking as she tries to discern her ethical duties within the context of the specific circumstances of caring for Mar-jorie and her parents. Is disclosure truly in the best interests of *these* parents and *this* patient at *this* time?

Dr. D focuses primarily on the negative consequences that a full disclosure might have: increased anxiety for the parents, their possible mistrust of this particu-lar emergency room (ER) and its staff, delayed treatment for the baby if the par-ents travel to another ER, their discovery that HCPs are fallible, and potential legal repercussions. Dr. D's dilemma can be framed by the question: are the envisioned negative consequences sufficient to trump the principle-based duty to be honest with the parents?

Both ethics and law recognize exceptions to truth-telling. One exception is "therapeutic privilege" which supports nondisclosure of information when, in the professional's judgment, disclosed information would have significant and harmful consequences to the patient's well-being. Yet, appeals to therapeutic privilege should be rare and should not be used to rationalize avoiding difficult but essential conversations with patients.

But Dr. D's dilemma is not adequately solved by such an appeal. Dr. D cannot and should not depend on a "code of silence" among all the professionals who now know about the medical mistake. Further, because the administered morphine dosage and the narcotic antagonist should be part of the Marjorie's medical record, this information may be disclosed to or discovered by the parents at some future time. Discovery of such a "cover-up" could increase the parent's distrust of HCPs and could put Dr. D and the hospital at greater risk of a lawsuit than immediate truthful disclosure. These additional negative risks and consequences are too sig-nificant to be set aside or ignored by an appeal to therapeutic privilege leading to nondisclosure.

Significant for this case is that "Dr. D knows the parents well." Presumably the parents trust her because she has previously provided effective ER treatment and resuscitation. Dr. D should use this trusting relationship as a context for an imme-diate and honest conversation with the parents about the mistaken dose of mor-phine.[4] She should apologize for the error and assure the parents that the respira-tory arrest is not necessarily a sign that Marjorie is getting worse. Although it is impossible to predict with certainty how these parents will respond to honesty and an apology, most persons do respond favorably to such an approach.[5] Dr. D should proceed with some degree of confidence that this approach will likely enhance and strengthen—rather than harm and hinder—these parents' trust in her.

Further, because similar mistakes could have serious consequences for future patients and even for Marjorie, Dr. D should assure the parents that the ER staff will engage in a process of root-cause analysis aimed at changing the ER systems so that similar errors can be prevented in the future. Dr. D should offer to inform the parents about system changes that are eventually made. Such analyses, as part of an overall commitment to quality improvement, are essential for all hospitals, but especially smaller ones. Small hospitals—often serving smaller, tight-knit communities—can more easily increase public trust if quality improvement processes are transparent and visible to the community.

Next, Dr. D should not be afraid to note that HCPs are not infallible and that mistakes do happen in hospitals.[6] Such a frank admission clashes with the myth of a "perfectibility model" of health care, that is, error-free health care is possible if all professionals were properly educated, trained, and motivated. This myth and model contribute to unattainable expectations and standards for patients, families, and professionals, and aim to fix blame and punish individuals as the first and sometimes exclusive response to mistakes. Dr. D, the ER staff, and the hospital have an opportunity to provide a corrective for these parents and perhaps the wider community by adopting a routine practice of disclosing mistakes, admitting their fallibility, and focusing on improving systems and creating safeguards so that such mistakes will be difficult to make in the future.

Finally, Dr. D should restate the ER team's commitment to promoting Marjorie's survival, communicate her fears that travel to another ER may put Marjorie at additional risk due to delayed treatment, yet be prepared to respect the parents' decision should they seek medical care for their daughter at another hospital.

Notes

1. Committee on Quality of Health Care in America, Institute of Medicine, *To Err is Human: Building a Safer Health System*, eds. Linda T. Kohn, Janet M. Corrigan, and Molla S. Donaldson (Washington, DC: Institute of Medicine, The National Academies Press, 2000).
2. American Medical Association, Council on Ethical and Judicial Affairs, *Code of Medical Ethics: Current Opinions with Annotations* (Chicago: American Medical Association, 1997) § 8.12: 125.
3. American College of Physicians, *Ethics Manual*, 4th ed., *Annals of Internal Medicine* 128 (1998): 576–94.
4. "Guidelines for Disclosure and Discussion of Conditions and Events with Patients, Families and Guardians," *Kennedy Institute of Ethics Journal* 11 (2001): 165–68.
5. A. B. Witman, D. M. Park, and S. B. Hardin, "How do Patients Want Physicians to Handle Mistakes? A Survey of Internal Medicine Patients in an Academic Setting," *Archives of Internal Medicine* 156 (1996): 2565–69.
6. Martin L. Smith and Heidi P. Forster, "Morally Managing Medical Mistakes," *Cambridge Quarterly of Healthcare Ethics* 9 (2000): 38–53.

An Ethicist's Analysis

John D. Banja, PhD

So, 7-month-old Marjorie was erroneously given a morphine overdose that caused her respiratory arrest. If Marjorie's physician, Dr. D, would consult the American Medical Association's *Current Opinions on the Code of Ethics*, § 8.12, she would discover:

> It is a fundamental ethical requirement that a physician should at all times deal honestly and openly with patients. Patients have a right to know their past and present medical status and to be free of any mistaken beliefs concerning their conditions. Situations occasionally occur in which a patient suffers significant medical complications that may have resulted from the physician's mistake or judgment. In these situations, the physician is ethically required to inform the patient of all the facts necessary to ensure understanding of what has occurred. Only through full disclosure is a patient able to make informed decisions regarding future medical care.[1]

Furthermore, Dr. D. would find standard RI.1.1.2 of the Joint Commission on the Accreditation of Healthcare Organizations (JCAHO) stating that "patients, and when appropriate, their families, are informed about the outcomes of care, including unanticipated outcomes."[2]

While the AMA Code or the JCAHO standards would warrant consideration of whether Marjorie's respiratory arrest should be understood as an "unanticipated outcome" or a "complication," I would wager that Dr. D might be thinking along different lines. I suspect that Dr. D would be drawn to the fact that the effects of the morphine overdose appear to have been successfully reversed, and that Marjorie neither appears to be experiencing any lasting harm nor to require further care. Because Marjorie's parents won't have to make any further treatment decisions in response to the error and Marjorie appears to be recovering nicely, why disclose the error? And if at some future time Marjorie does exhibit some cognitive or cardiac dysfunction, who could ever say with any certainty that the dysfunction was caused by the morphine overdose? After all, since Marjorie had to be rushed to the emergency room "approximately once a week since she was born," she experienced over 20 hypoxic episodes plus at least one other resuscitation effort, any one of which could explain some future disability.

In fact, though, at least three problems would be raised by Dr. D's concealing this error. First, Dr. D's hospital employs at least one nurse who is "inexperienced . . . rarely works in the ER and has never worked with critically ill children." Furthermore, one should ask why an adult-sized vial was within this nurse's reach for a pediatric patient *in extremis*. No matter how inexperienced this nurse may have been, any nurse in the heat of such an emergency could have made a similar error.

To the extent, then, that Dr. D's hospital allows such "latent system failures" to occur, some such error was probably going to happen sooner or later.

Consequently, there is reason to disclose this error to Marjorie's parents since, per the AMA's Current Opinions, they should have the option of considering where to take Marjorie for her future care. While using another hospital farther away may indeed be a danger, Marjorie was subjected to considerable peril at Dr. D's hospital and nearly killed. Her parents might be poorly educated, but their decision to risk an additional 30-minute drive to another, possibly safer, hospital, would not necessarily be irrational. But they can only make that decision if they are informed.

Second, and adding insult to injury, one would strongly suspect that if Marjorie's parents are not told of the error, they will also be billed—or have to pay some kind of co-payment—for Marjorie's resuscitation. This is so intuitively wrong that it requires little comment.

A third problem is that there is no way to ensure that Marjorie's parents will never learn of this error. The nurse who was the primary "error operator" or another staff member may experience unbearable pangs of conscience and tell them. If the error was noted in Marjorie's medical record and later read by another health provider, he or she might tell Marjorie's parents. While it is impossible to know how they might respond upon finding out, they may feel profoundly misled because concealing the error might encourage them to believe that Marjorie's arrest was somehow her fault or perhaps their fault. To the extent that Dr. D knows what happened but does not take steps to eradicate the possibility of this misbelief and the painful feelings that might be associated with it, she betrays Marjorie's parents' trust and compromises their psychological welfare. That is clearly a serious ethical breach and the ethical nub of this case.

Still, disclosing harm-causing error is one of the most anguishing experiences a health provider can have. Assuming she is certain that the morphine overdose caused Marjorie's respiratory arrest and after assuring her parents that Marjorie is recovering and apparently out of danger, Dr. D. should say, "I do need to tell you, however, that an error occurred as we were treating Marjorie, and I wonder if you'd like to know what happened." If Marjorie's parents want to know, Dr. D should calmly and slowly say, "Well, this is hard for me tell you, but we gave Marjorie too much of a particular kind of medicine when she came in, and that's what caused her breathing to stop. We quickly discovered our mistake and were able to give her some different medicine to get her breathing again. But I want you to know that her breathing problem was not because of anything she did or you did. It was because of something we did. Thank goodness, she seems to be doing fine right now. And, by the way, you certainly won't be billed for anything connected with that mistake we made."

How Marjorie's parents react to the news will depend on factors too numerous to discuss. But by first giving Marjorie's parents the option of hearing what happened and then following their lead, Dr. D. does as much as anyone could to respect them and maintain their trust. By doing the most difficult thing—telling the truth and admitting that an error occurred—Dr. D might also take giant steps toward averting a lawsuit. In any event, she should take pride in summoning the moral courage to do the right thing when her psychological defenses and inclinations may be pulling her in a very different direction.

RECOMMENDED READINGS:

Smith, Martin L. and Forster, Heidi P., "Morally Managing Medical Mistakes," *Cambridge Quarterly of Healthcare Ethics* 9 (2000): 38–53.

Notes

1. Council on Ethical and Judicial Affairs, American Medical Association, *Code of Medical Ethics: Current Opinions with Annotations*, 1998–1999 ed. (Chicago: American Medical Association, 1999).
2. Joint Commission on Accreditation of Healthcare Organizations, *CAMH: Comprehensive Accreditation Manual for Hospitals: The Official Handbook* (Oakbrook Terrace, IL: Joint Commission on Accreditation of Healthcare Organizations, 2001).

Further Reflections

General

1. This case takes place in a small community hospital where experienced personnel are in short supply. What role should this fact play in determining the physician's duty to tell the truth? Would the morally appropriate response differ in an urban center with easier access to more emergency rooms and qualified medical personnel, etc.?

Consequences

2. If health care professionals (HCPs) educate the public in general and their (wrongly treated) patients in particular about their fallibility, what consequences to patients, families, HCPs, health care institutions, and insurance companies might result? Would they be better or worse than the consequences of deception?

3. Smith suggests that "therapeutic privilege" justifies lying to patients in some cases (though not this one). Lindberg and Iserson argue that therapeutic privilege is a "discredited reason" for lying. What moral principles *might* support therapeutic privilege? Would they justify lying in this situation?

Autonomy

4. As Smith notes, patients need accurate and complete medical information to make good present *and* future health care decisions. But if HCPs suspect good

information will be misunderstood, misinterpreted, or misapplied; or if they believe the persons who have the right to the information will *not* make good use of it, are they justified in withholding that information?

5. What does respect for autonomy require of HCPs who disagree with their patients' choices?

Rights

6. Do patients (or, in the case of children, their parents) have a right to the truth about medical mistakes? If so, why? If not, why not?

Virtues

7. The virtue of fidelity requires HCPs to work for the welfare of their patients. The virtue of honesty requires HCPs to tell their patients the truth. What is the relationship between these virtues and the morally appropriate action in this case? (All commentators)

8. Several commentators suggest that truth-telling is a responsibility of HCPs and cite material from various professional codes of ethics to support this claim. However, the Hippocratic Oath did not require truth-telling of physicians; in fact, truth-telling was typically discouraged as an undue burden on the sick. Why, in your estimation, has the duty of truth-telling evolved as is has?

9. Should medical education promote the development of certain character traits so that HCPs will typically possess certain virtues (perhaps those described by Douglas in "The Truth")? If so, what character traits are most desirable in an HCP? If not, what steps should be taken to ensure that HCPs (usually) tell patients about medical mistakes? Do health care institutions have a role to play?

Equality/Fairness (Justice)

10. Justice allows persons who are unequal in morally relevant ways to be treated unequally. Do Marjorie's parents possess any characteristics that make them unequal when compared to the typical patient/parent who should be told the truth? If so, what are these traits and why do they imply moral inequality?

11. Is the fact, discussed by Banja, that the error was successfully treated, a morally relevant reason regarding withholding information from some patients/families?

Chapter 7

Who Makes Decisions in Family-Centered Health Care?

Univille is a town of 20,000 located in a Midwestern state. The population is largely engaged in agriculture or agricultural support services, although it also supports a community college serving 4000 students. For the last decade the college has made a concerted effort to enroll more minority students and has had modest success in attracting African American, Hispanic American, and Vietnamese American students. The presence of non-Caucasian students has generated some hostility among the townspeople. In addition to the usual "town-gown" conflicts, local citizens resent the introduction of "foreigners" and often treat them rudely or (at best) not in a friendly or courteous fashion. Not surprisingly, the minority students resent this treatment.

Univille has a small community hospital whose staff, reflecting the demographics of the general community, are all white. In response to increasing numbers of unwed mothers, with a concomitant lack of responsibility for children on the part of unwed fathers, the hospital began a family-centered pregnancy program. This program, initiated in hope of encouraging family bonding and shared responsibility for pregnancy, labor, delivery, and child care, advocates (though does not require) participation in and joint decision making by both partners regarding prenatal classes, physician visits, labor and delivery, and well-baby follow-up care. Although not specifically aimed at minority populations, the program has served some minority couples from the community and the college.

Ms. N is a 19-year-old pregnant woman due to deliver her first child in one week. She and her partner, Mr. J, both African American students at the college, have been enthusiastic participants in the family-centered pregnancy program. Ms. N and Mr. J have jointly attended classes, kept doctor's appointments, studied normal pregnancy processes, and considered several labor and delivery options. They have opted for natural labor and delivery in a birthing room, have toured the facilities, and are prepared for "the big day."

When Ms. N presents to the hospital with ruptured membranes, attempts are made to notify Mr. J of her admission (his roommate is uncertain of his whereabouts, but promises to track him down). During the admitting evaluation, Ms. R, the labor and delivery nurse, examines Ms. N and notes a labial lesion. Upon questioning, Ms. N states that she has recently had burning and pain in the labial area, typical signs of an acute episode of genital herpes simplex virus (HSV) infection. Ms. R asks about a history of HSV, and Ms. N admits that she was treated for an HSV infection a few years ago, prior to meeting Mr. J.

Transmission of HSV to a newborn can result in severe complications, such as respiratory distress, seizures, coma, and even death of the infant. To decrease the risk of transmission to the infant during vaginal delivery, women with acute HSV infections are typically delivered by caesarean section (C-section). Ms. N agrees to the C-section but informs Ms. R that Mr. J is not aware of her history of herpes and that she does not want him to know.

Ms. R questions Ms. N about this decision. She points out that participants in the family-centered program are expected—and expect—to share decisions about the labor and delivery process, as well as about choices that will have an impact on their child. The decision to have a C-section is a momentous decision that has significant risks for both Ms. N and her child. Mr. J will naturally expect to be consulted about this decision, and Ms. R, the obstetrician, and, soon, the nursery personnel are being asked to either ignore or deceive him. Ms. R points out that they will have to give him some explanation about the change in plans and wonders what they should say. Ms. N, in tears, replies that she has no idea what they should say—only what they should not say.

Mr. J arrives after Ms. N has been taken into surgery and is informed of the pending C-section. He becomes quite upset and demands to know why she is having surgery and why he was not consulted before surgery began. Ms. R explains that Ms. N is doing just fine, that she consented to the surgery, and that the surgery is to decrease risk to the baby. Mr. J, clearly frightened, asks what is wrong with the baby. Ms. R assures him that the baby is fine. Mr. J retorts, "If my baby and girlfriend are just fine, why are you doing a C-section?" When Ms. R replies that she cannot give him any further information, Mr. J replies, angrily, "You'd tell me if I were white, right?"

From a moral point of view, what should Ms. R tell Mr. J?

Introduction

This case raises four inextricably intertwined moral issues:

1. Who is the appropriate decision maker when decisions will have significant impact on persons other than the patient?
2. When, if ever, may patient confidentiality or privacy be breached?
3. Do new paradigms—here, about who is the patient—require revising established moral obligations of health care providers (HCPs)?
4. What role does race play in HCPs' moral obligations?

The AJ Method

Step 1: Information Gathering   What facts are relevant to this dilemma? How likely is it that Ms. N will be helped or harmed if the nurse tells Mr. J? if the nurse does not tell him? What would be the implications of this choice for the child's future welfare? for Mr. J's and Ms. N's relationship? Who else might be helped or harmed, depending upon the nurse's response? What motivates Mr. J's charge of racism? Why was Ms. N reluctant to reveal her HSV? What did the hospital indicate about decisional authority for participants in the family-centered program? Does the nurse have any familiarity with African American history?

Three other important factual issues contribute to this dilemma: (1) Strong evidence indicates that children raised in two-parent families have a better chance of living a good life;[1] (2) The health care system historically has treated and often continues to treat African Americans badly;[2] and (3) Our health care system neither readily nor explicitly recognizes interests of family members in medical decision making.[3] The family-centered pregnancy program aims generally to address the first issue. Their success in this—and perhaps future—dilemma(s) will depend, at least in part, on their appreciation of and responses to the second and third.

Step 2: Creative Solution   Any creative solution would have to respect Mr. J's request without violating Ms. N's confidentiality.

Step 3: Pros and Cons   Survey CARVE principles to identify important moral reasons that support conflicting options for resolving this case.

Consequences   What would be the immediate effects of failing to tell Mr. J? of telling him? How likely would the effects be? Who would be affected? What would be the longer-term effects of failing to tell Mr. J? of telling him? (Reverby)

Some HCPs may worry that women's voices will be lost if women are not seen as the ultimate decisional authority about their health care. This is an empirical issue about which one might make predictions, but not assurances. If the program does subordinate the interests of women to those of the family unit, should it be abandoned? Or might family interests or welfare outweigh those of individual women? Women are, after all, members of families whose welfare they may be presumed to desire.

Autonomy   Who has decisional authority in this case? (All commentators) Is Ms. N capable of an autonomous choice in this situation?

Western medicine prioritizes *individual* decisional authority. Barring incompetence or explicit instructions to the contrary, patients are considered the *only* appropriate persons to (1) receive information regarding and consent to treatment (confidentiality), and (2) consent to access to their bodies (privacy). A traditional response to Ms. R's dilemma would take the following form: the person who will physically undergo and who is most at risk from the C-section is Ms. N; therefore she—and she alone—possesses decisional authority for surgery.

The autonomy-based position has received support from feminist scholars as one means of enabling women to take responsibility for and control of their lives. Historically, women have deferred to or had decisional authority usurped by men, long thought to be more rational and less emotional, thus better able to make difficult choices.[4] Limiting womens' autonomy has not infrequently placed them at great(er) risk, often over their expressed objections (e.g., forced C-sections for fetal distress, drug testing during pregnancy).[5]

On both traditional and feminist accounts, decisional authority depends on and is protected by commitments to patient privacy and confidentiality. Patients are more likely to share sensitive information with HCPs if assured it will go no further. As appropriate therapy—and the confidentiality on which it depends—require sensitive information, HCPs have long taken confidentiality to be an important moral cornerstone of the patient-professional relationship. And, speaking practically, others are less likely to thwart a woman's choice if they lack information on which to base effective objections.

Nonetheless, commitment to *individual* autonomy and confidentiality (like all moral commitments) is not absolute. At least two conditions for overriding individual autonomy—and, derivatively, confidentiality—have been posed: (1) Those who will be significantly affected by a health care decision (e.g., family members) should have some say in it;[6] and (2) Many cultures, of which African Americans are but one, embrace a communal approach to decision making.[7] For such communities, exclusive focus on the individual as the locus of decisional authority and the exclusive recipient of beneficent actions may be misplaced. Thus race may be relevant, not because HCPs are racist, but because race may signal alternative assumptions and problem-solving approaches.

If Mr. J or the soon-to-be-born child will be affected significantly by Ms. N's decision, consent by both parents may be desirable. If Ms. N and Mr. J share a cultural, race-related tradition that makes unilateral consent aberrant, that tradition may provide sufficient reason to override Ms. N's explicit request.

Rights Parents have the right of self-determination for their minor children. Does this right extend to Mr. J, as the father of the child? (Chervenak and McCullough; Rasmussen) Within the patient-professional relationship, Ms. N has a right to be aided. Does this right extend to Mr. J? All parties—including Mr. J and the soon-to-be-born child—have a right to not be harmed. (Chervenak and McCullough) Ms. N has rights to self-determination, privacy, and confidentiality. (Chervenak and McCullough; Rasmussen)

Virtues How should the professional virtue of fidelity—particularly to patient self-determination—be exercised here? (Chervenak and McCullough; Rasmussen) Does fidelity require maintaining cultural competence (in addition to technical competence)? (Reverby) Are the virtues of tolerance and curiosity relevant? What role does honesty play? (Rasmussen)

Beyond self-interested or cultural justifications for sharing information with Mr. J, does the hospital's commitment to family-centered care generate a fidelity-based obligation to inform him? After all, the program in which Ms. N and Mr. J have both been faithful participants purports to treat the *family* as the patient. If this commitment is taken seriously, the family unit is the appropriate decisional authority. The rationale for this shift is that families do better if they see themselves as interdependent and if particular members eschew unilateral problem solving. To *be* a unit, the family must *act* as a unit. But if the commitment to family-centered decision making is merely metaphorical, many of the program's anticipated benefits may be threatened or precluded entirely. Will fathers' bonding with and assuming responsibility for their children be undercut if HCPs revert to the autonomy model when complications arise?

Equality/Fairness (Justice) Is Mr. J being treated unfairly because of his race? Is justice served by treating him the same as (equality) an Anglo father would be treated? by treating him differently (fairness)? (Chervenak and McCullough; Reverby)

What role does race play in this dilemma? Nurse R might have been surprised at Mr. J's charge of racism, and might believe she is treating Mr. J as she would treat any father in these circumstances. But *is* Nurse R acting with Mr. J as she would act with a white father? Might she consider decisional authority more fluid or a breach of confidentiality more justified if the distraught father were white? Does she subconsciously question Mr. J's decisional capacity because he is black? The case provides insufficient information to answer these questions but, given the history of strained relationships between the health care system and African Americans, and the often hostile reception of minorities by Univille citizens, they are worth raising.

On a related note, even if Nurse R is treating Mr. J precisely as she would treat a white father, might the history of poor treatment of African Americans justify treating Mr. J differently, perhaps as a means of repairing or compensating for earlier damage to African Americans (even if not to Mr. J personally)? Put another way, as a means of improving race relations, at least in Univille, might Mr. J's race justify breaching confidentiality in this case even if the breach would not be generally justified?

The Law   The following legal considerations are relevant to this case: (1) Who, legally, has decisional authority? Does participation in the hospital-sponsored program count as an implied contract that extends joint decisional authority to partners of pregnant women? (2) Would the nurse breach Ms. N's confidentiality by discussing her case with Mr. J? (3) Does Mr. J have legal decisional authority for the fetus that would justify his inclusion in decisions regarding the C-section?[8]

The following commentaries examine the application of various moral principles to this dilemma, thereby assisting the reader to undertake *Step 4: Analysis* and *Step 5: Justification.*

Notes

1. Judith Wallerstein, *The Unexpected Legacy of Divorce: A 25 Year Landmark Study* (New York: Hyperion, 2000); Suet-Ling Pong, *The Educational Success of Children in Nonintact Families: Do Ethnicity and the School Matter?* Grant funded by American Educational Research Association, 1994–1996; n.d., http://www.aera.net/grantsprogram (25 Mar. 2004); Henry N. Ricciuti, "Single Parenthood and School Readiness in White, Black, and Hispanic 6- and 7-Year-Olds," *Journal of Family Psychology* 13, no. 3 (1999): 450–65; Gunilla Ringbäck Weitoft et al., "Mortality, Severe Morbidity, and Injury in Children Living with Single Parents in Sweden: A Population-based Study," *Lancet* 361, no. 9354 (2003): 289–95.

2. Annette Dula, "African American Suspicion of the Healthcare System is Justified: What Do We Do About It?" *Cambridge Quarterly of Healthcare Ethics* 3 (1994): 347–57; Susan M. Reverby, "More than Fact and Fiction: Cultural Memory and the Tuskegee Syphilis Study," *Hastings Center Report* 31, no. 5 (2001): 22–28; eds. Marsha Lillie-Blanton, Wilhelmina Leigh, and Ana Alfaro-Correa, *Achieving Equitable Access: Studies of Healthcare Issues Affecting Hispanics and African Americans* (Lanham, MD: Joint Center for Political and Economic Studies/University Press of America, 1996); E. R. Brown et al., *Racial and Ethnic Disparities in Access to Health Insurance and Healthcare* (Menlo Park, CA: UCLA Center for Health Policy Research and Kaiser Family Foundation, 2000), 31 Jul 2000, http://www.kff.org (24 Mar. 2004); Karen Scott et al., *Diverse Communities, Common Concerns: Assessing Healthcare Quality for Minority Americans: Findings From the Commonwealth Fund 2001 Health Quality Survey* (New York: Commonwealth Fund, 2002), http://www.cmwf.org/publist/publist2.asp?CategoryID=11 (24 Mar. 2004); Arden Handler and Kristiana Raube, *Patients' Satisfaction with Prenatal Care* (Chicago: The Center for Health Administration Studies/University of Chicago, n.d.) http://www.chas.uchicago.edu/projects/patientssat.html (24 Mar. 2004).

3. John Hardwig, "What About the Family?" *Hastings Center Report* 20, no. 2 (1990): 5–10; James Lindemann Nelson, "Taking Families Seriously," *Hastings Center Report* 22, no. 4 (1992): 6–12; Jeffrey Blustein, "The Family in Medical Decisionmaking," *Hastings Center Report* 23, no. 3 (1993): 6–13.

4. Carol Gilligan, *In a Different Voice* (Cambridge: Harvard University Press, 1982).

5. Susan Irwin and Brigitte Jordan, "Knowledge, Practice, and Power: Court-Ordered Cesarean Sections," *Medical Anthropology Quarterly* 1, no. 3 (1987): 319–34; Lawrence O. Gostin, "The Rights of Pregnant Women: The Supreme Court and Drug Testing," *Hastings Center Report* 31, no. 5 (2001): 8–9; ed. Patricia Boling, *Expecting Trouble* (Boulder, CO: Westview Press, 1995).

6. Leslie J. Blackhall et al., "Ethnicity and Attitudes toward Patient Autonomy," *JAMA: Journal of the American Medical Association* 274 (1995): 820–25; Lawrence O. Gostin, "Informed Consent, Cultural Sensitivity, and Respect for Persons," *JAMA: Journal of the American Medical Association* 274 (1995): 844–45.

7. Robert F. Murray, "Minority Perspectives on Biomedical Ethics," in *Transcultural Dimensions in Medical Ethics*, eds. Edmund Pellegrino, P. Mazzarella, and P. Corsi (Frederick, MD: University Publishing Group, 1992), 39–40; Godfrey B. Tangwa, "The Traditional African Perception of a Person: Some Implications for Bioethics," *Hastings Center Report* 30, no. 5 (2000): 39–43; Jeffrey T. Berger, "Cultural Discrimination in Mechanisms for Health Decisions: A View from New York," *The Journal of Clinical Ethics* 9, no. 2 (1998): 127–31; Insoo Hyun, "Waiver of Informed Consent, Cultural Sensitivity, and the Problem of Unjust Families and Traditions," *Hastings Center Report* 32, no. 5 (2002): 14–22.

8. Jessica Berg, Paul S. Appelbaum, Charles W. Lidz, and Lisa S. Parker, *Informed Consent: Legal Theory and Clinical Practice*, 2nd ed. (New York: Oxford University Press, 2001), esp. part II: "The Legal Theory of Informed Consent," 41–164. See also American Medical Association, Council on Ethical and Judicial Affairs, *Code of Medical Ethics: Current Opinions with Annotations*, 2000–2001 ed. (Chicago: American Medical Association, 2000), § 8.08 "Informed Consent," 165–69; § 8.12 "Patient Information," 174–75.

An Historian's Analysis

Susan M. Reverby, PhD

This case illustrates some of the historically created tensions that shape the experiences of African Americans with the health care system. Mr. J is not told why his parturient girlfriend has been given a caesarean section (C-section). His angry response, "you'd tell me if I were white, right?" is his logical rejoinder to a situation he evaluates as illogical.

Having participated in the hospital's family-centered prenatal program, Mr. J has every reason to expect to be included in the birthing decisions as an equal. Now he faces what seems patently unfair. His retort in all probability reflects experiences of dealing with slights, hostilities, and possibly even physical threats throughout his life and in this white, rural enclave.

Well-meaning white health care providers and workers often bristle with defensiveness when an African American patient or family member raises racism as the reason for a decision. Ms. R, the nurse, is trying to respond reasonably to Ms. N's request to keep the knowledge of her herpes from her boyfriend and to respect confidentiality. But the nurse may have no understanding of what either Ms. N or Mr. J has experienced individually or carries as part of the collective memorial of African Americans.

Ms. R should begin by not assuming that Mr. J's response is ridiculous because her own motives are sensible and honor her promise to her patient. Without being either defensive or paternalistic, she should attempt to assure Mr. J that she could understand that he might think race was the reason in this case, but that there are medical exigencies that required the C-section as quickly as possible. He should be told that this is a standard of practice. She should not expect immediately that this will mollify Mr. J, but her calmness and acceptance of his viewpoint will help defuse the tension.

Both Mr. J and Ms. N bring stories from their own racial backgrounds into this encounter. This is as much a part of their family as their own relationship. New to the area, they have only the brief prenatal program from which to judge the all-white hospital personnel. Ms. R has no way of knowing what stories about the hospital have already circulated among the black students, even if Mr. J and Ms. N have been pleased by their personal experiences to date. One person's bad experience can become the subject of rumor in a community that is racially marginalized. But even if nothing happened at this hospital there can still be mistrust.

Studies have shown that African Americans bring to their encounters with the health care system what can be labeled "mistrust baggage" created by a history of experimentation without explanations, substitution of research for treatment, and denial of care.[1] They have substantiated reasons to be fearful. Mr. J may know about the Tuskegee Syphilis Study, the longest running (1932–1972) nontherapeutic experiment in American history when nearly 400 African American men in Alabama with late latent syphilis were followed, but not treated, for their disease.[2] He may have relatives who were sterilized without consent, friends whose dignity was compromised for teaching purposes or whose needs were ignored, or heard the rumors about AIDS as an experiment gone awry and targeted at the black community.[3] He may harbor a possible fear that his girlfriend and child are being used in some nontherapeutic manner or for teaching purposes because they are black.

Ms. R's acknowledgment that she also knows some of this history would help. If she does not know anything about these experiences, she might consider discussing this with nurse managers. In-service education on the experiences of African Americans with American health care should be provided, given the changes in the population the hospital now serves.

The fact that Mr. J did not know in advance about either his girlfriend's herpes history or that if it were active it might lead to a C-section raises questions about the prenatal program and its failure to prepare couples for this possibility. The Centers for Disease Control (CDC) does not require contact tracing or reporting of herpes; this is determined on a state-by-state basis. With all the focus on HIV/AIDS and the mandates to report syphilis and gonorrhea, this hospital's staff may have little experience with other sexually transmitted infections (STIs) such as chlamy-dia, human papillomavirus, and herpes. The prenatal program should use the health consequences of STIs to try and explain as nonjudgmentally as possible the reasons to be honest with partners about sexual histories and should assume most patients, regardless of race, may have had more than one sexual partner. If the prenatal pro-gram had taught about the consequences of herpes, Ms. N might not have had to face this dilemma at the time of delivery.

In this case the nurse might want to allow Ms. N a chance to talk about why she did not tell Mr. J about her history. Ms. N should be reassured that herpes affects 45 million people, or one out of five in the adolescent and adult populations, across race, class, and gender lines.[4] Ms. R should try and understand that it may be Ms. N's need to appear "respectable" to her boyfriend that is affecting her willingness to explain her sexual history. If she comes from a strict religious background, she may not want her boyfriend, her family, or the nurse to know about any previous sexual activity. In a small town, and with the pressure at the college to be the best possible representative of other African Americans, Ms. N may also feel she has let every-one "down."

Family-centered care is an important way to encourage support for single mothers and their children. But the hospital needs never to forget that the people it is serving from a minority community are both individuals and seen as representa-tives of their community at one and the same time. They carry the burden of their own histories and the memories of their community with them into every health care encounter. Trust has to be built, not assumed.

Notes

1. W. Michael Byrd and Linda A. Clayton, *An American Health Dilemma: Race, Medicine and Health Care in the United States, 1900–2000* (New York: Routledge, 2002); eds. Annette Dula and Sara Goering, *"It Just Ain't Fair": The Ethics of Health Care for African Ameri-cans* (New York: Praeger Press, 1994).
2. Susan M. Reverby, ed., *Tuskegee's Truths: Rethinking the Tuskegee Syphilis Study* (Chapel Hill, NC: University of North Carolina Press, 2000).
3. See notes 1 and 2, above.
4. Centers for Disease Control, "STD Prevention, Genital Herpes," June 2001, http://www.cdc.gov/std/Herpes/STDFact-Herpes.htm (24 Mar. 2004).

A Philosopher's Analysis

Lisa Rasmussen, PhD

This case illustrates an omnipresent tension between the general moral duty to tell the truth and the specific moral duty in the medical setting to respect and protect a patient's confidentiality. It is further complicated by the hospital's encouraging, but not mandating, family decision making.

On first glance at least two features of the case might lead one to think Ms. R should tell Mr. J the truth. First, many hold that each individual has a general moral duty to tell the truth. On this account Ms. R owes Mr. J an honest answer to his question. Second, the hospital places great emphasis on family decision making as a means of encouraging joint responsibility for pregnancy and child rearing. Based on this reasoning, Mr. J might have as much right to the information as does the patient herself.

Other considerations mitigate this first impression, however. While many do recognize a general moral duty to tell the truth, they also hold that this general duty can be overridden by other specific duties. In this case the duty to protect patient confidentiality overrides the duty to tell the truth. Patient confidentiality is important in medicine for at least three reasons. First, in order to treat a patient, a physician may need to know personal facts about her which she might not reveal if she thinks this information will be shared with others. Second, patients should be able to make decisions for themselves, which in this setting means that a patient should have the right to determine who may know her personal information.

A third, more subtle, reason for maintaining patient confidentiality is particularly important in this case. While the hospital's emphasis on family-centered decision making may be laudable, this emphasis can inappropriately override an individual's right to make decisions for herself. Many argue that women are socialized to put others' interests before their own, or to prefer that a male make "important" decisions (e.g., a decision regarding appropriate treatment). Society may also expect this. Especially in the case of pregnancy, where the well-being of mother and child may at times clash, health care professionals (HCPs) must be cautious about assuming that the child's interests outweigh the mother's or that the father is the appropriate decision maker. It is important for Ms. R to remember that the mother is the patient and, unless the mother agrees he may be told, the father has no right to the information.

In a case like this, it is also worth reflecting on how such problems could have been averted. The hospital's policy of encouraging family-centered decision making will likely encounter similar conflicts in the future. Such policies should be reviewed and strategies for handling future conflict should be discussed. For example, the hospital should stress to participants and HCPs alike that while it encourages family-centered decision making, an individual still has a right to determine who has access to his or her medical information.

One might also wonder what could have been done to prevent this particular source of tension. For example, what else might have been said to the mother regarding disclosure of her herpes simplex virus (HSV) infection to the father? The doctor or nurse should gently stress that the hospital is required by law* to report

---

*Editor's note: Reporting requirements for particular sexually transmitted diseases vary among states.

this sexually transmitted disease, and that the father will learn the truth eventually. The doctor or nurse might also explain to her that though disclosure will be difficult, the outcome is likely to be preferable if she tells him herself, in a controlled setting with someone else present. A doctor's presence would be beneficial in a number of ways. First, if either party has medical questions, he or she will be able to answer them. Second, since the situation will be emotional, the presence of an additional person may help to mitigate the father's reaction. Third, and importantly, any young couple in this situation is under a variety of pressures, and emotional volatility is a real possibility for both of them. If the doctor mediates the meeting, he or she will be in a position to observe how the father reacts to the news and how the couple interacts with each other. In this way, he or she may be able to help both parties better cope with their new circumstance and direct them to appropriate counselors.

Finally, the hospital's focus on fostering family bonding and shared decision making also commends this course of action. Family bonding is most tested in times of stress, and the program's focus on families suggests that they should provide guidance and counseling in situations like this.

An Obstetrician's and an Ethicist's Analysis

Frank A. Chervenak, MD, and Laurence B. McCullough, PhD

This case raises ethical issues concerning both informed consent and confidentiality and their implications for an organizational policy of family-centered pregnancy care and decision making. Because unexamined organizational policy can unintentionally create the potential for ethical conflicts, a preventive ethics approach to organizational policy is essential, as this case powerfully illustrates.[1]

One of the main purposes of the informed consent process is to respect the patient's autonomy—her right to make decisions about her medical care with her physician and other members of the health care team. The patient is the best judge of her own interests and therefore should be the primary decision maker about which forms of clinical care will support and implement her values and preferences.[2] While the partner or husband of a pregnant woman may have a legitimate stake and therefore interest in decisions about the clinical management of her pregnancy, his role in such decisions is the prerogative of the pregnant woman.[3] An organizational policy of family-centered pregnancy care should therefore not assume that the pregnant woman's partner or husband is a co–decision maker, but should explicitly inform pregnant women and their partners/husbands and other family members that the pregnant woman is the primary decision maker about her clinical care, and involvement of others in her decisions will occur only with her express permission. Such a policy should be implemented by explaining to patients, at their very first visit, the nature of informed consent, the woman's primacy as decision maker, and her right to decide on the role of others in decisions about her clinical care. When the woman has had the opportunity to make her decision about the role of others, they should then be informed about her decision and asked to respect and support it. After all, the primary moral relationship of family members to the woman is respect for her autonomy, not paternalistic attempts to coerce or even substantially control her decisions.[4]

Confidentiality is the obligation of health care professionals (HCPs) and organizations to protect information about patients from unauthorized access by individuals or entities other than the patient, her HCPs, and authorized personnel of health care organizations. This obligation is founded in both beneficence (i.e., the benefit for patients that follows from their confidence that their secrets will not be revealed to others with no authorized access to them) and respect for autonomy (i.e., the patient's right to control access to health care information about herself).[5]

The results of clinical examinations and tests should therefore be disclosed only to the pregnant woman and may not be revealed to others without her express consent.[6] Ethically justified exceptions to this obligation are recognized and include the following jointly sufficient and individually necessary conditions: "when (1) there is a high probability of harm to a third party, (2) the potential harm is a serious one, (3) the information communicated can be used to prevent harm, and (4) greater good will result from breaking confidentiality than from maintaining it."[7] With respect to this woman's decision to accept cesarean delivery to minimize the chance of exposure to her baby to herpes simplex virus (HSV), none of these conditions applies. There is therefore no ethical justification to violate the team's and organization's obligation of confidentiality to her.

Once the baby has been delivered and Ms. N has recovered from surgery, her physician should meet with her and discuss the need to inform Mr. J that he may have HSV and should be tested. Given the implications of HSV for Mr. J's health (and that of his potential future sexual partners and their possible pregnancies), the first three conditions above for limiting confidentiality are met. With the physician's and team's support, Mr. J can be informed with the goal of achieving the fourth condition. These conditions create an ethical obligation on Ms. N to see to it that Mr. J learns of his need to be examined and tested, either directly from her or, with her permission, from her physician.

Had Univille Hospital's family-centered pregnancy program taken a preventive ethics approach, the limitations on Mr. J's involvement in decisions about the management of Ms. N's pregnancy could have been negotiated and explained in advance and justified as sound ethical practice for all patients, regardless of race, ethnicity, etc. In this way, he would not have been surprised by Ms. N's having made a unilateral decision, and the suspicion that excluding him has a racially biased motivation would be nipped in the bud. The ethical response in this actual case to

Mr. J's concern about racial bias is clear: explain that Ms. N's decisions about the clinical management of her pregnancy are protected by a professional obligation of confidentiality, which is completely independent of the race of pregnant women and their partners. If Mr. J insists on learning more, it would also be justified to explain that he has an obligation, as a family member and not as a patient (as explained above) to respect and support Ms. N's decisions. Such respectful enforcement of the ethical obligations of interested and concerned partners, husbands, or other family members is an important preventive ethics strategy for protecting Ms. N's privacy until she has had time to recover and consider her obligation to ensure that Mr. J learns about his need for testing for HSV.

Notes

1. Frank A. Chervenak and Laurence B. McCullough, "Clinical Guides to Preventing Ethical Conflicts Between Pregnant Women and Their Physicians," *American Journal of Obstetrics & Gynecology* 162 (1990): 303–7.
2. American College of Obstetricians and Gynecologists, "Ethical Decision Making in Obstetrics and Gynecology," *Ethics in Obstetrics and Gynecology* (Washington, DC: American College of Obstetricians and Gynecologists, 2002), 1–6; American College of Obstetricians and Gynecologists, "Ethical Dimensions of Informed Consent," *Ethics in Obstetrics and Gynecology* (Washington, DC: American College of Obstetricians and Gynecologists, 2002), 19–27.
3. Laurence B. McCullough and Frank A. Chervenak, *Ethics in Obstetrics and Gynecology* (New York: Oxford University Press, 1994).
4. Ibid.
5. See note 3, above, and "Ethical Decision Making," note 2, above.
6. American College of Obstetricians and Gynecologists, "Ethical Guidance for Patient Testing," *Ethics in Obstetrics and Gynecology* (Washington, DC: American College of Obstetricians and Gynecologists, 2002), 32–34.
7. Ibid., 33.

Further Reflections

General

1. What moral principles and health care goals support a "family-centered health care" (FCHC) approach to health care delivery? How does FCHC differ from regular health care? How does it differ in terms of:
   A. Types of treatment, care, and support provided to patients?
   B. The definition of who is the patient?
   C. The way in which information is communicated to patients and their families?
   D. The way patients are socialized and HCPs are trained in the delivery of health care?

E. The moral values it supports (e.g., joint responsibility in pregnancy and child rearing)?

F. The nature and locus of health care decision making?

G. Consideration of the interests and desires of family members in treatment decisions?

2. How might the small-town and a generally racially homogeneous environment either complicate or facilitate the delivery of good health care to this family? What role is race *perceived* to play in this dilemma? What role *does* race play in this dilemma?

Consequences

3. Identify and evaluate the consequences of withholding *and* of giving the information to Mr. J.

Autonomy

4. If FCHC urges couples to share decision-making responsibilities and authority for health care decisions that will affect the entire family, does it compromise respect for autonomy? Can FCHC successfully negotiate this middle ground between these two approaches to morality? Compare the assumptions and responses of Rasmussen and Reverby.

Rights

5. Parents have a well-recognized right to make decisions regarding health care of their minor children. What does this right imply about giving Mr. J the information he requests?

6. Does Mr. J have a right to make decisions regarding his child, who is currently a fetus? If he does have this right, how can it be balanced against the right— strongly supported by Rasmussen and by McCullough and Chervenak—of the pregnant woman to control information about her health status?

Virtues

7. If FCHC urges couples to share decision-making responsibilities and authority for health care decisions that will affect the entire family, does it compromise professional promises of confidentiality and responsibility to the patient?

8. If honesty is a virtue, why—from a moral point of view—shouldn't Ms. R tell Mr. J the truth?

9. Reverby suggests that one way of reducing the sorts of misunderstandings cited in the case is to support professional and patient education. Rasmussen, on the other hand, suggests the tensions in this case result from misguided

decision-making policies. What implications do these claims have for professional integrity?

Equality/Fairness (Justice)

10. Given the legacy of racism and discrimination toward African Americans in our culture in general and in the delivery of health care in particular, might unequal treatment (i.e., telling Mr. J the truth) be more just than treating him like all expectant fathers?

Border Crossings*

Mrs. Y, a Hmong woman in her mid-40s, brings her 7-year-old son to the county health clinic for a scheduled well-child appointment and for routine childhood vaccinations (required by the local school district before a child can be enrolled each year). The nurse practitioner (NP), Ms. O, notes immediately that the boy is not a well child, is in fact pale, trembling, and very warm to the touch. His temperature is 104 degrees Fahrenheit.

Mrs. Y speaks no English and the NP speaks no Hmong. Both adults must rely on Mrs. Y's 12-year-old daughter to interpret. The NP ascertains that the boy has been listless for about two days, but only felt this warm this morning. The boy complains of generalized aching (worse in his head), a stiff neck, photosensitivity, and feeling hot. The NP fears the child has meningitis (two cases have been recently diagnosed in the area), and recommends the child be taken to the nearest hospital emergency room (ER) for evaluation and probable admission. Mrs. Y appears reluctant to do this.

Mrs. Y and her family are members of a Hmong community of approximately 1000 members in the central California valley. Most of the adults came to the region in the mid-1980s as refugees, lack Western-style education, and speak little English. They support themselves through agriculture—selling their produce at roadside stands, at farmers' markets, and to local independent grocers and restaurants. They have strong memories of war and persecution from the Indochina conflict in Southeast Asia, and are wary of outsiders. They function as a self-contained social unit with only minimal interaction with members of the "Anglo" culture, exceptions being the sale of their produce, the education of their children in the pub-

---

*Thanks are due to Donald Heinz, PhD, for "naming" this case.

lic school system, and the infrequent use of local health care clinics to obtain care required by the public school system or for the occasional treatment of discrete, acute illnesses.

While the NP is explaining (via the daughter's translation) why it is necessary for the child to go to the hospital, the boy has a grand mal seizure. The NP immediately provides supportive care and an ambulance is called.

The child is taken to the ER of the local hospital. Mrs. Y does not accompany her son in the ambulance. However, she soon arrives at the ER with her daughter, husband, several members of an extended family (including adults), and a woman identified as a Hmong shaman. The father of the child can speak and understand some English, but a young Hmong man in his early 20s acts as interpreter for the parents and the health care providers. He explains that the parents insist on being present in the treatment room along with the Hmong healer. The parents, the Hmong healer, and the family interpreter are allowed to enter the treatment room. An intravenous (IV) line is in place; the boy is receiving fluids and antibiotics through the IV, and is being sponged to reduce the fever. Blood samples are being drawn as they enter the room. The Hmong healer opines that the child's hot and cold humors are out of balance, that the fever is causing too much heat to be lost. This heat must be preserved for the balance to be restored. Thus, the father objects to both the sponging and the IV fluids, indicating (now through the hospital's interpreter) that these modalities interfere with the body's efforts to conserve heat. He requests that these interventions be discontinued and that the boy be covered with warm blankets. He also is upset that blood has been drawn and objects to a planned spinal tap, expressing concern that removing these body fluids will further throw the body out of its natural humoral balance. The father will not sign the consent form for the spinal tap.

The ER personnel explain that the body is too hot, that cooling is necessary to prevent a recurrence of seizures (which they believe are caused by the high temperature). They indicate that the blood and spinal fluid are needed both to diagnose the cause of the seizure, and to determine which antibiotic(s) will be most effective against the (presumed) infecting agent.

Further treatment has come to a standstill as the ER personnel and the father of the child (and the other Hmong who are at the hospital) each believe that what the "opposition" defines as appropriate treatment will, in fact, make the child worse.

From a moral point of view, what should the ER personnel do at this point?

Introduction

Joel Zimbelman, PhD, Kristin Lundberg, RN, MA, PhD(c),
and Bee Lo, ND

On first blush, this case pits the values of patient-centered beneficence against respect for autonomy and the right to self-determination. Beneficence morally compels health care professionals (HCPs) to pursue efficacious treatment, while respect for autonomy recognizes that competent parents are legitimate surrogates for their children. Thus, two very broad issues form the moral center of this dilemma:

1. Whose conception of benefit should determine care?
2. Whose autonomy is paramount?

The AJ Method

Step 1: Information Gathering   What facts are relevant to this dilemma? How likely is it that the child will be helped *or* harmed by following the suggestions of the emergency room (ER) personnel? the Hmong healer? What would be the implications of this choice for the child's future health? Who else might be helped or harmed, depending upon the response of ER personnel? (Heinz; Lundberg) What motivates the plan of care suggested by the ER personnel? the Hmong healer/family? (Lundberg; D. Damazo; R. Damazo) Why was the mother reluctant to bring the child to the ER? (Lo)

The Hmong are one of several Southeast Asian ethnic peoples who, starting in the mid-1970s, emigrated as refugees from various conflicts in Indochina. The Hmong practiced a subsistence way of life in Laos, and were geographically and culturally isolated from modern societies. They have been portrayed in the press as initially baffled by toilets, electricity, and kitchen appliances. Despite this image, they possess an uncanny ability to adjust to mainstream society while maintaining conventional beliefs, values, and practices anchored by their worldview. Their practices are being reshaped—without being entirely abandoned—by their encounters with American educational, religious, sociopolitical, and economic systems.

Perhaps no domain so strongly demonstrates the influence of society and culture in people's lives than illness or injury. A people's worldview is their way of knowing about the world and their place in it. In the Hmong holistic belief system, the soul and the flesh are not separate entities. This system, grounded in the concepts of life force, balance, and harmony, underlies Hmong explanations of illness, injury, health, and healing practices.[1] The Hmong believe that communicable diseases, body aches, allergies, and injuries are best treated by physical remedies, such as the setting of bones and the use of herbs. Their first line of home therapy includes physical, herbal, and spiritual medicine. They understand that proper nutrition and herbs contribute to health. Yet the Hmong also regard physical ailments as the manifestation that the soul is not well, requiring attention to the spiritual aspect of existence.

At the same time, the Hmong respect systems and philosophies of medicine other than their own. They are familiar with many causes of illness, including germs (though they do not quite understand microscopic agents like bacteria and viruses that cause illnesses such as meningitis), and their pragmatic approach to life is to utilize whatever intervention works best.

Specific Hmong health practices may seem exotic and initially provoke unfavorable comparisons to Western medicine. For example, the Hmong believe that cutting or puncturing the skin allows a person's soul to escape and evil spirits to enter, and provokes an imbalance in a person's temperature. The Hmong also believe that life is in the blood, so when Western diagnostic procedures require several blood draws, the Hmong are very uncomfortable. As a result, Western treatments such as shots, intravenous lines (IVs), and surgery are seen as very invasive, and many Hmong will reserve these treatments as a last resort. Thus, the Y family would fear that the IV and the spinal tap would put their child at grave risk.

Further, the Hmong culture is a patriarchal-based clan system where male clan members, leaders, and elders come together to make decisions. Sometimes this is a lengthy process that requires long conferences. When a Hmong person is seriously ill, immediate and extended family members come to show support and comfort. A shaman, who is the primary caregiver and healer in the Hmong culture and whose status equals that of a physician in Western medical culture, is asked to treat the sick person.

Such cultural information has both psychological and practical import. HCPs who understand how people perceive, feel, think, and are motivated are more likely to construct *workable* plans of care. But for many Western thinkers an action's moral rightness or wrongness requires balancing moral principles. Yet to insist exclusively on this approach will make cross-cultural communication either impossible or irrelevant, and any attempt at resolving differences is doomed to fail. From this perspective, cultural sensitivity is largely irrelevant—except, perhaps, as an obstruction—to ideal health care.

Step 2: Creative Problem Solving   Any creative solution would have to respect the beliefs—which are at least partially incompatible—of both communities. (All commentators)

Step 3: Pros and Cons   Survey CARVE principles to identify important moral reasons that support conflicting options for resolving this case.

Consequences   What would be the immediate effects of following the advice of the ER personnel? of the Hmong family/healer? How likely would the effects be? Who would be affected? What would be the longer-term effects of overriding the requests of the family? (D. Damazo; R. Damazo; Lo)

Autonomy Recall that autonomy, most broadly understood, applies to choosing the values in terms of which to live one's life, as well as the means to achieve those values. Who has decisional authority in this case? Are the parents capable of an autonomous choice in this situation? Are the Western HCPs? (R. Damazo; Heinz; Lo; Lundberg)

As the Ys appear to have their child's best interests at heart, they have the right to choose among treatment alternatives. Thus, their autonomous decision to pursue (from their perspective) a time-tested efficacious treatment should be respected by the HCPs. But the child's HCPs believe this approach would not help—and may actually harm—the child.

Can one affirm both beneficence and autonomy *without* explicitly attending to the cultural dissonance, misunderstanding, and Western medical hegemony that saturate this case? The history of tension between HCPs and Jehovah's Witnesses suggests a creative solution: As the child is at significant risk of harm (death) by being held hostage to cultural beliefs he has not (yet) autonomously embraced, HCPs could obtain temporary custody, treat the child until he (hopefully) recovers, then release him to his (hopefully grateful) family. Saving the child's life meets the obligation of beneficence while simultaneously protecting *the child's future* autonomy.[2]

This approach, while theoretically satisfying, is practically problematic, not least because it will likely generate similar dilemmas in the future. Cross-cultural health care is challenging because cultures diverge, often dramatically, in their conceptions of "... the roles and responsibilities of the patient, the family, and the health care professionals involved, and of what it means to treat patients and families with respect."[3] Crucial to the success of clinical encounters is appreciating differing conceptions of the causes and appropriate treatment of disease,[4] as well as disparate ideas about *who* should treat the patient.[5] Western physicians typically focus on *curing* a discretely defined pathological condition; many other healers focus instead on *alleviating* the patient's symptoms or functional limitations.[6] In any case, a focus on the child's future autonomy ignores the parents' present autonomy and the Hmong conceptions of harms and benefits. Further, it practically (if not theoretically) ignores, rather than addresses, the distinctive cultural issues from which the conflict arises.[7]

Rights The parents have the right of self-determination, here extended to decisional authority for their minor child. (Heinz; Lundberg) Within the patient-professional relationship, the child has a right to be aided. All parties have a right to not be harmed.

Virtues How should the professional virtue of integrity—particularly the commitments to patient welfare and decisional authority—be exercised here? (D. Damazo; Heinz) Is the virtue of curiosity relevant? (Heinz) Courage? (Heinz) Tolerance? (All commentators)

Equality/Fairness (Justice) Are the parents being treated unfairly because of their non-Western beliefs? (Lo) If so, is this treatment justified? If so, why? If not, why not? Is justice served by treating the child the same as (equality) a Western child would be treated?

Without repudiating moral principles as generally helpful tools, all our commentators most prominently focus on whether cross-cultural communication is both possible and desirable. They advocate an approach that will illuminate the varying perceptions of what is going on; analyze the larger issue of inter-cultural communication and understanding; and grapple with the pragmatic concern of how to provide beneficent health care to persons from non-Western communities.

We might think about context-sensitive questions that must be answered if we hope to successfully care for people from diverse cultures. At the very least, HCPs will need to be cognizant of disparate values and worldviews, views of medical care, designation of appropriate care providers, and the relative roles of HCPs and family members in decision making. As a first step, HCPs might look to other disciplines—the humanities, cultural anthropology, social psychology, history—to acquire information about worldviews: basic values, concepts of health and illness, and culturally sensitive approaches to problem solving.

Cultural anthropology, for example, has long advocated "thick descriptions"—locating persons in a rich and very detailed cultural context, as necessary for understanding people's interpretation of and response to situations.[8] Such an approach has not been the hallmark of most ethical case analysis in the past, though it is growing in importance. Lundberg argues for broadening this understanding by examining concepts of knowledge, power, and authority as ways to think about and bridge cultural differences and similarities. Limiting our analysis (as medicine has typically done) to a functional, categorized system (i.e., the food they eat, the way they dress) will only serve to reify, rather than bridge, differences.

That said, Heinz reminds us that connections between individuals and not just cultural systems are crucial.[9] His personalist approach suggests that the virtue of self-deprecation—the willingness to assume that one may not have all the answers—is a necessary component of cross-cultural problem solving.

Perhaps more important than self-deprecation is the virtue of imagination. This virtue—the commitment to see a problem in terms of the values, worldview, and particular perspective of the Other—may provide the best hope for resolving moral disagreement.

Nonetheless, humans on both sides of the cultural divide often share some values that can serve as the foundation for communication. Lo, R. Damazo, and D. Damazo argue that all parties in this case share at least one common desire, value, and commitment: restoring the child's health. This shared sense of purpose makes possible a mutually beneficial and respectful resolution.

The desired outcome in this case is certainly to promote the best interests of the child. But beyond seeking greater understanding among the parties, what actions should be taken? All commentators endorse critical self-awareness; a willingness to question the dominance of one's own (and in this case the Western medical) view; a call to imaginative exploration of themes and perspectives; and the need to respond sympathetically *and* empathically.

As a strategy for preventing such dilemmas in the future, these suggestions are commendable. But bacterial meningitis is a life-threatening condition. If untreated, the mortality rate is virtually 100 percent. Treatment is most effective if started early (within hours), though still carries a mortality risk of 15 percent. Bacterial meningitis also may cause brain damage, loss of hearing, blindness, paralysis, and learning disabilities. It is most reliably diagnosed with a spinal tap, necessary to identify the infecting organism and the correct antibiotic for treatment.

Can this child afford to wait? If the HCPs treat over the parents' objections, what is gained? The child may still die or be permanently disabled. What is lost? Does the possibility of intercultural cooperation die under a banner of medical hegemony? What should be done with *this* child?

The Law   The following legal considerations are relevant to this case. (1) What legal obligations attach to public health clinics with respect to the provision of qualified translators—when such *are unavailable?* (2) Under what conditions may HCPs legally usurp decisional authority of a (presumably) competent parent regarding care of a minor? If HCPs treat over the parents' continued objections, are they guilty of assault and battery? (3) Are parents and/or HCPs guilty of child endangerment, abuse, or medical malpractice if they consent to unorthodox or "unscientific" therapies? if they do not? (4) Does respect for First Amendment religious freedoms have a role in determining the legally permissible course of action in a case such as this?[10]

The following commentaries examine the application of various moral principles to this dilemma, thereby assisting the reader to undertake *Step 4: Analysis* and *Step 5: Justification.*

Notes

1. Attajinda Deepadung, "The Interaction Between Thai Traditional and Western Medicine in Thailand," *Transcultural Dimensions in Medical Ethics*, eds. Edmund Pellegrino, Patricia Mazzarella, and Pietro Corsi (Frederick, MD: University Publishing Group, 1992), 197–212.
2. Dena S. Davis, "Genetic Dilemmas and the Child's Right to an Open Future," *Hastings Center Report* 27, no. 2 (1997): 7–15.
3. Kathleen A. Culhane-Pera and Dorothy E. Vawter, "A Study of Healthcare Professionals' Perspectives about a Cross-Cultural Ethical Conflict Involving a Hmong Patient and Her Family," *The Journal of Clinical Ethics* 9, no. 2 (1998): 179–90, 187.
4. M. Margaret Clark, "Cultural Context of Medical Practice," *The Western Journal of Medicine* 139 (1983): 806–10.
5. Arthur Kleinman, Leon Eisenberg, and Byron Good, "Culture, Illness, and Care: Clinical Lessons from Anthropologic and Cross-Cultural Research," *Annals of Internal Medicine* 88 (1978): 251–58. For a rich discussion of the long-standing history of the cultural tugs-of-war in U. S. health care, see Alan M. Kraut, "Healers and Strangers: Immigrant Attitudes toward the Physician in America: A Relationship in Historical Perspective," *JAMA: The Journal of the American Medical Association* 263, no. 13 (1990): 1807–11.
6. See Kleinman, Eisenberg and Good, note 5, above, 252–53.

7. Edmund G. Howe, "Commentary: 'Missing' Patients by Seeing Only Their Cultures," *The Journal of Clinical Ethics* 9, no. 2 (1998): 191–93; Nancy S. Jecker, Joseph A. Carrese, and Robert A. Pearlman, "Caring for Patients in Cross-Cultural Settings," *Hastings Center Report* 25, no. 1 (1995): 6–14.

8. Clifford Geertz, *The Interpretation of Cultures* (New York: Basic Books, 1974).

9. See note 7, above.

10. Legal issues related to language access responsibilities under federal and state law are discussed in Jane Perkins, Mara Youdelman, and Doreena Wong, *Ensuring Linguistic Access in Health Care Settings: Legal Rights & Responsibilities* (Los Angeles: National Health Law Program, 2003). See also Jessica Berg, Paul S. Appelbaum, Charles W. Lidz, and Lisa S. Parker, *Informed Consent: Legal Theory and Clinical Practice,* 2nd ed. (New York: Oxford University Press, 2001), esp. part II: "The Legal Theory of Informed Consent," 41–164; American Medical Association, Council on Ethical and Judicial Affairs, *Code of Medical Ethics: Current Opinions with Annotations,* 2000–2001 ed. (Chicago: American Medical Association, 2000), § 8.08 "Informed Consent," 165–69; and § 3.01 "Nonscientific Practitioners," 87–89; and Lainie Friedman Ross, *Children, Families, and Health Care Decision-Making* (Oxford: Clarendon Press, Oxford University Press, 1998), chap. 7, "The Child as Patient," 131–51, and discussion of relevant court cases, 134–35.

The issue of whether a First Amendment right should be recognized that allows parents to legally withhold medical care from their children (and thus provide parents with either a religious exemption from child abuse and neglect charges; or allow a religious defense to a criminal charge) is growing in public interest. See 1996 Federal Child Abuse Prevention and Treatment Act (CAPTA, P.L. 104–235) and Keeping Children and Families Safe Act of 2003 (P.L. 108–36) and analysis at http://nccanch.acf.hhs.gov/pubs/factsheets/about.cfm (26 Mar. 2004). While opposing such exclusions, William Harwood provides an insightful discussion of the conceptual, constitutional, and practical issues at stake in the debate at William Harwood, "Religion, Death, and the Law," *Free Inquiry Magazine* 23 (Summer 2003) at http://secularhumanism.org/library/fi/harwood_23_03.htm (26 Mar. 2004). Children's Health Care is a Legal Duty (CHILD) surveys the religious exemptions by state for specific public health and treatment requirements at http://www.childrenshealthcare.org (26 Mar. 2004).

An Anthropologist's Analysis

Kristin Lundberg, RN, MA, PhD(c)

Social and cultural factors give context and meaning to health, illness, and injury. The experience is more than that of the patient. It also reflects the worldview of the individuals helping the person in distress. Health care encounters, for this reason, are prime opportunities to understand the Other, as well as reflect on ourselves. By doing so, we work toward bridging our differences in relating to each other.

Our efforts to understand people different from ourselves focus on describing and explaining their particular beliefs and practices. A more productive approach explores the concepts of power, authority, and knowledge because it examines dimensions persons and cultures have in common.

All cultures have processes by which people interpret, understand, and give meaning to human experience. These processes yield knowledge. Everyone has knowledge. One person's having knowledge does not mean another person lacks it. Our modern world recognizes two types of knowledge—one is associated with Western science, the other is a practical type based in experience. People from different cultures may find they "know" different things, for example, what causes a particular illness.[1]

When people from different cultures meet, particularly when Western medicine is involved, we find power and authority mediating knowledge. *Power* is the ability to manipulate or exercise control over others. *Authority* is the exercise of that power granted by consent of those involved. The power becomes legitimate through the consent of authority. Disparate beliefs regarding knowledge and authority may tempt representatives from both cultures to resort to power to resolve their differences.[2]

The concepts of knowledge, authority, and power can help us understand what is going on in this case. Mrs. Y brings her son for his scheduled appointment because she recognizes the *authority* of the school and health systems to set conditions for her son's education. She understands what these systems require, and agrees sufficiently to comply with the requirements. While the mother is willing to recognize the nurse practitioner's (NP's) authority *in this context,* she may not accord the NP authority regarding her son's illness. This reluctance stems, in part, from their differing *knowledge* about diseases and their causes. Mrs. Y's knowledge of her son's illness takes on a new meaning for the mother as she encounters the NP's concerns, because she recognizes the NP has an expertise. While both the mother and the NP know the child is in danger, their interpretations of the symptoms differ. The NP *knows* an electrical dysfunction in the child's brain threatens the child's ability to breathe. Mrs. Y *knows* that her child's soul has left the body, an equivalent threat to life. The mother *knows* her son needs help when he seizes. The NP *knows* the expected and required intervention within her profession and acts accordingly. The mother processes the meaning and nature of the event, then acts consistent with Hmong cultural convention. She rushes home to summon the proper *authority* to deal with this crisis and to gather the necessary relatives to support the afflicted person.

The defining moment of this case arises when the Hmong "object" to additional emergency intervention. The health care professionals (HCPs) encounter an obstacle with which they are ill-equipped to deal: the Hmong do not afford them the *authority* or blanket *power* that is a usual part of their practice. The HCPs probably believe the Hmong are rejecting their expertise; the Hmong experience the same kind of affront. Hmong respect Western healers and realize that they have an expert knowledge. They are not objecting to the HCPs' assistance so much as asserting the legitimacy and authority of their own knowledge and their right to participate both in decision making and in the provision of efficacious health care. The HCPs' assertion of authority does not intimidate the Hmong. They have a long history of successfully dealing with persons and entities who attempt to exert power over them.

The reader enters this case study essentially where the Hmong do. The child has already received initial emergency care, including the venapuncture. This is of concern, yet the Hmong can accept such initial expert interventions. What is important *now* is for the HCPs to solicit the Hmong opinion of the incident. Determining proximate and ultimate cause for events is very important in Hmong diagnosis and treatment decisions. Soliciting their input also demonstrates respect for and recognizes the authority of the parents and the shaman, and initiates a consensual process between the two parties.

First, the lead medical person needs to introduce the HCPs and then acknowledge the Hmong by asking his or her name and relation to the child, starting with the person thought to be the father. Next, the HCP should ask questions whose utility has been established in cross-cultural medical care: (1) What do the Hmong call this problem; (2) What do they think caused the problem; (3) Why do they think the problem started when it did; (4) How do they think the sickness works; (5) How severe do they believe it to be; (6) What main problems do they think the sickness has caused; and (7) What do the Hmong fear most about the sickness?[3] Finally, the HCP needs to ask what kind of treatment the Hmong think should be used and what results are hoped for from that treatment. Through these actions, the Hmong and the HCPs have begun discussion and negotiation of care, and the Hmong will know their knowledge is valued. The Hmong and the HCPs will find that between them they will figure out how to render both Hmong and biomedical kinds of care to mutual satisfaction.

As this case shows, averting antagonism and alienation does not happen solely by HCPs knowing different cultural practices and beliefs. The Hmong demonstrate masterful intuitive perceptions and impressions of people and are far more adept in these skills than most Anglos. Intent is everything. If HCPs embody a sincere willingness to respect Hmong knowledge and authority and afford participation, the Hmong will reciprocate. But this only comes about by balancing the forces of power and authority. HCPs learn in school and the current system reinforces just the opposite: a noncollegial relationship between patient and healer. Yet, successful health outcomes depend on cooperative attributes as much as on technological skill and biomedical knowledge of practitioners. Rather than compromising care, shared decision making enhances it.

Notes

1. Stephen A. Marglin, "Losing Touch: The Cultural Conditions of Worker Accommodation and Resistance," in *Dominating Knowledge: Development, Culture, and Resistance*, Wider Studies in Development Economics, eds. Frederique Apffel Marglin and Stephen A. Marglin (New York: Oxford University Press, 1990), 231–43; and Mark Hobart, "Introduction:

The Growth of Ignorance?" in *An Anthropological Critique of Development: The Growth of Ignorance,* ed. Mark Hobart (London: Routledge, 1993), 1–30.

2. Brigitte Jordan, *Birth in Four Cultures: A Cross-cultural Investigation of Childbirth in Yucatan, Holland, Sweden, and the United States,* 4th ed. (Prospect Heights, IL: Waveland Press, 1993); Ellen S. Lazarus, "Theoretical Considerations for the Study of the Doctor-Patient Relationship: Implications of a Perinatal Study," *Medical Anthropology Quarterly* 2, no. 1 (1988): 34–58; Carolyn F. Sargent and Grace Bascope, "Ways of Knowing about Birth in Three Cultures," in *Childbirth and Authoritative Knowledge,* ed. Carolyn F. Sargent (Berkeley: University of California Press, 1997), 183–206; and Max Weber, *The Theory of Social and Economic Organization,* ed. Talcott Parsons (London: Collier-Macmillan Limited, 1964).

3. Arthur Kleinman, L. Eisenberg, and B. J. Good, "Culture, Illness, and Care: Clinical Lessons from Anthropological Cross-Cultural Research," *Annals of Internal Medicine* 99 (1978): 25–58.

A Religious Ethicist's Analysis

Donald Heinz, PhD

This case initially presents itself as a clash—almost a contest—between two approaches to healing, two cultures, even two belief systems. The emergency room (ER) staff find themselves at a dangerous intersection where moral theory, their own professional obligations, and multicultural disparity collide.

In recent decades patient autonomy has risen to the top of any hierarchy of medical values. In this case of a minor child, self-determination is claimed by the family. There is little doubt, morally or legally, about a patient's (or his surrogate's) right to refuse treatment. The hospital will be aware it could be sued for assault and battery if it treats without consent. But there are competing values. Beneficence obligates the health care team to do good by the patient, to offer the best medical care of which they are capable. Because the patient is a minor, they may feel their professional obligations all the more keenly, including any reporting responsibilities they may have to social service agencies. Surrendering a child with possible meningitis to his family's demands for nontreatment, if not a transgression of that most basic value, *primum, non nocere* (first of all, do no harm), is certainly a failure of beneficence (acting to prevent harm).

But it is not some family idiosyncrasy that occasions this clash of competing values and professional obligations; it is a cultural disparity of views about the cosmos, the soul, and the meaning of health and disease. Around the world many voices are raised on behalf of cultural survival and autonomy. Their echoes inescapably enter the ER.

Even the most well-intentioned and sympathetic medical personnel are likely to see their own medicine and culture as superior. The Hmong, many of whom speak little or no English, may appear unsophisticated or backward. They seem to have chosen to adapt themselves to this country, to learn English, and to comply with public school regulations, including required vaccinations. Should it be assumed they will take the additional step of bowing to Western medical practices, which they probably have come to see as impressive?

The ER staff may believe they hold the trump cards. They could refer the sick little boy and his recalcitrant family to child protective services. They could hint at child abuse. They could probably get a court order authorizing appropriate medical treatment. Must it come to this? If they back off, momentarily, to consider alternative strategies and approaches, it might be possible to cross this intersection without a crash.

Alliances can be made. Border crossings between cultures and beliefs are possible. Definitional boundaries may, on examination, be permeable. The 12-year-old daughter is, after all, an American. She goes to school, speaks English, was born here. She knows more about this country and this culture than she does the Hmong society from which her parents emigrated. She lives, at least partly, in the world the ER staff inhabit. Can she also play a role beyond simply translating? Attentive medical personnel will try to find in this girl a bridge each group can cross. What about the young Hmong male interpreter? He was probably quite young when his own family emigrated. He has learned to swim in this culture. His role here is to interpret the family's concerns and wishes to the medical staff. The nurses and physicians should try to enlist him as an ally, carrying messages of concern and care back to the family. If taken seriously, he could reduce mutual suspicion, stand for each community, give American medicine—and this strange Hmong extended family—a human face.

Finally, there are the Hmong shaman and the authoritative father. The shaman appears to have opinions rooted in the spirit world that displays itself in household, village, and nature. She sees the soul of the little boy to be rooted in the Hmong cosmos. She herself is probably a "wounded healer," initiated as a shaman in the midst of her own illness, her own brush with death. Attuned to liminal experience, she moves back and forth across the threshold between material and immaterial reality. She is accustomed to turning her interpretive skills and her powers of divination to the diagnostic task in front of her. Perhaps in the hills of Thailand or Laos she has seen patients who have already been treated in lowland clinics (akin to Western medicine). But the case offers no evidence that she's been consulted previously regarding this child; we hear of no trance state, no authoritative divination. Indeed, she arrives at the hospital only after the child's fever is diagnosed at the clinic, the grand mal seizure has been suffered, and a diagnosis of meningitis looms. Should we not conclude that she is at the beginning of her relationship with this little boy? If so, her initial opinion should not be reified into a final pronouncement which then must be opposed. To take her first word as her last word is to set up an irreconcilable conflict.

How will the ER staff perceive the Hmong healer? Will they make the imaginative leap to see her as a fellow professional? A shaman, who combines the roles of spiritual advisor and healer, has no exact corollary in the West. Yet she brings together in her own self more than one valuable perspective. Surely the hospital's hospice unit and perhaps their own education or in-service training have taught the staff that the patient and family who stand before their eyes is a human complexity, deserving a deft, nuanced, multivalent response. It takes a whole armamentarium of values and beliefs to get a human being right. The staff can decide to consult with the Hmong healer, perhaps assisted by the daughter and the young man as translators. They can listen carefully to her worldview, her concerns, her instincts. They can share theirs. They can form a professional alliance. They can explain and urge their proposals, while validating her values and approaches. They can propose to do two things, rather than one thing. They can mediate two worlds; they can meet at the border and invite crossing into each other's territory.

The final border crossing is to the father. The father may have seized on the shaman's first word and, for his own purposes, turned her hunches into bad medical science. He brings his strong memories of war and persecution in his home country, perhaps a sense of betrayal and lingering anger, into this American ER. He may be adopting an adversarial position, defensively setting the shaman and his own cultural sensibilities up against the strange world of American medicine. At stake for him are his authority in this family, his need to be seen as making the hard judgment calls, not to be humiliated by the hospital staff, not to be treated like a barefoot hill tribesman, not to be humiliated by the fact that it is his daughter who can communicate best. Rather than perceiving the father as the immovable roadblock to proper medical treatment, the ER staff could invite him as an indispensable and appropriate ally in the treatment of his little boy. As the pivotal figure, he must be approached with respect and be allowed to maintain face, with no efforts to intimidate him with the power of the system. Together, ER staff and Hmong healer have a chance to ease the father's concerns, address the deepest values of both cultures, and get the child all the treatments he requires.

If this alliance is successful, family autonomy and health care beneficence will have come together. A border crossing between two cultures, two worldviews, and indeed two values in medical ethics will have resulted.

Fifteen years of experience on a bioethics committee have made me hopeful for solutions built on careful, patient, nondefensive, nonhierarchical communication. Should this all fail, I would reluctantly support getting a court order authorizing treatment of the child. Even granting the great significance recently won for the values of cultural autonomy, I do not believe they trump the child's life, especially when the value, in this case, seems somewhat indefinite, is not a decisively defined position like a Jehovah's Witness refusing a blood transfusion, and may be more a matter of the father's dignity in the family than of a Hmong religious worldview. I could not trade the child's possible death from meningitis for the father's dignity or for the sole integrity of a Hmong healing system.

RECOMMENDED READINGS

Fadiman, Anne. *The Spirit Catches You and You Fall Down,* (New York: The Noon-day Press, 1997).

Heinz, Carolyn Brown. "Hmong Shamanism," in *Shamanism: An Encyclopedia of World Beliefs, Practices, and Culture,* eds. Mariko Walter and Eva Fridman, (Santa Barbara: ABC-Clio Press, forthcoming Fall 2004).

A Nurse Practitioner's Analysis

Rebekah Damazo RN, PNP, MSN

The nurse practitioner (NP) who first encounters this family must grapple with many of the same ethical challenges faced by the health care professionals (HCPs) in the emergency room. The most crucial moral issue is obtaining informed consent for treatment and this requires competent communication with her patient. Without accurate and meaningful communication with this family, HCPs cannot guarantee that the child's illness is competently diagnosed and treated.

"Quality communication lies at the core of cultural competency."[1] HCPs should not have to rely on a 12-year-old child to interpret. Using a child as an interpreter is unfair to parent and child, placing enormous pressure on both at a time of family crisis, when neither may be emotionally able to handle it. Children are often embarrassed by the content of medical conversations or may feel worried about their ability to appropriately portray the severity of a medical situation to their parents. They typically do not understand the severity of medical conditions and, if outcomes are not positive, may develop guilt about their interpretation of medical procedures or treatments. Further questions of medical ethics also emerge: Can patients truly give informed consent when their interpreter has little or no understanding of the seriousness of an infection, the need for a medical procedure, or the importance of a specific treatment? Interpreters are not just translating words, but also the concept, theory, or idea that needs to be explained.[2]

Because of these considerations, federal law under Title VI of the Civil Rights Act of 1964 has been interpreted by the courts as requiring that HCPs have interpreters available. Unfortunately in health care settings ineffective communication between English-speaking HCPs and patients with limited English proficiency is a common cause of discrimination.[3] Ideally the NP would be able to make use of the professional interpretation services mandated for and provided by the clinic.[4] The seriousness of the NP's initial concerns would be professionally conveyed to the mother, and communication between family and NP would be improved. It is also important to inform the mother that the immunizations must be delayed until the fever is gone, since that is what brought the family to the clinic.[5]

However the case suggests that a professional translator is unavailable, which is a common problem for many smaller or remote clinics. In such cases, NPs must rely on the resources available—in this case a child who is able to serve as a translator.

In keeping with the commitment to competent communications, HCPs who regularly serve different cultural groups have a responsibility to become familiar with their cultural beliefs and health practices.[6] The fact that the family brought the child to the clinic for care and treatment shows they hold some respect for or basic trust in the clinic and Western medicine. That trust enables the NP to open up a conversation and to inform the family of the seriousness of their child's condition, specifically, that their child's life is in danger and that he needs emergency treatment.

Hmong families complain that not enough time is spent explaining diagnosis and treatment options.[7] In this case, the NP should explain the complexity of the situation and the events that are about to happen, especially the need to transfer the child in an ambulance to expedite treatment. She should add that effective, well-documented medications, common in traditional Western medicine, are readily available to treat this infection. Stating things positively is very effective in working with the Hmong.

Hmong patients have different conceptions of health, illness, and medicine. For example, while providers may feel that the principle of informed consent requires an explanation of possible negative outcomes, Hmong patients (in general) do not want to hear about risks of long-term morbidity or mortality and may take such explanations as deterministic predictions or "hexing."[8]

When the NP determines the child must be transported to the emergency department, she should encourage Mrs. Y to accompany her child in the ambulance. If she refuses, the NP should advise the family to proceed to the hospital immediately. She should be sure to let Mrs. Y know that she has confidence in the hospital where her child will be treated.

The NP is also morally obligated to protect the health of the clinic staff and family and community members that may have come in contact with the child.[9] This requires that the NP help identify the cause of the meningitis and determine if it is the type of infection that could be spread through person-to-person contact.[10]

In my experience as a pediatric nurse practitioner, I have worked with Hmong clients in various clinical and public health settings in northern California. I have found the Hmong are typically very concerned about the health of their children. If procedures are explained with appropriate translation, they are typically very agreeable to suggested treatments that will benefit their family.[11]

Attempts to deliver health care across cultural barriers can result in either conflict or collaboration. It is important to emphasize that this child's care is a collaborative effort between the family and HCPs that will be involved in their child's treatment.

If early medical treatments fail, Hmong may seek folk or herbal remedies in addition to those provided by Western HCPs. In extreme cases families may remove their children from the care of a specific provider, refuse care, or go somewhere else for treatment. This typically occurs in situations where a family feels conflict between their traditional beliefs and Western medicine.

To summarize: We know that culture is very important in determining health care practices. Legally, the clinic and hospital are required to provide appropriate professional translation services. In the situation described, the nurse practitioner is morally obligated to recognize the cultural differences among her clients and have a basic understanding of the belief systems that dictate health-seeking behaviors. Establishing trust and respect with the Hmong community will facilitate a cooperative relationship in the treatment of health concerns.

Notes

1. R. W. Putsch, "Language Access in Healthcare: Domains, Strategies and Implications for Medical Education," n.d., http://air/org/cccm/progress/putsch.pdf (8 Aug. 2003).
2. B. Barrett et al., "Hmong/Medicine Interactions: Improving Cross-cultural Health Care," *Family Medicine* 30, no. 3 (1998): 179–84.
3. According to Title VI of the Civil Rights Act of 1964, "all healthcare providers receiving federal financial assistance from the US Department of Health and Human Services are prohibited from conducting any of their programs, activities and services in a manner that subjects any person or class or persons to discrimination on the grounds of race, color, or national origin" (Office of Civil Rights, 2000).
4. *Federal Register* 67, no. 22 (2002): 4968–82, http://frwebgate.access.gpo.gov/cgi-bin/getdoc.cgi?dbname=2002_register&docid=02-2467-filed (26 Mar. 2004). Appendix B refers to the Title 22 California Code of Regulations, Section 73501: "California has a wide array of other laws and regulations that require language assistance, including those that require: (a) intermediate nursing facilities to use interpreters and other methods to ensure adequate communication with patients, (b) adult day care centers to employ ethnic and linguistic staff as indicated by participant characteristics, (c) certified interpreters for non-English speaking persons at administrative hearings, and (d) health licensing agencies to translate patients rights information into every language spoken by 1 percent or more of the nursing home population." From the United States Department of Health and Human Services, The Office of Civil Rights, Appendix B (2 Feb. 2001), http://www.hhs.gov/ocr/lep/appb.html (24 Mar. 2004).
5. Integrative Medicine Cultural and Medical Traditions, "Hmong Culture and Medical Traditions," 2002, http://xpedio02.childrenshc.org/stellent/groups/public/@xcp/@web/@integrativemed/documents/policyreferenceprocedure/web009310.asp (26 Mar. 2004).
6. Cross Cultural Health Care Program, "Interpreter Services: Code of Ethics," n.d., http://www.xculture.org/interpreter/overview/ethics.html (8 Aug. 2003); Department of Health and Human Services, Office of Minority Health; "National Standards on Culturally and Linguistically Appropriate Services (CLAS) in Health Care," *Federal Register* 65, no.

247 (22 Dec 2000): 80865–79, http://www.omhrc.gov/clas (18 May 2003); American Nurses Association, "Code of Ethics Working Draft #8 (rev. June 1998)," Washington, DC: American Nurses Publishing, American Nurses Foundation/American Nurses Association, http://home.cwru.edu/~pst/anaethics.htm (26 Mar. 2004).

7. See note 2, above.
8. Ibid.
9. See American Nurses Association, note 6, above, § 6.
10. S. I. Aronin and V. J. Quagliarello, "Bacterial Meningitis," *Infectious Medicine* 20, no. 3 (2003): 142–53.
11. See note 5, above.

A Naturopathic Doctor's Analysis

Bee Lo, ND

This case reveals many of the common problems that occur when doctor and patient don't see eye to eye. This incongruence occurs when doctor and patient come from different backgrounds, have different perspectives on health, and/or do not know, understand, or trust each other. Dealing with patient-doctor misunderstandings is not only an issue when working with new refugees or immigrants; language barriers and differences in cultural health beliefs often compound the problem. Establishing rapport and trust is difficult, but it is essential to providing effective health care services.

As a refugee, former interpreter, and physician, I have witnessed the health care process from many vantage points. For example, as a physician who specializes in alternative medicine, I see disagreements between my "American" patients and their Western-trained doctors about alternative medicine. Even though at least 42 percent of Americans use some form of natural therapy, their MDs often still oppose it.[1] This upsets patients who believe they have the right and responsibility to promote their own wellness.

This case—described from the perspective of the health care providers (HCPs)—demonstrates how these disagreements can unfold. If Mrs. Y could tell her side of the story, we would get a different perspective and perhaps better understand why everything happened the way it did. As a former interpreter, I felt frustrated. This case came across like the HCPs were the "good guys" trying to save the child's life, while the family members, in their ignorance, opposed the "expert" opinion. In reality, both parties were trying to do what was best for the child's health. Due to language and cultural barriers the problem escalated.

The case does not discuss the very sensible reasons *why* Mrs. Y was reluctant to comply with the referral to the emergency room (ER). Mrs. Y needed to consult with her family and was unable to comply with the nurse practitioner's (NP's) request to make an urgent decision. When pressed to make this decision on her own, she did what her culture dictated and ran home to get her husband, her son, and the shaman (an elder and healer) to help. The NP, who believed the child had all the signs of acute meningitis and needed urgent treatment at a local hospital, felt Mrs. Y was unreasonable to leave her child or to refuse treatment. But to Mrs. Y, consulting with her family was the most reasonable approach.

Even the perception of *what* was occurring differed among those involved. For the NP, the child's grand mal seizure suggested infection in the brain, requiring immediate ER attention. To Mrs. Y the seizure was caused by a spirit—*Dab Qaug Dab Peg*—and had nothing to do with infection.

Given their inexperience with Western medicine and doctors, Hmong family members normally want to be there to comfort the patient. They want the shaman—the primary care healer in their culture—present. In fact, for a shaman to come with Mrs. Y to the ER is a special privilege.

The traditional Hmong treatment of chills and fever is to wrap the person in blankets in order to raise the body temperature artificially for a couple hours. This treatment is often effective in combating the illness. Seeing HCPs sponging their child to reduce the body temperature was the exact opposite of what they believed would be helpful.

Hmong also believe parents have ultimate responsibility for their children. They believe that before any invasive treatment can be done on the child, the parents must give permission. When the family saw their child hooked up to an intravenous line (IV), they didn't like it because they had not been informed of its purpose nor given an opportunity to consent to treatment. The Hmong would consider the IV and spinal tap to be very invasive procedures. The father would require a full explanation of their purpose and significance (that the procedure could save the child's life) before giving approval.

The best way to prevent anything like this from happening in the future would be to educate HCPs about the cultural backgrounds, differing beliefs, and healing systems of their patients so they can better understand how to deal with patients who are not accustomed to allopathic healing ways. The health care system should also offer education to immigrant patients about Western healing arts, including an opportunity for questions and answers regarding commonly used diagnostics and treatment procedures, to help patients new to Western medicine understand why doctors do what they do in the hospital.

In conclusion, I must say that there was a feeling of anger inside me toward our health care system for not educating HCPs to better equip them to meet the needs of diverse patients in their communities. It is not only ethical but practical for clinics, hospitals, and medical schools to train HCPs to better meet their patients' needs. This is especially true since the Western way is the dominant health care system in this country and the only one fully covered by insurance. Since we have assumed this position of dominance, it is our responsibility to provide adequate interpretation for the patient.

As a former interpreter, I know that many misunderstandings would have been avoided if the county health clinic had had an interpreter to explain the situation to Mrs. Y before referring her child to the hospital against her will. As a doctor, I know that cultural education can build better patient-practitioner rapport and provide better health care services to all patients.

Notes

1. David M. Eisenberg et al., "Trends in Alternative Medicine Use in the United States, 1990–1997: Results of a Follow-up National Survey," *JAMA: Journal of the American Medical Association* 280 (1998): 1569–75.

An Emergency Room Physician's Analysis

David Edwin Damazo, MD

The fact that the mother did not travel with the child to the hospital complicates this case and seems unlikely based on my experience treating children from the Hmong culture. However, if an ambulance is called to an emergency and a child is transported "lights and sirens" to the emergency room (ER), arriving before the family, the spinal tap would already have been performed, blood would already have been drawn, intravenous (IV) medications would have been administered, and the fever would be in the process of being controlled before the family arrived to express their wishes or concerns relative to the child's medical treatment.

The Hmong traditionally treat fever with cold compresses and would be allowed to do this in the ER after their arrival.[1] Hmong also accept blood tests, but they may question why blood must be taken more than once in one visit or why a large volume of blood is needed.[2] Fadiman states the Hmong believe they have a finite amount of blood which can't be replaced, so blood should be taken sparingly.[3]

Western health professional schools do an excellent job of teaching the diagnosis and treatment of clinical disease, but sometimes they fail to prepare future physicians to incorporate psychosocial and cultural factors, and to overcome personal biases in the care of patients. Ideally, encounters between Hmong patients and their health care providers (HCPs) would have the luxury of a significant period of time during which Western medicine could work in tandem with traditional Hmong healing practices. But in an emergency this is not often practical.

The special circumstances of emergency medicine give rise to distinct ethical concerns. This situation, involving a child in crisis, requires quick action. In an emergency situation, such as the one described, the physician's first duty is to the child. The Emergency Physicians Code of Ethics has as its first obligation the duty to "embrace patient welfare as a primary responsibility."[4] Often, the emergency physician cannot rely on earned trust or prior knowledge of patients' beliefs, values, or wishes related to their care. Those are luxuries of the primary care provider.

Informed consent can ethically be waived when a child arrives unaccompanied and the urgency of the situation demands an immediate response. Thus, the main ethical concern for HCPs in the ER would be to communicate clearly and comprehensively about what has already occurred, the expected results of treatment, the need for hospitalization, and perhaps the need for prophylactic treatment of other children in the family to avoid the spread of infection.[5]

In my practice I have found little resistance to the use of medical tests as long as the family understands their nature and their importance to the child's health. Allowing time to explain the gravity of the situation, giving the family a history of the problem within our community and what they can expect from usual treatment is typically rewarded with compliance with Western medical procedures. I also support the use of spiritual treatments and herbal remedies, as long as they do not undermine or inhibit other treatments the patient is receiving or negatively impact the course of the disease. Even Western medicine supports the use of prayer in connection with medical treatment.[6]

In 22 years of practice as an emergency physician, I have never had a family bring a shaman to the ER nor begin an argument about a course of treatment. My experience with the Hmong in the ER has been one of respect for my medical advice and treatment. Hmong families I have worked with frequently seek the advice and interventions of a shaman, who may sacrifice an animal or provide special ceremonies on behalf of the child outside the hospital. In some cases they may ask permission to perform ritual healing treatments within the hospital. Where time allows, traditional Hmong healing practices may continue in tandem with Western medicine. The importance of thorough, concrete explanations using only skilled professional interpreters can't be overemphasized.[7] Where possible, Hmong families should be allowed to make decisions in traditional ways, allowing extended family members, clan leaders, and a shaman to be present when discussing and explaining diagnosis and treatment options.

That said, if I encountered a family, regardless of culture, that attempted to block or interfere with recommended emergency procedures for care in a life-threatening situation, I would immediately call the police and have them removed from my ER so I could perform my moral obligation to the patient: providing appropriate emergency medical treatment in an effort to preserve life. Emergency physicians are bound by a code of ethics which recognizes the obligation to treat patients with all the skills and knowledge gained from their training.[8]

However, it should be recognized that when the emergency medical system is activated, emergency physicians respond based on the urgency of the patient's condition. Physicians should, when the situation is under control, indicate to the family what was done and why.

Notes

1. Patricia Nuttall and Filomena Flores, "Hmong Healing Practices Used for Common Childhood Illnesses," *Pediatric Nursing* 23, no. 3 (1997): 247–51.
2. Integrative Medicine Cultural and Medical Traditions, "Hmong Culture and Medical Traditions" (27 Nov 2002), http://xpedio02.childrenshc.org/stellent/groups/public/@xcp/@web/@integrativemed/documents/policyreferenceprocedure/web009310.asp (26 Mar. 2004).
3. Anne Fadiman, *The Spirit Catches You and You Fall Down* (New York: Farrar Straus & Giroux, 1998).
4. American College of Emergency Physicians (ACEP), "Code of Ethics for Emergency Physicians" (approved June 1997, reaffirmed Oct. 2001), http://www.acep.org/1,1118,0 .html (26 Mar. 2004).
5. S. I. Aronin and V. J. Quagliarello, "Bacterial Meningitis," *Infectious Medicine* 20, no. 3 (2003): 142–53.
6. T. J. Kaptchuk and D. M. Eisenberg, "Varieties of Healing. 2: A Taxonomy of Unconventional Healing Practices," *Annals of Internal Medicine* 135, no. 3 (2001): 196–204.
7. B. Barrett et al., "Hmong/Medicine Interactions: Improving Cross-cultural Health Care," *Family Medicine* 30, no. 3 (1998): 179–84; R. W. Putsch, "Language Access in Healthcare: Domains, Strategies and Implications for Medical Education," n.d., http://air.org/cccm/progress/putsch.pdf (13 May 2003).
8. See note 4, above.

Further Reflections

General

1. What is the central moral dilemma in this case? What accounts for or is the cause of this moral dilemma?
2. Different cultures affirm different *metaphysics*—views of the way the world hangs together and functions. As a result, cultures affirm different conceptions of health and healing. What should be the response of health care professionals (HCPs) in the dominant Western culture, which has developed a disease-based health care system, to those who wish to forgo standard treatments for other options, especially if HCPs believe these other options are ineffective in treating a patient?
3. How would one determine whether a set of health care practices "works"?
4. Bee Lo is much more optimistic about rapprochement and intercultural communication than the other commentators. Why might this be?

Consequences

5. Identify and evaluate the consequences of acceding to *and* of ignoring the request of the family.
6. Define the benefits and burdens—from the perspective of *both* the Hmong family and the HCPs—that are possible in this case.

7. Is Lundberg's concern with "averting antagonism and alienation" sufficiently important to risk harmful outcomes in the treatment of this patient, about which D. Damazo and Heinz worry?

Autonomy

8. Our pluralistic society recognizes that its members affirm and structure their lives in terms of a wide array of belief systems. Does this freedom extend to beliefs about health and freedom to pursue any approaches to healing that they desire, even if their efficacy has not been established to Western medicine's satisfaction?
9. How would knowledge of Hmong culture improve HCPs' ability to adequately care for this child? Does such knowledge help in decision making? in determining potential appropriate treatments? in the ability of the HCPs to work with (control?) the parties involved? in some other way?

Rights

10. Parents have a well-recognized right to make health care decisions for their minor children. Does this right extend to refusing Western health care and pursuing culturally distinct therapies?

Virtues

11. If treatments are not equally efficacious, should HCPs relinquish control to patients or families who want to practice such health care on themselves or their family members? If HCPs do this, have they violated professional integrity?
12. If we are honest, might we have to suspect that attempts at intercultural communication are simply strategies to convert others to the Western way of thinking?

Equality/Fairness (Justice)

13. HCPs often ignore patients' requests when they believe them to be misguided. Is doing so in cross-cultural encounters more, less, or equally unjust—or not unjust at all?
14. R. Damazo and Lo make a strong case for qualified translators in clinics frequented by non-English-speaking clients. Is provision of such services, given rising medical costs—especially if non-English-speaking clients constitute a very small portion of the community served—unjust?

Chapter 9

Why Should We Have to Shoulder This Burden Alone?

Ms. H is a 23-year-old unmarried mother of a 3-year-old son, Jason, who was born 7 weeks prematurely. After birth, Jason was slow to gain weight and continues to be a small and somewhat frail child who requires regular medical care for frequent infections. Ms. H herself suffers from asthma. When she develops an acute respiratory infection, she requires oxygen, nebulization every four hours followed by postural drainage and chest percussion (to loosen and remove the thick and sticky mucus that obstructs her airways), and a bronchodilator every six hours to open her airways. In addition, she requires antibiotics to fight the infection and a steroid to reduce the swelling in her airways. Each year Ms. H is typically treated three to five times in the emergency room (ER); she responds well to these treatments, so has not been hospitalized. After each ER visit, she is discharged with prescriptions for nebulizer treatments every six hours, and an oral antibiotic and an oral bronchodilator four times a day.

Ms. H is self-employed; she provides janitorial services to several local businesses. She is a hard worker whose employers are quite satisfied with her work. Her monthly income is insufficient to enable her to afford insurance, yet sufficient to disqualify her for Medicaid. As a result, Ms. H cannot afford the prescriptions or equipment (she has been using a vaporizer instead of a nebulizer) she needs. When she has any extra money, she does purchase the drugs, but always discontinues their use earlier than is ad-

vised—hoping that one prescription will get her through two, or even three, crises. Nor can Ms. H afford regular (nonemergent) medical care. Having no proof of payment (insurance or Medicaid), she has been unable to find a local physician who will accept her as a patient.

In an attempt to pay off her medical debts, Ms. H added seven new of-fices to her workload. (She anticipated this would net her an additional $700 each month.) After one month, however, she was too exhausted to do her job and care for Jason. In addition, she had three asthma attacks dur-ing the month—more than she has had previously in so short a time—so she reluctantly resigned her new clients.

In the last three years, Ms. H has received approximately $30,000 worth of care for which the hospital has not been reimbursed. Ms. H tries to pay $50 each month against what she owes, but she is often unable to make a payment and, in any case, her payments are a drop in the bucket. Given her precarious financial circumstances, her debt to the hospital will surely increase. This is especially worrisome as the small hospital (20 beds) is the only acute facility for several small regional ranching and farming communities. The hospital has lost money for the last three years and if this trend is not reversed may have to close. The hospital's closure will leave its patients without convenient access to either emergency or acute in-patient services.

Mr. M, the hospital administrator, meets with the four local family practice physicians. He describes Ms. H's situation. Mr. M argues that Ms. H's condition could be much better managed with regular physician over-sight. Ms. H, like many medically indigent persons, usually only comes to the hospital when she is in deep distress—that is, after home remedies have failed. If Ms. H had a physician, she could go to her own doctor's of-fice for earlier (and cheaper) intervention. Too, a regular physician could prescribe and monitor compliance with a treatment regimen, thereby avoiding many of her acute episodes altogether. Mr. M offers to purchase a nebulizer that Ms. H can keep at home, as well as have his staff instruct her in its proper use. The hospital pharmacy will provide—free of charge—whatever regular medications a physician orders for her; but he can do this only if Ms. H has a physician. He requests that one of the physicians assume responsibility, on a pro bono *(free of charge) basis, for her regular care. Under this arrangement most of Ms. H's visits to the ER could be avoided.*

The physicians agree with Mr. M's assessment, but are nonetheless reluc-tant to welcome Ms. H into their practices. All report that an overabundance of their patients have some difficulty paying their health care bills. Most of their clients are small farmers or ranchers who, like Ms. H, are uninsured or underinsured. Few of their patients pay their bills in full at the time of service. As the doctors see it, the hospital is no worse off than they are. True, the debt is greater, but so is the hospital's budget.

Are the physicians, individually or collectively, morally obligated to assume ongoing responsibility for Ms. H's care?

Introduction

This case raises three important moral issues:

1. Does Ms. H have "a right to health care" and if so, who is obligated to provide it to her?
2. What moral obligations, if any, do the physicians have to Ms. H, and what strategies for dealing with her problem are morally justified?
3. How should the provision of health care access to all citizens be balanced with the need to keep costs contained?

The AJ Method

Step 1: Information Gathering   What is the nature of the tension between the hospital and physicians? What harms will Ms. H suffer if the physicians refuse to assume responsibility for her care? the hospital? What harms will the physicians suffer if they assume responsibility for Ms. H? Is Ms. H genuinely unable to afford health care? What motivates the administrator's request? What motivates the physicians' reluctance to care for Ms. H?

The dilemma faced by Ms. H, the hospital administrator, and the physicians is a recurrent scenario in this country. Over forty million Americans have no health insurance; an equal number are underinsured; and these numbers have grown steadily over the past several years.[1] As costs for health care rise; as lack of health insurance becomes catastrophic for even middle-class families; and as the benefits of early medical interventions are clearly seen to improve quality of life, the moral and political costs of not addressing the access issue increase.[2]

Step 2: Creative Problem Solving   A creative solution would have to meet the patient's and hospital's needs without unduly burdening the physicians. (Gannett; Sahadevan)

Step 3: Pros and Cons   Survey CARVE principles to identify important moral reasons that support conflicting options for resolving this case.

Consequences   Who will be harmed if the physicians reject this offer? What will be the nature of those harms? Who will benefit if they accept the offer? What will be the nature of those benefits? What might appeal to the principle of utility advise? (Gannett; Kronick; Westbie)

Autonomy   Whose autonomy is relevant here? Whose should predominate?

Rights   Does Ms. H have a right to be aided? Does she have a right to health care? (Gannett) If so, who has the duty to aid? The physicians have a right to not be harmed. Is Ms. H's right of self-determination relevant to this dilemma?

Do individuals have a right—a moral claim against other persons or institutions—to *individualized* (i.e., not population-based) health care? The argument for a right to health care is developed in many ways: a religious grounding in the moral principle of love for or a duty to seek the welfare of neighbors;[3] a liberal theory of substantive justice;[4] or a theory of human rights. The latter is given broad support in the UN Universal Declaration of Human Rights.[5]

Some individuals have argued that the nature of illness (e.g., its unpredictability and high cost), the status of health as a primary human good (necessary to all goals that humans might aspire to), and our commitment to justice support a right to health care that citizens of a society can claim—similar to freedom of speech or assembly—from their government.[6]

Others have argued against a moral right to health care.[7] If one believes that health care is no different from other goods one might pursue—cars, clothes, a college education—health care will be understood as something one freely chooses to purchase in the consumer-driven marketplace. Then, people who want health care can purchase it; while those who would rather spend their money on other goods will forgo health care. Those who cannot pay "cash on the barrel head" are free to bargain for health care, for example, trading their goods or services for medical attention.

Of course nations may decide—based on utilitarian grounds—to confer statutory rights to (some) health care as a matter of a national policy. Here, the argument would be that a right to health care maximizes the aggregate good (stability, security, quality of life) of society.[8] If societies affirm health care as a basic or a political right, they must be committed to mechanisms (e.g., taxation, limiting freedom of association for HCPs) required to provide that care.

Virtues   What does professional integrity or fidelity to patients advise? (Kronick; Westbie) Is compassion relevant?

Even if Ms. H has no right to health care, do the health care professionals (HCPs) in this case have any moral obligation to advance her welfare and provide nonemergency treatment? Or are patients like Ms. H no more than an opportunity for charitable care—laudable, generous, and praiseworthy, but not morally *required*? When physicians and patients have not established formal clinical relationships; or when patients are unable to claim—based on a contractual or fiduciary relationship—a right to care, an obligation on individual physicians seems dubious.

Moreover, when ongoing *pro bono* support for indigent patients might undermine the financial integrity of a medical practice; and when continuing unreimbursed care for some jeopardizes the provision of health care for many (particularly salient to members of small communities who lack alternatives), concerned citizens must face the utilitarian question of whether the needs of the many outweigh the needs of the one or the few. Although Ms. H is but one patient, she is one among many, similarly situated, who collectively threaten to overwhelm the medical system in her small town. While the hospital, as an institution, is theoretically (and legally) committed to all who need urgent care, meeting this commitment in the short run may obliterate its ability to meet it over time. If the hospital closes, Ms. H—and all future patients—will suffer. Thus, an appeal to consequences (if not fidelity) suggests that some accommodation must be reached.

Equality/Fairness (Justice) If the physicians reject Mr. M's offer, is Ms. H unjustly burdened? If the physicians accept the offer, are they unjustly burdened? What role does equality—for example, equal access—play here? Should greater society play a role? (All commentators)

The moral principle of justice is often used to argue for a system that would provide universal health care. Justice-based arguments stress the unfairness of denying care to persons who, through no fault of their own, need health care: their employers do not provide insurance, their minimum wage jobs make individual purchase impossible, or they are born with or acquire diseases or disabilities that they were powerless to avoid. Given these needs, a just system would provide health care that is cost-effective, accessible to all citizens, and of consistently high-quality. But full realization of all three criteria is probably impossible. As our commentators note, at least some compromise in one or two criteria must be made in order to attain a political and socially acceptable balance of access, cost-effectiveness, and quality/comprehensive coverage. As a result, *all* health care systems must ration care—by limiting access, expenditures, or quality or comprehensive coverage. The present hybrid fee-for-service, managed care, and government subsidized programs in the United States have limited access (e.g., to specialists, some drugs). Other nations and states, including most importantly Oregon, offer less comprehensive programs, limiting access to certain diagnoses or treatments.[9] Various arrangements to balance access, quality, and cost-effectiveness against freedom of choice of caregivers, types of care, or sites for care have been proposed.[10] All such arrangements incorporate some sacrifices in quality, costs, and coverage for some individuals and groups.

The Law The following legal considerations are relevant to this case. (1) What are the legal obligations of institutions to treat those who cannot pay? (2) What are the legal obligations of independent providers to treat those who cannot pay? (3) Is there a difference in the legal status (with respect to claims for the provision of health care) of patients who have established relationships with physicians or health care institutions and those who have not?[11]

Ms. H's plight gives these theoretical issues a human face. Public health care policy must consider fundamental principles and commitments, previous legal and policy decisions, and economic costs and benefits of various policies. But for most consumers, HCPs, and health care administrators, the theoretical decisions and concerns with "statistical lives" are inevitably supplanted by the individual stories and sufferings of patients—often children, the indigent, the old, and, with increasing frequency, working parents—who are either unable to gain access to the health care system, or who fail to receive the optimum treatment for their problems. These "identified lives" provide a stark and vivid entry into the debate on rights and access to health care.

The following commentaries examine the application of various moral principles to this dilemma, thereby assisting the reader to undertake *Step 4: Analysis* and *Step 5: Justification*.

Notes

1. Congressional Budget Office, "How Many People Lack Health Insurance and For How Long?" May 2003, http://www.cbo.gov/showdoc.cfm?index=4210sequence=0 (26 Mar. 2004); U. S. Census Bureau, "Health Insurance Coverage: 2001," http://www.census.gov/prod/2002pubs/p60-220.pdf (26 Mar. 2004); Kaiser Commission on Medicaid and the Uninsured, *Health Insurance Coverage in America: 2001 Data Update* (Washington, DC: Kaiser Family Foundation, 2003).

2. J. Michael McWilliams et al., "Impact of Medicare Coverage on Basic Clinical Services for Previously Uninsured Adults," *JAMA: Journal of the American Medical Association* 290 (2003): 757–64.

3. Philip S. Keane, *Catholicism and Health-Care Justice: Problems, Potential, and Solutions* (Mahwah, NJ: Paulist Press, 2002); B. Andrew Lustig, "Reform and Rationing: Reflections on Health Care in Light of Catholic Social Teaching," in *Secular Bioethics in Theological Perspective*, ed. Earl E. Shelp (Dordrecht: Kluwer Academic Publishers, 1996), 31–50.

4. Michael J. Sandel, *Liberalism and the Limits of Justice*, 2nd ed. (Cambridge: Cambridge University Press, 1997); and John Rawls, *A Theory of Justice* (Cambridge: Harvard University Press, 1971).

5. United Nations, "Universal Declaration of Human Rights," Adopted and proclaimed by General Assembly resolution 217 A (III) of 10 December 1948, http://www.un.org/Overview/rights.html (26 Mar. 2004).

6. Gene Outka, "Social Justice and Equal Access to Health Care," *The Journal of Religious Ethics* 2, no. 1 (1974): 11–32; Allen Buchanan, "The Right to a Decent Minimum of Health Care," in *Contemporary Issues in Bioethics*, 5th ed., eds. Tom L. Beauchamp and LeRoy Walters (Belmont, CA: Wadsworth Publishing, 1999), 374–79.

7. Robert Nozick, *Anarchy, State, and Utopia* (New York: Basic Books, 1974). The implications of Rawls's and Nozick's theories to the challenge of access to health care are rendered in H. Tristram Engelhardt, Jr., "Rights to Healthcare, Social Justice, and Fairness in Healthcare Allocations: Frustration in the Face of Finitude," chap. 8 in *The Foundations of Bioethics*, 2nd ed. (New York: Oxford University Press, 1996), 375–410.

8. The Physicians Working Group for Single-Payer National Health Insurance, "Proposal of the Physicians' Working Group for Single-Payer National Health Insurance," *JAMA: Journal of the American Medical Association* 290 (2003): 798–805.

9. Henry J. Aaron and William B. Schwartz, *The Painful Prescription* (Washington, DC: The Brookings Institute, 1984); Martin A. Storsberg et al., *Rationing America's Medical Care: The Oregon Plan and Beyond* (Washington, DC: The Brookings Institute, 1992); Oregon Department of Human Services, Oregon Health Plan, n.d., http://www.dhs.state.or.us/healthplan (26 Mar. 2004).

10. Two very different but influential and important reform proposals representative of the range of options being proposed are John C. Goodman and Gerald Musgrave, *Patient Power: The Free Enterprise Alternative to Clinton's Health Plan* (Washington, DC: Cato Institute, 1994) and The Physicians Working Group for Single-Payer National Health Insurance, note 9, above, and http://www.pnhp.org, or http://www.physiciansproposal.org (26 Mar. 2004).

11. See E. Haavi Morreim, *Balancing Act: The New Medical Ethics of Medicine's New Economics* (Washington, DC: Georgetown University Press, 1995), chap. 6, "The Obligations and Limits of Fidelity: Physicians' Professional Services," 105–32; and American Medical Association, Council on Ethical and Judicial Affairs, *Code of Medical Ethics: Current Opinions with Annotations*, 2000–2001 ed. (Chicago: American Medical Association, 2000), § 2.03, "Allocation of Limited Medical Resources," 7–10; § 2.095, "The Provision of Adequate Health Care," 28; and § 9.065, "Caring for the Poor," 209–10.

A Patient's Analysis

Mikki Westbie

Physicians take a vow to alleviate pain and suffering. Doesn't that extend to all members of the community in which they practice? I understand that I do not yet have a primary care physician and the assumption of my health care should not take away care given to existing patients.[1] I am not requesting preferential treatment, or services that would bankrupt a doctor's office. But I am a hard-working member of this community—a place where these professionals chose to practice—who merely needs medical supervision so I can receive necessary medication the hospital is willing to donate. Isn't that worth a few minutes of someone's time? Furthermore, the hospital said preventive care would reduce the costs of illness. Isn't cost what the doctors said they were concerned about when they declined to treat me?

I recognize our local practitioners already have a large base of nonpaying or underpaying patients and I understand their reluctance to add another. After all, diagnostic equipment, treatment supplies, overhead, and staff are significant expenses. If clinics are not paid for office visits or reimbursed for their expenses, they will eventually have to close. Then the entire community will suffer.

From a patient's perspective, however, such monetary concerns should be secondary to helping people. Illness or injury can produce catastrophic losses for individuals and their families. Medical professionals are the gatekeepers of access to treatment; only by virtue of their expertise can patients receive optimal health care. There is no alternative. Therefore, the medical profession must be held to a higher standard than are other types of businesses.

Yet patients feel that their health care is treated as a privilege tied to their purchasing power. Those with a great amount of money have access to the best medical resources; those with little or no money are tolerated—so long as they do not take too many resources or accumulate too much medical debt. The costs associated with my treatments are prohibitive; nonetheless, I must receive preventive, routine, or emergency care to remain healthy enough to support my son and myself. To pay for those services I have added clients, only to develop a respiratory crisis due to overwork and stress. I have delayed treatment due to lack of funds and have instead accrued tremendous medical debt from emergency treatment. And I have discontinued medications early to save money—only to be lectured not to do that. What else can I do? The hospital has offered an alternative, but only in conjunction with medical oversight. My future health care is tied to my pocketbook, and that is empty.

Unfortunately my financial status is not unique within this region. Our community is in a precarious economic condition that extends to the medical clinics and the hospital. It is clear that this area is in need of outside assistance. According to the American Medical Association physicians are expected to provide patient advocacy when local resources are inadequate or exhausted.[2] This is a reasonable stipulation, as those professionals benefit from the ability to practice in local hospitals and clinics. However no expectation is placed on the greater society to help local communities. Why should local practitioners be the only ones expected to solve such a problem?

Under our current social policy Americans do not have the right to basic health care. This makes the United States the only industrialized nation that does not guarantee its citizens nonemergent medical treatment.[3] Given the nation's wealth and cutting-edge medical technology, how can this be a just policy?

Nearly every inhabitant of the United States contributes to our national tax base; certainly I do. Even those who do not pay income taxes still pay sales tax, usage fees, and so on. A sizeable portion of those taxes is used to fund medical research, student financial aid, and health care facilities. Most medical students rely on financial aid to complete their education. Many are given the opportunity to train at public health clinics frequented by poor patients. And all medical practitioners utilize information about the causes and treatment of disease gained from publicly funded biomedical research. Since all Americans contribute to funding medical education and health care, doctors are as beholden to the poor as to the rich for their professional training and subsequent careers. It is therefore unjust to exclude some people, individually or collectively, from the benefits of the health care system they helped to create—and continue to support—simply because they lack private resources to pay for health insurance or medical treatment.

Those of us considered the working poor comprise the group usually associated with inability to pay; however, a growing population of uninsured or underinsured Americans are having to decide between paying for shelter or for insurance, buying food or purchasing medication. We are now joined by employees whose employers have abandoned coverage, retirees whose company benefits have been lost to corporate bankruptcy or whose Medicare coverage excludes necessary (but expensive) medications, and the poor or disabled, whose Medicaid benefits have been slashed in response to our faltering economy. Since this constitutes a growing nationwide problem, the nation needs to respond. Why should physicians alone be expected to solve the problem?

Given these deteriorating conditions, it is obvious that the current health care system is inadequate. Furthermore, previous "solutions" have merely compounded the problem: Fee-for-service medicine and traditional health insurance exclude those unable to afford the cost. To combat this inequity, government programs were implemented. But those are plagued with overcharging, duplication-of-service, and bureaucratic inefficiency. So Health Maintenance Organizations (HMOs) were introduced to curtail wasteful spending. Unfortunately, they have often undermined a patient's right to informed consent and the doctor-patient relationship by restricting information about treatments not covered. Furthermore, organizations that require physicians to put their patients' welfare second damage the fundamental trust society has placed in the medical profession.

The difficulties I have had receiving treatment locally are mirrored in the larger society. It is time that the nation establishes a universal health care system, so that everyone can acquire appropriate treatment. We need to rethink the whole system when any member of society has to choose between seeing a doctor and feeding a child.

Notes

1. American Medical Association, "Potential Patients" (Policy E-10.05, 17 July 2002), http://www.ama-assn.org/ama/pub/category/8327.html (26 Mar. 2004).
2. American Medical Association, "Caring for the Poor" (Policy H-160.961, 3 April 2003), http://www.ama-assn.org/ama/pub/category/8327.html (26 Mar. 2004).
3. K. Terrell, "Koop Discusses Barriers to Right to Healthcare" [Electronic version], *Rice News* 11, no. 14 (Nov. 29, 2001), http://www.rice.edu/projects/reno/rn/20011129/Templates/Koop.html (15 June 2003).

A Philosopher's Perspective

Lisa Gannett, PhD

Ms. H is one of an estimated 48.6 million Americans who, over a two-year period, will be without medical insurance for at least six months.[1] Like 80 percent of uninsured individuals, Ms. H belongs to a family where at least one member works full- or part-time, but where the family income is too much to qualify for Medicaid and too little to afford insurance premiums. Like many uninsured individuals, Ms. H is self-employed and forced to pay full premiums without benefit of negotiated group discounts, and suffers from a "preexisting condition" that drives up premium costs further.

Uninsured Americans are four times more likely than insured Americans to use hospital emergency rooms as regular places of care, contributing to a 10 percent to 15 percent higher mortality rate. Lack of access to ongoing primary and preventive care results in failure to detect diseases like hypertension or cancer at early stages and to manage chronic conditions like asthma or diabetes. This lowers quality of life and increases the eventual burden on publicly funded programs like Medicare.[2]

Reliance on emergency care in place of less costly primary and preventive care saddles patients with bills they cannot pay and strains hospital resources. This 20-bed acute care hospital is at risk of closure if the trend of financial loss is not reversed. Unreimbursed treatment provided to uninsured (and underinsured) patients like Ms. H contributes to its budget deficit. Once a rural hospital closes, it is unlikely to reopen, and the whole community loses: family support during hospitalization becomes difficult, continuity of care suffers, and increased travel time in emergencies may make the difference between life and death.

Mr. M recognizes the inefficiencies of a "system" of health care delivery that fails to intervene when care will be most medically and economically effective. Should Ms. H receive regular, ongoing attention from a primary care physician, her health and the hospital's fiscal health would be the better for it: pro bono primary care for Ms. H will improve her health, contain treatment costs, and protect a vital resource for residents of the surrounding rural communities.

This reasonable suggestion tempts us to believe that the four primary care physicians are acting selfishly in rejecting the proposal. But moral kudos are not tantamount to moral duties. The physicians may be morally commended for assuming medical responsibility for Ms. H, but they are not morally obligated to do so. Physicians are obligated to treat people only in emergencies; they are otherwise free to choose whom to serve.[3] The physicians quite correctly point out that Ms. H's situation is hardly unique. Fairness requires that pro bono care be offered to others who find themselves in similar straits, and this would simply displace the hospital's reimbursement difficulties onto the physicians. Mr. M's solution, though reasonable, is no more than a stopgap measure.

The particularities of this case are symptomatic of widespread problems with health care access in the United States that demand structural redress. Unlike other industrialized nations, the United States has no laws that guarantee health care for its citizens or residents. Is the government morally obligated to intervene when differences in economic means, medical status, or geographic location prevent individuals from obtaining care?

Article 25 of the UN's Universal Declaration of Human Rights states that health care is a right:

Everyone has the right to a standard of living adequate for the health and well-being of himself and of his family, including food, clothing, housing and medical care and necessary social services, and the right to security in the event of unemployment, sickness, disability, widowhood, old age or other lack of livelihood in circumstances beyond his control.[4]

Presumably the United States is committed as a nation to the right to health care, as it was one of 48 member states of the UN General Assembly voting to adopt the Declaration on 10 December 1948. Though not legally binding, the Declaration does comprise a moral standard agreed upon by the world's nations. The International Covenant on Economic, Social, and Cultural Rights (ICESCR), adopted by the UN General Assembly on 16 December 1966 and effective on 3 January 1976, makes rights recognized by the 1948 Declaration legally binding on nations. Article 12 recognizes "the right of everyone to the enjoyment of the highest attainable standard of physical and mental health," and supports "[t]he creation of conditions which would assure to all medical service and medical attention in the event of sickness."[5] Although President Carter signed the treaty on 5 October 1977, it is not yet in force within the United States because Congress has not ratified it.

Theories of distributive justice differ in their assessments of whether governments are bound by duty to "create conditions" consistent with rights to "the highest attainable standard of physical and mental health" for everyone. Libertarians oppose any restriction on individuals' freedom to contract for health care services. This applies to patients' abilities to secure whatever kind and quality of care they can afford, and providers' abilities to practice wherever they please, regardless of rural-urban disparities in access to care. For libertarians, charity is the only morally permissible way to remedy inequalities of access to health care; taxation for this purpose constitutes theft.[6] Socialists and some liberals believe a single-tier system committed to the "highest attainable standard of physical and mental health" for everyone respects the ideal of moral equality (the lives of all people matter, and matter equally).[7] Other liberals support a multitier system that guarantees a decent minimum, but is not committed to "the highest attainable standard." The decent minimum might be defined in terms of a standard of care that permits normal functioning and therefore equality of opportunity.[8]

These theories of justice support such different positions because they assume different concepts of rights, freedom, and equality—noninterference vs. entitlement rights; positive vs. negative freedom; and abstract vs. concrete equality. This is not the place to debate theoretical foundations, and it may well be that there is no universal standard of justice that *requires* the United States to respect the UN Declaration and ratify ICESCR or enact legislation that guarantees health care for all Americans. In a sense, we are joining a conversation of more than 225 years' duration in the United States about what those truths "self-evident" to the authors of the

Declaration of Independence—that "all men are created equal" and in possession of "certain inalienable rights" including "Life, Liberty and the pursuit of Happiness"—ought to mean.

We might join this discussion by asking why the United States is the only Western and industrialized nation to fail to guarantee health care for its citizens or residents. There is no paucity of economic resources: to the tune of $3 billion a day, the United States far exceeds the rest of the world in per capita health care spending. Nor are scientific know-how or technological wherewithal lacking; again, in these areas, the United States leads the world. In other words, this is not an overcrowded lifeboat sort of moral dilemma. Rather, the moral justification called for is analogous to refusing to distribute life vests to all ship's passengers when there are plenty to go around.

The failure to ensure universal health care cannot be explained by a lack of value attached to life, or even just some lives, given that the right to life is fundamental. Nor can this failure be explained by conceiving the right to life solely as a right of noninterference. Tax dollars pay firefighters and police officers to save and protect lives, and we believe ourselves entitled to their interventions on our behalf. Why is the use of tax dollars to pay physicians and nurses to save and protect our lives disanalogous? Much antipathy is expressed toward "big government," yet the government spends hundreds of billions of tax dollars annually on "national security." The government is maligned for "bureaucratic inefficiency," yet corporate administrative costs far exceed those for public health care. Capitalism is valued in the United States, but its viability is surely not threatened by recognizing that health care is not a commodity like DVD players and jet-skis, and may be therefore subject to different social priorities and even market forces. Opponents of single-payer health care who decry restrictions on the freedom of physicians to contract their services need to be asked why the freedom of workers to change jobs without fear of losing health care matters less. Is equality merely formal, resting in equal application of the law? Or is equality something morally more substantial, involving the recognition that, in a wealthy society, the pursuit of happiness should not be made difficult or impossible by poor health and lack of access to care, because the lives of all people matter?

Notes

1. Families USA Foundation, "Going Without Health Insurance: Nearly One in Three Nonelderly Americans," *Families USA Publication No. 03-103*, prepared for Cover the Uninsured Week, March 2003, http://www.familiesusa.org/site/PageServer (24 Mar. 2004).

2. American College of Physicians–American Society of Internal Medicine (ACP–ASIM), "No Health Insurance? It's Enough to Make you Sick–Scientific Research Linking the Lack of Health Coverage to Poor Health," 2000, http://www.acponline.org/uninsured/lack-contents.htm (26 Mar. 2004).

3. American Medical Association, *Principles of Medical Ethics*, June 2001, http://www.ama-assn.org/ama/pub/category/2512.html (26 Mar. 2004), Principle VI.

4. United Nations, "Universal Declaration of Human Rights," Adopted and proclaimed by General Assembly resolution 217 A (III) of 10 December 1948, http://www.un.org/Overview/rights.html (26 Mar. 2004).

5. United Nations, "International Covenant on Economic, Social and Cultural Rights," Adopted and opened for signature, ratification and accession by General Assembly resolution 2200A (XXI) of 16 December 1966; entry into force 3 January 1976, in accordance with article 27, http://www.unhchr.ch/html/menu3/b/a_cescr.htm (26 Mar. 2004).
6. H. Tristram Engelhardt, Jr., "Rights to Healthcare, Social Justice, and Fairness in Healthcare Allocations: Frustration in the Face of Finitude," chap. 8 in *The Foundations of Bioethics*, 2nd ed. (New York: Oxford University Press, 1996), 375–410.
7. Kai Nielsen, "Autonomy, Equality and a Just Healthcare System," *The International Journal of Applied Philosophy* 4 (1989): 39–44.
8. Norman Daniels, *Am I My Parent's Keeper?* (New York: Oxford University Press, 1988).

A Health Policy Analysis

Richard Kronick, PhD

As a society we have failed in our moral obligation to create a system of health care financing that provides affordable access to high quality care. More than forty million Americans, most of them workers or their dependents, are uninsured. A system of coverage that relies on a patchwork of public programs for the elderly and subsets of the poor, and voluntary, employer-sponsored insurance for most Americans is inequitable and immoral because it allows tens of millions of hard-working adults and their children to suffer financial and medical care catastrophes when they become ill. In addition to federal and state government support for Medicare and Medicaid, the federal government subsidizes coverage for workers whose employers provide insurance. The cost of that insurance is not considered taxable income, a tax deductible expenditure that costs the federal and state governments approximately $150 billion per year. This subsidy is concentrated on those who need it least—the relatively well paid who are in higher tax brackets and receive larger employer contributions—while denying assistance to many of those who need it most.

As a result people suffer. Being uninsured is bad for one's health, though existing research does not provide a precise answer to the question: How bad is it?[1] Even in the absence of a precise answer, mortality and morbidity rates are clearly higher for the uninsured than the insured. The case of Mrs. H provides a poignant example of the mechanism of effect.

Finding the technical means to create an equitable financing system is not a mystery. There is no shortage of proposals for financing reform that would lead to universal coverage and a more equitable distribution of the financing burden.[2] To date, however, we have been unable to assemble, at state or federal levels, a winning political coalition to enact any of the technically feasible solutions.

In an immoral world, what is the obligation of moral physicians? Prior to the enactment of Medicare and Medicaid in 1965, the moral obligation of physicians was well defined: provide one-half day per week of services at a free hospital-based clinic.[3] Further, physicians commonly charged patients according to their ability to pay (charging wealthier patients more and poorer patients less). It is not clear how many physicians did donate one-half day per week of their time, but enforcement mechanisms existed to support the norm: hospital staff privileges were contingent on membership and good standing in the local medical society, and medical society membership could be denied to physicians who were not good colleagues.

Subsequent to the enactment of Medicare and Medicaid and the expansion of private insurance to cover more physician services, the physician's moral obligation became less clear. Fueled by public sector payments, free clinics were transformed into hospital revenue centers. The norm that physicians should provide one-half day per week of unpaid work atrophied as most free clinics disappeared. Rhetorical responsibility for financing care for the medically indigent shifted from the medical profession to the government. And today physicians who serve Medicare and Medicaid patients for what might be considered inadequate payment may feel that they have already "given at the office."

If the physicians in this case are like most physicians in rural America, their net income is at least five times the annual income of the average person in the community in which they live. Should they agree, collectively, to provide care to Mrs. H and figure out some method of determining which physician will care for her? Certainly they should. The physicians should figure out a way of making this work for Mrs. H, and they probably can do so without making life unbearable for any of them.

But while it seems clear that the physicians should agree to care for Mrs. H, can they promise to do so for Mrs. I and Mr. J and all of the other hard-working but uninsured persons in their community? Unfortunately not. In most communities with large concentrations of low-income uninsured persons, it is simply not possible for physicians, either individually or collectively, to agree to provide all persons with all the care they need. And even if the physicians were able to provide care to uninsured persons and maintain the net income they "needed," the organizational resources required to figure out how to share the burden of delivering care to the uninsured and to assure that hospital, prescription drugs, and other ancillary services (including the services of specialists in other communities) were available would create a substantial additional burden. Physicians are trained to provide health care and should concentrate their talents on doing so; it does not make sense to expect physicians to invest substantial organizational energy in trying to make an inherently immoral system slightly less cruel.

The larger problem of creating an equitable and moral financing system can only be solved through political action. I am heartened that, for example, the California state legislature is currently considering a series of bills that would move toward universal coverage in California. One of these bills would require employers either to provide health insurance to their employees or pay a fee to a state fund. The state fund would then use the fee revenue, along with matching federal payments for those persons eligible for Medicaid or Healthy Families, to provide health insurance to all workers covered by unemployment insurance. While none of these bills is perfect and the prospects for enactment are uncertain, it is encouraging that some legislative attention is being devoted to the problem. It is also encouraging that the California Medical Association, in an uncommon alliance with the California Labor Federation, supports constructive change. In addition to urging moral physicians to collaborate in their efforts to provide what care they can to those in need, I urge them to attend to legislative activity, to contact their representatives, and to encourage their state medical associations and other organizations to which they may belong to support progressive legislation.

In the United States we have a time-honored tradition of considering the uninsured as "them," and separating them from "us." Ever the optimist, I continue to hope that someday soon we will recognize our common interests, and that moral physicians will no longer be faced with immoral choices.

Notes

1. J. Hadley, "Sicker and Poorer—The Consequences of Being Uninsured: A Review of the Research on the Relationship Between Health Insurance, Medical Care Use, Health, Work, and Income," *Medical Care Research and Review* 60, no. 2 (2003) (Supplement): 3S–75S; Richard Kronick, "Commentary," *Medical Care Research and Review* 60, no. 2 (2003) (Supplement): 100S–112S.
2. See, for example, ed. E. K. Wicks, *Covering America: Real Remedies for the Uninsured* (Washington, DC: Economic and Social Research Institute, 2001); ed. E. K. Wicks, *Covering America: Real Remedies for the Uninsured*, Vol. 2 (Washington, DC: Economic and Social Research Institute, 2002).
3. R. A. Kessel, "Price Discrimination in Medicine," *Journal of Law and Economics* 20, no. 1 (1958): 20–53; Paul Starr, *Social Transformation of American Medicine* (New York: Basic Books, 1982).

A Physician/Organizational Ethicist's Analysis

Suresh Sahadevan, MD, FRCP, DGM, FAMS

What is striking about this case is how Ms. H's recurrent illness remains a predicament as long as all the individual parties (Ms. H, the physicians, and Mr. M) see the problem only from their own perspectives. Each party is worried about his or her own rights and responsibilities (albeit of differing magnitude and practical import), and each is unable to see how Ms. H's problem can be solved.

One unique consequence of an organizational ethics approach is that it offers the opportunity for all relevant parties or stakeholders to discuss problems together. In this case, the relevant stakeholders include prospective patients, physicians, and the hospital. The opportunity to consult together may enable stakeholders to see each other's perspective and to appreciate how often problems are mutual. For example, in addition to the direct negative effects on the hospital's employees (should the institution close), physicians would have to find admitting privileges elsewhere—probably much farther away—which would pose hardships on patients and physicians alike. An organizational ethics program offers participants a venue to reflect on their own roles, responsibilities, and values, as well as those of the organization.

An effectively functioning organizational ethics committee can create a far better chance of collectively resolving what only appear to be individual dilemmas of the three main stakeholders of this community hospital. At a minimum the committee should have representatives of prospective patients, physicians, and the hospital administration to voice the concerns and interests of each stakeholder, as well as the difficulties and objectives of others.

How do these points apply to the case at hand? The four family practice physicians, Mr. M, and organization ethics program members could meet. At the meeting the hospital's dire financial straits—as well as the consequences of its closure—can be openly shared. Physicians, through this information sharing, may better appreciate the gravity of the problem and its genuine nature (e.g., it is not a result of financial mismanagement). Likewise, the hospital's administrators may become more aware of the dilemmas facing the physicians, should they make an exception by seeing Ms. H pro bono in a community where many others are also uninsured or underinsured and having difficulties paying health care bills. Representatives of prospective patients can become more informed about the fragility of their health care system and, in turn, more aware of their general responsibilities for maintaining good health and the importance of considering various ways to help each other out in this area.

A meeting of this sort could also engender a reflection on the community-driven mission of the hospital and what values this mission represents. The physicians may realize that it is in their interests to help ensure that the hospital remains financially viable. After all, their own ability to continue with their practices certainly requires the existence of the hospital. Additionally, knowing that the hospital is willing to purchase a free nebulizer and its pharmacy's offering medication free of charge to Ms. H should encourage the physicians to review their initial reluctance to see the patient pro bono, given the seriousness of her problems. The hospital, in turn, may become aware of the limits of expecting any single doctor to look after Ms. H free of charge. This expanded awareness may prompt physicians, Mr. M, and organization ethics members to identify resources and ways of solving the problem—ways that probably would not have been considered by the individuals involved.

For instance a social worker could be asked to identify resources, like churches or volunteer groups, that may be in a position to help Ms. H. Possibly the physicians could agree to cooperate with Ms. H's care by rotating her visits amongst themselves and making arrangements (with the patient's permission) to share her medical records so that the continuity of her care would not be compromised in the process. Similarly, both physicians and administrators may want to jointly review various aspects of the existing health care delivery at the hospital to see whether strategies actually exist where the quality of health care delivery by the hospital can be retained (or even improved) while reducing the operational costs of that care (e.g., reviewing whether the length of hospital stay of various inpatients can be appropriately reduced and more care transferred to less costly outpatient settings).

In the process of managing these difficulties effectively—and most importantly, ethically—an organizational ethics approach can engender goodwill and trust that will be invaluable for addressing future challenges.

Further Reflections

General

1. Kronick argues that "as a society we have failed in our moral obligation to create a system of health care financing that provides affordable access to high quality care." Is that claim correct? If not, why not? If so, what is the basis for that moral obligation?
2. What, in your mind, are the greatest successes and the greatest failings of American health care?

Consequences

3. Identify and evaluate the consequences of the physicians' taking on Ms. H's care.

Autonomy

4. Sahadevan suggests that the only way to resolve the challenges of this case is to bring the "stakeholders" together to discuss their (assumed to be freely chosen) roles and responsibilities. Specify their obligations and the moral values that support them. Indicate whether these obligations were autonomously undertaken.

Rights

5. Gannett and Westbie discuss the notion of "a right to health care," grounding it in human need and in political contracts. Discuss this purported right to health care—its moral and legal foundation(s), its substance, and who is obligated to provide and pay for such care.

6. If the physicians accept Ms. H as a patient, does she have an individual right to health care? Does the fact that Ms. H would be a pro bono patient limit the physicians' obligations (or Ms. H's right, if she has one) in comparison to the obligations to (rights of) paying patients?

Virtues

7. Physicians espouse moral obligations to their *own* patients, but not to those with whom they have no preestablished relationship. What moral principles could justify this disparity?
8. Regardless of whether physicians have a professional obligation to care for the medically indigent, do individual citizens, communities, or the government— to be called virtuous—have obligations to assist their neighbors or citizens achieve access to health care?

Equality/Fairness (Justice)

9. Kronick suggests that the United States has been unable to develop a sustainable health care system because we lack the "winning political coalition" essential to its acceptance and implementation. Discuss whether justice requires such a system and, if it does, what would be required politically to enact the health care plan based on "an equitable and moral financing system."

Chapter 10

Dollars or Drugs?

Mr. H is a 52-year-old former employee of a regional manufactured home builder who lives with his wife and two teenage sons. He has suffered for several years from idiopathic pulmonary fibrosis. After years of worsening respiratory function, Mr. H became totally disabled. Over the years Mr. H had become increasingly anemic, short of breath, and weak. In spite of continuous use of supplemental oxygen, he lacked the energy to do everyday activities like making his bed, walking his dog, and doing yard work. The family had health insurance from his wife's job (she was an elementary school teacher), and Mr. H was able to get good care under that policy, though the deductibles and co-pays on the policy were quite steep, and the policy only had limited coverage for prescription drugs (co-payments were typically 50 percent of drugs' costs).

Two years ago Mr. H was evaluated at the regional transplant center to determine if he might be an appropriate candidate for a lung transplant. He was found to be a very good risk for this sort of a procedure: he still exercised regularly, did not smoke, and had a good cardiac reserve (that is, his lung disease had not injured his heart). In addition, he and his wife and sons were enthusiastic about having a transplant, and were willing to undertake the extensive and rigid rehabilitative and medication regimens that were required after surgery. The transplant staff was delighted with his excellent prognosis for two reasons: (1) Their goal is to save lives and (2) They are not yet a Medicare-approved transplant center; that approval depends on (among other things) 69 percent first-year and 62 percent second-year survival rates; excellent candidates such as Mr. H

185

improve the program's statistics and, hence, its chance for Medicare approval.

When a donor lung became available a year ago, Mr. H underwent the lung transplant. His recuperation has been free of complications. He is active again, is able to engage in increasingly rigorous exercise, has had no shortness of breath, and tolerates his eight medications without appreciable side effects. His transplant surgeon and pulmonologist, based on periodic checkups, have given him an excellent prognosis. While he has not yet been able to return to work, he is hopeful that, should his condition continue to improve, he will be able to at least begin building some custom pieces of furniture again.

In the year since his transplant Mr. H's out-of-pocket expenses have exceeded $10,000. His drugs are especially expensive, costing $1346.95/month. As Mr. H's insurance only covers half of prescription costs, his out-of-pocket drug costs are $673.48/month.

Recently Mr. H stopped by his local pharmacy to pick up his next month's supply of medications. As the pharmacist began packaging the medications, Mr. H asked him to omit the prescription for Cellcept, a crucial immunosuppressant and the most expensive medication ($779/month). Mr. H indicated that he couldn't afford all the drugs on this visit, but hoped to be able to resume the full regimen of drugs next month. The pharmacist reminded Mr. H that his survival depends directly on the immunosuppressant drugs. Mr. H indicated that he understood that his future health depends on protecting his transplanted lung, and that protecting his transplanted lung depends on his taking these medications. But the family also has a mortgage and a car payment, needs to buy groceries and clothe the kids, etc. Mr. H says he just hopes the other immunosuppressants will "pick up the slack" until next month.

The pharmacist recognizes that many of his clients cannot always afford to purchase medications that their doctors have prescribed. However, in Mr. H's case, the failure to take the immunosuppressant not only puts Mr. H's health at dire risk; it also affects the statistical success of the regional transplant center. His death will have an effect on the aggregate mortality rates of the program, possibly jeopardizing both access to and continuing insurance coverage for regional patients who need transplants. That is, omitting the immunosuppressant puts both Mr. H and future transplant patients at significant risk of early death.

How should the pharmacist respond to Mr. H?

Introduction

This case incorporates all major moral principles.[1] We must investigate the consequences to all involved, whether Mr. H's past and present choices were/are autonomous, whether Mr. H's right of self-determination trumps the right of others to be aided, if professional integrity requires the pharmacist to intervene or accept Mr. H's decision, and whether justice requires protecting a scarce resource one has been fortunate enough to receive.[2] Nonetheless, the case can be distilled to a single moral question:

Are recipients of scarce health care resources morally obligated to protect and preserve them?

AJ Method

Step 1: Information Gathering   What facts are necessary for resolving this case? What are the likely effects on Mr. H of forgoing one of his immunosuppressants for a month? on his family? on the transplant center? What motivates Mr. H's decision?

Organ transplantation is truly life-saving. Persons who would once have died from organ failure now live longer.[3] This blessing, however, comes with costs. First, patients trade one chronic disease (end-stage organ failure) for another (chronic immunosuppression).[4] Second, transplant patients often feel an enormous (and sometimes burdensome) obligation to live up to their health care professionals' (HCPs') expectations.[5] Third, the "gift of life" binds patients in gratitude to strangers (donor families)—bonds they are sometimes reluctant to accept.[6] Must transplant patients assume these burdens?

Step 2: Creative Problem Solving   Any creative solution would have to relieve Mr. H's financial strain without violating the pharmacist's professional responsibility.

Step 3: Pros and Cons   Survey CARVE principles to identify important moral reasons that support conflicting options for resolving this case.

Consequences   Who will be harmed by Mr. H's decision? How? Who will be benefited? (All commentators)

We begin with chronic immunosuppression. Transplants succeed because drugs prevent the body's rejection of the foreign organ. Without these drugs, the body would destroy what it perceives to be an outside invasion (much like the body fights off invasion by germs). These powerful drugs have multiple effects. In addition to preventing the rejection, immunosuppressants can cause Parkinson-like tremors (try drinking coffee or eating soup!), liver or kidney damage (which, if severe enough, may require a liver or kidney transplant), excessive weight gain (grocery and clothing bills grow by leaps and bounds), irritable personality, depression, and increased risk of various cancers. Add to this having to pay the not-insignificant sum of $1350 each month—money that could pay the mortgage, car insurance, day care, college tuition. Given these common consequences, we should not be surprised if patients—or their families—sometimes question the wisdom of the transplant and are tempted to omit their drugs.[7]

Patients' choices to abandon post-transplant care affect HCPs: they must ensure that the patients understand the likely implication of this choice is death;[8] and they may be obliged to limit future care to comfort measures only, so as to minimize further waste of valuable resources—both of which may be psychologically burdensome to the HCPs.

Autonomy   Under what circumstances may patients autonomously revoke an earlier (presumably autonomous) decision? (Kaatz) Might transplant recipients autonomously (perhaps only implicitly) consent, at the time of transplant, to do whatever is necessary to preserve the organs they receive? (Hoso and Allen)

Still, patients are not wait-listed for a transplant without their consent. Moreover, the relationship of transplant team members and patients and their families typically exemplifies the type of relationship most patients and providers aspire to. HCPs know their patients and significant others intimately. Clinic visits are frequent and unhurried. Pretransplant interviews with the pulmonologist, surgeon, social worker, psychologist, pharmacist, respiratory therapist, nurses, and insurance clerk are required. HCPs spend as much time as is necessary to ensure that patients and families know exactly what is involved and what behavior is necessary and expected. This relationship is truly teamwork at its finest. As a result, decisions to undergo organ transplantation are likely to be autonomous, and postoperative surprises would seem unlikely.

And yet a posttransplant patient's life is full of surprises, for *knowing* that one might be depressed is a quite different subjective experience from *being* depressed. Knowing potential side effects from drugs is not the same subjective experience as living them, day in, day out. Expenses may exceed expectations, especially for patients who have multiple rejection episodes (requiring rehospitalization) or chronic complications (e.g., steroid-induced diabetes) which increase physical, emotional, and financial burdens. As it happens, forewarned is often not forearmed. At what point may patients say "enough"? Is a decision to have a transplant a type of "Ulysses contract" which may not be reconsidered, regardless of the patient's experiential evolution?[9]

Rights   Does Mr. H have a right to be aided financially? Is his right to self-determination intact, or has it been restricted by his earlier choices? Do future patients have the right to not be harmed (e.g., by loss of access to transplants)? (Hoso and Allen)

Virtues   Does Mr. H owe compliance (fidelity) to the system? (Hoso and Allen) How might the pharmacist, or the transplant professionals, best demonstrate compassion for Mr. H? (Hoso and Allen; Kaatz) Does fidelity rule out or require any particular actions on the part of the HCPs? (Kaatz; Siminoff and Morse) Is sacrificing other needs to pay for his medications an opportunity for courage on Mr. H's part? his family's part?

Continual pleas are made to the public to "give the gift of life." But the metaphor of a "gift" may be inapt.[10] A gift, purely speaking, comes with no strings attached. Yet on receiving even ordinary gifts, many people feel obliged to "return the favor," perhaps by giving the giver a gift of similar value or significance at some future time (e.g., the giver's birthday). Such reciprocity is impossible for organ recipients. How can one possibly repay the gift of life?

The metaphor may fail to hold in another way: an ordinary gift not to one's liking can be recycled to someone else or donated to the Salvation Army; but one is stuck with the gift of life (odd as that sounds). As a result, one cannot divest oneself of expectations that come with the gift: giving meaning to the donor's death, easing the sadness of the donor's family, contributing to the transplant center's success. Most organ recipients gladly assume these roles, but some do not. Do those who find their new burdens difficult to bear fail to demonstrate the virtues of courage, honesty, or fidelity if they reject the gift—and all expectations attached to it? Do HCPs fail to demonstrate professional integrity if they accept patients' choices to forgo after-care?

These issues are not merely of personal interest. If organ recipients can, morally speaking, reject the gift, they can reject medical regimens necessary to preserve it. Derivatively, HCPs—whose codes of ethics without exception pledge to support patient autonomy and self-determination—must allow patients to abandon therapy, unless some compelling moral argument can be made for why *personal* autonomy does not hold for transplant patients.

One such argument is that every recipient owes compliance to the person who would have preserved the gift, had she or he been lucky enough to receive it. The need for organs far exceeds the supply.[11] A donated organ can be used by only one recipient and roughly 3.6 persons "compete" for each donated lung. Each recipient effectively (though not, of course, intentionally) deprives 2.6 other persons of a lifesaving resource. Do the lucky few owe it (based on fidelity or keeping one's promise) to the unlucky many not to waste the gift?

Perhaps the lucky few owe fidelity, manifested in postoperative compliance, to the system generally. The AMA believes that scarce resources should be distributed so as to "maximize the . . . three primary goals of medical treatment: number of lives saved, number of years of life saved, and improvement in quality of life."[12] Failure to follow through with the treatment regimen violates at least the first two criteria in terms of which one qualified as a recipient.

Further, transplant centers cannot operate without federal approval, but federal approval is granted only to centers that demonstrate good survival rates. Each patient's death worsens his or her center's survival statistics, thereby threatening the program's viability and availability to future patients. Most patients gladly comply with even quite burdensome posttransplant routines, but do patients *owe* future patients a chance—by not unnecessarily reducing positive outcomes?

But if patients are not allowed to give up on their transplants, are HCPs obligated to help them shoulder their burdens, including financial burdens? After all, no one can be expected to do the impossible.

Equality/Fairness (Justice)   Is requiring transplant patients to assume the financial burden for posttransplant care unfair? (Siminoff and Morse) Does this assumption differ from (i.e., is it unequal with) assumptions about other patients with chronic illnesses?

The Law   A number of legal considerations are relevant to this case. (1) Do HCPs in general and pharmacists in particular have a legal obligation to prevent foreseeable harms to their patients that may result from the patients' own choices? (2) Under what conditions may HCPs legally override the decisional authority of a competent patient? (3) What is the extent of a pharmacist's legal obligation of confidentiality with respect to persons to whom they are dispensing drugs?13

The following commentaries examine the application of various moral principles to this dilemma, thereby assisting the reader to undertake *Step 4: Analysis* and *Step 5: Justification*.

Notes

1. For a thorough examination of the ethical issues surrounding organ transplantation, see Robert M. Veatch, *Transplantation Ethics* (Washington, DC: Georgetown University Press, 2000). For a shorter discussion, see Ake Grevnik, "Ethical Dilemmas in Organ Donation and Transplantation," *Critical Care Medicine* 16, no. 10 (1988): 1012–18.
2. For an excellent justification of the moral obligations of pharmacists to clients, see Richard M. Schulz and David B. Brushwood, "The Pharmacist's Role in Patient Care," *Hastings Center Report* 21, no. 1 (1991): 12–17. Though dated, in that it argues for obligations that have subsequently been adopted, its presentation of the moral reasoning for pharmacists as patient advocates and educators is excellent.
3. Survival statistics vary with the organ transplanted; 64 percent of heart-lung transplants to 97 percent of pancreas transplants were still alive one year after transplant. The one-year survival rate for lung transplants is 77 percent ("About Transplants: Fast Facts," n.d., http://www.ustransplant.org/facts.html [26 Mar. 2004]; see also United Network for Organ Sharing, http://www.unos.org [26 Mar. 2004]).
4. Ann Mongovern, "Sharing Our Body and Blood: Organ Donation and Feminist Critiques of Sacrifice," *Journal of Medicine and Philosophy* 28, no. 1 (2003): 103.
5. Laura A. Siminoff and Kata Chillag, "The Fallacy of the 'Gift of Life,'" *Hastings Center Report* 29, no. 6 (1999): 34–41.
6. Renée C. Fox and Judith P. Swazey, *Spare Parts: Organ Replacement in American Society* (New York: Oxford University Press, 1992).
7. Approximately 25 percent of posttransplant patients fail to comply with their *prescribed* medication schedule (Deborah L. Shelton, "Problem of Noncompliance Affects Transplant Patients Too," 4 May 1998, http://www.ama-assn.org/ama/pub/category/8538.html [26 Mar. 2004]).

8. But see Thomas E. Starzl, MD, PhD, and Rolf M. Zinkernagel, MD, "Antigen Localization and Migration in Immunity and Tolerance," *New England Journal of Medicine* 339, no. 26 (1998): 1905–13 in which Starzl, the pioneer of immunosuppressive therapy, suggests that some patients do quite well with no, or few, antirejection drugs.

9. Rebecca Dresser, "Bound to Treatment: The Ulysses Contract," *Hastings Center Report* 14, no. 3 (1984): 13–16.

10. See notes 4, 5, and 6, above.

11. See note 3, above. Further, from 1997 to 1999 only 42 percent of potential organ donors donated (though 54 percent of families asked consented); see Ellen Sheehy et al., "Estimating the Number of Potential Organ Donors in the United States," *New England Journal of Medicine* 349, no. 7 (2003): 667–74.

12. Council on Ethical and Judicial Affairs, American Medical Association, "Ethical Considerations in the Allocation of Organs and Other Scarce Medical Resources Among Patients," *Archives of Internal Medicine* 155 (1995): 29–40.

13. Most helpful in grappling with these issues is Richard R. Abood and David B. Brushwood, *Pharmacy Practice and the Law,* 3rd ed. (Gaithersburg, MD: Aspen Publishers, 2004), chap. 3, "Federal Regulation of Medications," and Chap. 16, "Legal Issues with Ethical Implications."

A Transplant Team's Analysis

Andrea D. Hoso, RN, CCTC, and Roblee P. Allen, MD

Mr. H has been the beneficiary of a scarce medical resource. As of 30 June 2002, 3757 patients were awaiting lung transplantation. From 1 July 2001 through 30 June 2002, 1076 (28.7 percent on the list) received transplants and 463 persons (12.3 percent of those waiting) died before a suitable graft became available.[1] In accepting such a rare gift Mr. H assumed a moral responsibility to maximize its benefit for him.

Successful transplantation depends on patient compliance with medications and medical follow-up. Mr. H made the commitment to follow the medical plan needed to maintain his new lung. He committed himself to a lifelong program of strict adherence to care for himself and the graft. This program encompasses a holistic approach with dietary modifications, regular exercise programs, scheduled laboratory and diagnostic procedures, routine medical follow-up, and avoidance of known toxins that would compromise the graft or personal longevity (e.g., substance abuse). By accepting this organ Mr. H also made a promise to his family, the donor family, the transplant center, the community at large, and other potential transplant recipients not to minimize the sacrifices made by all concerned. Thus he cannot ignore the potential impact of his death or graft failure if he does not comply with his commitment to utilize his new lung to his maximum potential.

In deleting one of his immunosuppressants, Mr. H is putting himself at great risk for graft rejection, complications (e.g., an opportunistic infection associated with treating acute rejection, anaphylaxis from medications needed to treat a rejection episode), and possibly death. While this decision would satisfy the patient's right to exercise his own autonomy, he has a moral obligation to consider the impact of this decision on his family, the transplant center, and the community at large. Certainly mitigating circumstances might modify this commitment (e.g., developing metastatic cancer, or a devastating stroke); decisions regarding any modifications of this lifelong commitment cannot be made in a vacuum. But absent mitigating circumstances, patients' decisions cannot be made without due consideration of the consequences to all concerned.

Many transplant recipients are plagued by survivor's guilt. In one sense this stems from the issue of the donor's death in order that Mr. H might continue to live. In another sense Mr. H's continued survival places a huge economic burden on his family. His concern over the family's financial situation may represent a misplaced sense of moral obligation to unburden the family unit of these expenses. This concern does not, however, address the emotional impact of family grief in the event of Mr. H's demise, or the physical and emotional hardships the family would face if his quality of life declined.

Furthermore, since the viability of the medical center's transplant program hinges on patient outcomes, Mr. H is putting not only himself at risk, but future patients as well. To receive Medicare funding for transplantation, a medical center must meet strict objective outcome criteria. These criteria are based solely on patient survival. Medicare guidelines do not take into account any subjective data (i.e., patient financial status, time and distance the patient lives from the transplant center, family obligations, etc.). One patient's death could literally mean the demise of the center. If a regional transplant center closes (for lack of Medicare approval), other patients would face hardships in attaining transplants and follow-up care.

Medicare approval of a center generally marks the turning point in the financial viability of the transplant program. This is in large part because a significant number of lung transplant recipients are Medicare beneficiaries (due to disability rather than advanced age). Also, Medicare certification serves as a benchmark for negotiations with private insurers for Center of Excellence status. Center of Excellence status enables a facility to secure contracts with these insurers to provide transplant care to its members. This gives the center further financial stability by expanding the pool of patients eligible for treatment by that center.

If a center closes, patients currently wait-listed at the center would need to be referred to another facility. Since each center has its own specific acceptance criteria and expertise (e.g., the lung transplant center at Chapel Hill, North Carolina, has the most U.S. cystic fibrosis transplant experience and is therefore willing to accept more difficult cases), patients are not automatically accepted for transplantation at another center. Even though waiting times are transferable, patients could face much longer waiting times if the number of patients already listed at another facility is longer—and the longer the wait, the greater likelihood a patient will die waiting.

When Mr. H chooses to not comply with his medical therapy, he jeopardizes the lives of others.

The number of patients in a geographic area and the resources required (e.g., transplant immunologist, transplant pathologist) for a lung transplant program mandate that these facilities are located in large metropolitan areas. To make transplantation more widely accessible, many transplant centers establish outreach clinics in remote communities. In addition, with the advent of telemedicine, ultraspecialized care can be delivered at a local level. In communities that lack such arrangements, primary health care providers assume a greater role in providing transplant care. But often these providers do not have the extensive specialized knowledge to provide the complex medical management required by transplant patients.

Conversely, local providers may be more aware of unique opportunities that exist in smaller communities for assisting the transplant recipient. These may include support groups, financial aid, respite care for caregivers, transportation services, and in-home help. The pharmacist, for example, may be able to exploit a personal relationship with the pharmaceutical representative to enroll Mr. H in a medication assistance program or to arrange for samples of medication at no (or reduced) cost.

The pharmacist has a duty because of the requirements of his scope of practice to counsel Mr. H about the erroneous assumption that the other immunosuppressants will "pick up the slack." Failure to do so would make the pharmacist liable for negligent practice. Similarly, he also has an obligation to educate Mr. H about other alternatives to noncompliance that he can then discuss with his transplant physician. Though the pharmacist's legal liability extends primarily to the patient, his ethical liability is more encompassing. It embodies all of the tenets of medical ethics (beneficence, nonmaleficence, autonomy, and justice) and their application to the community, family, transplant center, etc.

Finally, Mr. H's decision has the potential for generating negative responses when families are approached for consent to organ donation. If donor families believe recipients will not take care of themselves after transplantation, the rate of donations may decline. This, of course, will adversely affect the already inadequate availability of organs needed for patients awaiting lung transplantation. As a member of the health care team, the pharmacist should work to avoid this harmful outcome.

RECOMMENDED READINGS

Lawrence, E. Clinton. "Ethical Issues in Lung Transplantation." *American Journal of Medical Science* 315, no. 3 (1997): 152–55.

Loewy, Erich H. *Textbook of Healthcare Ethics.* New York: Plenum Press, 1996.

Mekneally, Martin F. et al. "Bioethics for Clinicians: 13. Resource Allocation." *Canadian Medical Association Journal* 157 (1997): 163–67.

Note

1. Scientific Registry of Transplant Recipients, Health Resources and Services Administration (HRSA), "About Transplants: Fast Facts," n.d., http://www.ustransplant.org/facts.html (1 Aug. 2003). The statistics are based on data available from the Organ Procurement and Transplantation Network as of 31 October 2002.

An Ethicist's Analysis

Laura A. Siminoff, PhD, and Richard E. Morse, MA

Like many issues in bioethics, organ transplantation involves obligations both to individual patients and to society at large. Both of these obligations, however, depend on the way we conceive of our obligations to one another, to our community, and in turn what we expect our community owes to us as individuals. The dilemma faced by the pharmacist exemplifies a conflict of obligations. The pharmacist's response may have definitive consequences for Mr. H's immediate health, as well as for the continued survival of many in need of a transplant within the community. Therefore, we are left with several fundamental questions: What obligation does the pharmacist have to Mr. H? What responsibility, if any, does Mr. H assume by virtue of accepting a lung transplant? What role should the community play in ensuring Mr. H's continued health? Finally, how do we reconcile the conflicting commitments that arise within these obligations?

The Obligations of the Health Care Professional (HCP)

Transplantation is a complex enterprise that involves many areas of expertise. As such, successful transplantation relies on a myriad of health care professionals (HCPs). All have some responsibility in ensuring the continued success of the transplant system. In many situations, HCPs are confronted with dual obligations to individual patients and to the community, including other patients who have received a transplant and those who are still awaiting transplantation. Faced with these kinds of ethical dilemmas, HCPs are effectively asked to decide between the needs of patients and of the community.

In this case, the pharmacist is clearly cognizant of Mr. H's financial situation, but he is nonetheless concerned about the viability of the regional transplant center. Indeed, if Mr. H fails to take the prescribed immunosuppressants, it may seriously threaten the success of the transplant center and thus deny access to transplants for others in need. How then can the pharmacist serve his duty to Mr. H and still commit himself to the success of the transplant center?

First, the pharmacist has a professional obligation to inform and educate Mr. H of the potential consequences of his decision.[1] Mr. H holds unrealistic expectations about his ability to forgo his medications and still avoid graft rejection. The pharmacist has a duty to ensure that Mr. H appreciates the significance of his action. It may also be advisable to enlist the help of Mr. H's physician, who may be able to reinforce the pharmacist's message and may also be able to alter his drug regimen to include less expensive medications. In this way, it may be possible to meet both the needs of Mr. H and still preserve the success of the transplant program.

The Obligations of the Transplant Recipients

By all indications, Mr. H appears to have been an ideal candidate for the lung transplant. Indeed, during his first year after surgery, his progress has been good and he is tolerating his medications well. Mr. H appears to be a statistical success by those involved in his care. However, at some level, Mr. H's current failure to adhere to his medication regimen represents a threat not only to his immediate health, but also to those within the community who are concerned with the overall success of the transplant program. Therefore, to what extent should he be expected to adhere to his physician's recommendations, regardless of the social and financial costs to himself and his family?

Access to health care and related services in the United States has mostly relied on individuals' abilities to pay. Transplantation services and the prescription medications recipients rely on to maintain their grafts are poignant examples of health care costs because of the potential for death without continued expensive treatment, and because the patient has been the recipient of a scarce community good—the donor organ. Patients who are well insured and have considerable wealth have access to services to which many economically disadvantaged patients do not. Mr. H's dilemma in many ways is indicative of our society's priorities and commitments to those in need. Given his age and his family's financial situation, Mr. H fits within an unfortunate and growing subcategory of Americans who are neither wealthy enough to pay health expenses outright nor "unfortunate enough" to receive assistance under existing government-funded coverage systems.

While estimating the effects that his failure to adhere may have on his health is difficult, Mr. H's dilemma is not new nor unique to lung transplant patients. According to some estimates, nearly 50 percent of transplant patients have difficulty paying for prescription drugs.[2] On the other hand, data have shown that less than 10 percent of all graft failures result from patient nonadherence to drug therapy for any reason.[3] The extent to which impaired financial access leads to organ rejection is uncertain, as perfect adherence in no way guarantees success. Thus, the answer to the empirical (and utilitarian) question of whether to subsidize all prescription drug costs remains uncertain.

The Role of the Community

The role of the community in this case depends in large part on the perception of our obligations to one another. In the case of organ donation, the act of community members donating organs already speaks to some commitment on the community's part. Thus, it would seem that we have rejected the notion of community as merely individuals bound to one another by nothing more than an obligation of nonharm. Given the critical role of the community in providing transplantable organs, it would appear that the pharmacist has a significant obligation to ensure the future health of the community (in the form of the continuation of the transplant program). Moreover, Mr. H has already incurred a significant debt to the community that must be weighed along with his obligations to his family.

Conclusion

Transplantation evokes, as other health services have not, communitarian values.[4] The act of receiving and caring for a transplant must always be done with the realization that the community gave something to enable that transplant. Because of this, the health of the recipient is not simply one of concern about an individual patient, but that of the community. Thus, the pharmacist caring for Mr. H must not only act on behalf of the patient, but must also optimize strategies to ensure the continued interests of the community.

Notes

1. American Pharmacists Association, *Code of Ethics for Pharmacists* (adopted 27 October 1994), n.d., http://aphanet.org (at "About AphA"), (24 Mar. 2004).
2. American Society of Transplant Surgeons, "Survey of Present Status of Reimbursement for Immunosuppressive Drugs," Houston, TX, 1991, http://www.wws.princeton.edu/cgi-bin/byteserv.prl/~ota/disk1/1991/9133/913307.PDF (18 June 2003).
3. U.S. Congress, Office of Technology Assessment, *Outpatient Immunosuppressive Drugs Under Medicare* (Washington, DC: Government Printing Office, 1994).
4. James Childress, "Ethics and Allocation of Organs for Transplantation," *Kennedy Institute for Ethics Journal* 6 (1996): 397–401.

A Pharmacist's Analysis

Brian L. Kaatz, PharmD

The pharmacist in this scenario has an important role: providing the drugs and drug information related to a chronic and stable but very tenuous condition, namely lung transplant immunosuppression. Clearly, the therapeutic regimen in this case is critically important to the future well-being of Mr. H: mistakes or unwarranted changes in the way drugs are taken likely would have dramatically negative results, including organ rejection, which could be life-threatening. The pharmacist understands this, but Mr. H apparently does not.

Mr. H states he does not have the financial wherewithal to afford his entire regimen this month. His idea to modify the drug schedule to save money seems born more from of a lack of funds than any desire to compromise his own health or to be self-destructive. Although the natural progression of this increasingly common situation in the United States often ends in a fatality, there is no hint that this is Mr. H's intention. Simple education, then, will be the logical first step. It is imperative that Mr. H understands that any compromise in the prescribed drug regimen could be life-threatening, and the pharmacist must ascertain this understanding. In effect, this education will establish informed consent for the new (patient-initiated) regimen.

Should Mr. H persist in his plan to omit a key drug for a month, the pharmacist then must decide where his duty lies. He has a duty to two parties: the patient and the regional transplant center.

The pharmacist's duty to the patient is to maintain a covenantal relationship as outlined in the Code of Ethics for Pharmacists[1] and as developed in the concept of "pharmaceutical care."[2] Pharmacists have a moral obligation to be patient-centered and to actively promote optimal therapeutic outcomes on an individual basis. Thus, a pharmacist will not endorse a plan he knows will result in a poor outcome. There should be a bias for working to improve the patient's health care situation.

Complicating this, however, is a respect for autonomy. Appreciation for patient self-determination and the freedom to make one's own decisions is an important ethical mandate. This freedom has come to be regarded as an essential moral claim. It applies to a patient's decision to seek medical care in the first place, as well as choosing whether to adhere to recommended treatment, including medication therapy. Pharmacists and other health care personnel are trained to respect this mandate. If the pharmacist believes Mr. H clearly understands the ramifications of not taking Cellcept (the immunosuppresant) for a month, and that Mr. H has essentially given an "informed consent" for the consequences of his decision, the required action becomes less clear for the pharmacist. If Mr. H understands the likelihood of rejection and if he still maintains that his own best interest is to skip the drug, his decision is autonomous, if not entirely satisfactory from the pharmacist's viewpoint, and must be valued.

However, a second duty of the pharmacist is mentioned: the duty to the regional transplant center, which presumably is an important contributor to the health care needs of the area. Its longevity, in part, is dependent upon a statistical level of success which very well might be jeopardized by Mr. H's intent to modify his treatment.

Should the pharmacist notify the transplant center of Mr. H's apparent new plan? The answer to this question, from an ethical standpoint, has much to do with the pharmacist's motivation. If the reason to contact them is to shift the responsibility for what the patient does from the pharmacist to the transplant center, or if the reason is to increase pressure on the patient to do the "right thing," then the answer should be "no." The former reason abdicates the patient-pharmacist covenant and the latter violates the patient's autonomy.

On the other hand, if the reason to notify the center is to establish another means for obtaining positive patient-specific outcomes, then the rationale is ethically sound. Quite possibly the transplant center has resources to assist the pharmacist in his goal of improving the outcome for Mr. H. Indeed, in that respect the goals of the pharmacist and center are likely identical. However, the center's goals must be subordinated to *patient-specific* goals, should they conflict.

The pharmacist still should advocate for the patient's autonomous decision about whether to adhere to the drug regimen; but adding other pieces of information and another perspective might help him do that. The patient, however, should be told that the pharmacist is planning to notify the transplant center. Notification should not be done in a clandestine manner, working around the patient's wishes, but rather consistent with them.

Throughout all these transactions, the pharmacist's paramount goal should be to establish mutually acceptable goals with Mr. H, with his understanding and approval. The patient must completely understand the likely ramifications of his actions, and then be allowed to carry those out. Any measures taken by the pharmacist without a desire to fulfill the patient's best interests, both medically and ethically, are an *inappropriate* professional approach.

Notes

1. American Pharmacists Association, "Code of Ethics for Pharmacists" (adopted 27 Oct 1994), n.d., http://www.aphanet.org/pharmcare/ethics.html (26 Mar. 2004).
2. American Pharmacists Association, "Principles of Practice for Pharmaceutical Care" (approved August 1995), n.d., http://www.aphanet.org/pharmcare/princprac.html (26 Mar. 2004).

Further Reflections

General

1. Explicitly describe three actions the pharmacist could take to aid Mr. H. What moral principles support your recommendations?

Consequences

2. Commentators Siminoff and Morse and Hoso and Allen claim that Mr. H's noncompliance with his drug regimen jeopardizes not only his own life but the lives of others. What consequences to Mr. H, if any, might outweigh these negative effects to others?
3. Is patient survival the best criterion to use in determining whether a transplant center is eligible for Medicare funding? Why (not)?

Autonomy

4. Kaatz notes that ". . . freedom . . . applies to a patient's decision to seek medical care in the first place, as well as choosing whether to adhere to recommended treatment, including medication therapy." How does Kaatz's analysis

of the role of autonomy differ from that advanced by Siminoff and Morse and Hoso and Allen? Which analysis is more compelling? Why?

5. How should we understand the relationship of organ recipients to their health care professionals: as a nonbinding contract, the details of which are freely negotiated on an ongoing basis, or a binding contract where all parties have specific, particular, *nonnegotiable* obligations?

6. Hoso and Allen assert that "In accepting such a rare gift, Mr. H . . . committed himself to a lifelong program of strict adherence to care for himself and the graft." How is this responsibility justified? Is there any way for Mr. H to dispense with this obligation once the transplant occurs?

Rights

7. Do persons waiting for a transplant have a right to be aided? If so, what is it a right to? Do they have a right to not be harmed? Who has the responsibility to protect these rights? What is the relation of these rights to posttransplant patients' decisions to discontinue therapy?

Virtues

8. Siminoff and Morse claim that "the pharmacist has a significant obligation to ensure the future health of the community" [by doing what he can to increase patient compliance with the drug regimen]. Why does the pharmacist have this obligation? How might he ensure the health of the community?

9. Do transplant recipients implicitly promise to assume a "caretaker" attitude as a way of recognizing and thanking donor families? If so, what (if anything) might justify breaking this promise?

Equality/Fairness (Justice)

10. Many studies show that financially strapped people who are required to contribute a significant co-pay for medicines often simply forgo them. Is failure to provide ongoing financial support for posttransplant patients unjust? Would providing such support be unjust?

Chapter 11

Who Defines "Enough"?

Mr. and Mrs. N have been happily married for three years. They grew up in different Amish communities and married when they were both 19 years old. Both went to high school (somewhat unusual for Amish children, who often discontinue school after eighth grade) and had considered leaving the Amish faith to attend college. They had decided independently, however, that they were deeply tied to and identified by the Amish tradition. They valued the close, supportive community and its traditional way of life. They are now firmly entrenched in their culture and eagerly anticipate raising their children in its ways.

Mrs. N's first pregnancy was uncomplicated. Thus neither she nor her husband were prepared for the premature birth of their daughter. Mrs. N delivered their child after only 29 weeks of pregnancy. Tiny Anna was born weighing 1 pound, 3 ounces; she was quickly transferred to the Neonatal Intensive Care Unit (NICU) at the regional medical center.

Within the first 24 hours of her life, Anna suffered from respiratory arrest and a severe intracranial hemorrhage. Even with a ventilator, supplying Anna's vital organs (brain, kidneys, heart) with adequate oxygen was difficult. After one week she is deeply comatose and her kidneys are failing. Because infants are thought to be much more resilient to physiological insults (that is, better able to recover from trauma and disease) than are adults who face similar problems, Anna's physicians are unable to precisely predict the extent to which she will be incapacitated. Nonetheless, her physicians believe her prognosis is grave. Even if she survives, she is quite likely to be visually impaired (perhaps totally blind), unable to speak, to care for herself, perhaps even to recognize her parents. They are fairly certain she would require special schooling (not available in the

Amish community), and frequent medical care and hospitalization (also unavailable without traveling 50–75 miles—difficult for the Amish, who rely on horse-drawn carriages for transportation) to manage complications that are likely to result from the injuries resulting from her early birth. In any case, Anna will be hospitalized for several months, probably in the NICU or Pediatric ICU, until she is physiologically mature enough to go home.

Mr. and Mrs. N are devastated by the future Anna faces. They cannot imagine that they will be able to provide effectively for her needs. With an annual income of $3000 and no medical insurance (because the Amish faith rejects such things, including taking state Medicaid assistance), Mr. and Mrs. N despair of ever being able to afford the necessary care. Their community has rallied round them and will continue to support them and Anna in all ways possible; but the Ns fear that Anna's needs will exhaust the resources of their small colony (roughly 80 families). The cost of NICU alone, at $2700/day (not counting costs for medications, diagnostic tests, special equipment, physician's fees, etc.), is mind-boggling. The average cost of subsequent care for premature infants like Anna is roughly $100,000 per year—for each year of her life.

Mr. and Mrs. N discuss their plight with their community elders. The community has, on several previous occasions, raised thousands of dollars for medical bills of its members. Nor is the Amish community averse to the prospect of a severely disabled child in their midst; they have embraced disabled community members on many occasions. But in Anna's case the expenses are almost guaranteed to be overwhelming and Anna's disabilities threaten to be more so. Even if her current hospitalization could be covered, her continued care (if she lives) would far exceed communal resources, both financial and personal. Finally, rather than exhaust the community resources, Mr. and Mrs. N decide to forgo the medical treatment that might extend Anna's life. They request that all treatment, except medication to control any discomfort (e.g., pain, shortness of breath) Anna might experience, be discontinued. The community elders and dozens of community members are present and indicate their support for this request.

Several staff members wonder if the parents' request should be respected. They note that the parents are making this choice under extreme duress; that they were fully unprepared for this catastrophe, so are deciding "off the cuff" rather than as the result of cool-headed reflection. The staff also worry that the parents may be putting their own needs ahead of

Anna's. True, they seem fully focused on their daughter's needs, but virtually everyone would be daunted by the possibility of caring for a child with Anna's numerous (postulated) problems. Might they not be, if only unconsciously, trying to protect themselves from such a burden?

Other staff members wonder if cessation of treatment would violate the Americans with Disabilities Act or the Baby Doe Regulations (both of which forbid denying treatment solely on the basis of disability), or count as illegally endangering a child. They wonder if Child Protective Services, or perhaps the hospital's legal counsel, should be notified. After all, Anna's future condition cannot be predicted accurately. How, the staff wonder, can anyone say now that Anna's future life will be grim or unrewarding, or whether the community really will be unable to meet her needs?

From a moral point of view, should Mr. and Mrs. N's request be honored?

Introduction

This case raises three important moral issues:

1. Given the factual ambiguity surrounding Anna's prognosis, is a consequential analysis possible? If so, to whom may consequences legitimately be considered: the infant? the family? the Amish community? the disability community? health care professionals (HCPs)?
2. Who should have final decisional authority concerning treatment decisions of newborns: parents, the community, HCPs, society at large?
3. What criteria should form the basis for treatment decisions of high-risk newborns? In particular, should quality of life or economic costs ever be considered?

The AJ Method

Step 1: Information Gathering What facts are necessary for resolving this case? What are the actual deficits Anna currently faces? (Silvers) What is the future Anna will most likely face? (Silvers) Who is the appropriate decision maker about Anna's care? Are Anna's parents capable of autonomous decision making? What motivates their request to discontinue treatment? What motivates the HCPs to continue? What extended effects might this choice have (e.g., on persons with impairments)?

HCPs express great confidence regarding Anna's diagnosis, but virtually none about her prognosis. All parties deliberating Anna's plight have a moral obligation to "get the facts straight," but doing so may be impossible in this case. Anna's survival is uncertain, as are the nature, degree, and duration of the posited limitations—physical, cognitive, and emotional—she will experience if she does survive. The fact is, incontestible data are currently unavailable.

Step 2: Creative Problem Solving   Any creative solution would have to promote Anna's welfare and support the parents' autonomous choice.

Step 3: Pros and Cons   Survey CARVE principles to identify important moral reasons that support conflicting options for resolving this case.

Consequences   What are the effects of treatment on Anna, her parents, her Amish community, her HCPs, and society at large? (All commentators) Are these effects negative or positive? (Catlin, Settle, and Thiel; Gampel; Silvers) What are the effects of nontreatment on these parties? Are these effects negative or positive? What is the probability these outcomes will occur? (Silvers)

Effects of treatment choices are not limited to Anna. Parents of disabled children face significant burdens that not infrequently exhaust their physical and emotional resources. As a result, they forgo future opportunities, including having additional children. Are the Ns harmed if they cannot have the large family they desire and that is typical of the Amish? To whom do HCPs have obligations of beneficence and nonmaleficence? Surely to Anna, but what about her parents?[1] In making (non)treatment decisions should HCPs take account of the burdens of continuous child care and restricted future opportunity, transportation and separation from family and community, potential compromise of one's cultural and self-defining principles, forced and unwanted contact with the larger culture or the (perhaps unwanted) state support needed to provide care for the child Anna will become?[2]

What about the financial costs to a family and, by extension, to the close-knit community of which they are a part? Estimates of "average" costs vary and, in any case, have limited applicability to the costs of any particular child. What fiscal burdens can justifiably be placed on family and community members to save a child like Anna? Like others, the Ns and their community will have to forgo benefits—perhaps many or significant—to pay for Anna's needs.

What of the disability community? Does failing to treat newborns like Anna send a signal that disabled persons are "not worth saving"?[3] If so, are biases against disabled persons perpetuated, even aggravated, if HCPs cease treating any disabled newborn, such that they continue to be harmed by attitudes and obstructive social policies based thereon?

Finally, what of the HCPs themselves?[4] NICU nurses report "moral distress" from regularly participating in aggressive care for infants for whom they perceive care to be futile or cruel.[5] Which, if any, of these harms may be omitted from the consequential calculus undertaken in the NICU?

Autonomy   Who is the appropriate decision maker for Anna? (All commentators) Who is capable of autonomy? (Catlin, Settle, and Thiel; Harrison) Recall that autonomy protects not just discrete choices, but choices as means to promoting one's overall values and worldview. (Gampel; Girod)

When key facts are unavailable, decision makers must critically explore the ways in which information is gathered, communicated, and discussed. Thoughtful, well-informed, and morally satisfying decisions may require postulating—on the basis of best, if incomplete, information—multiple future scenarios to understand (non)treatment options. What information is essential to autonomous decision making? At the least, HCPs must articulate the *factual assumptions* about treatment outcomes (e.g., death or survival with mild, moderate, or profound disability). Informed consent must be educated consent; and educated consent requires as complete a picture, even if hypothetical, as possible of both future possibilities and their probabilities—as well as ensuring that decision makers appreciate that information.[6]

Equally important, all parties must consider a range of values and come to terms with their own value assumptions and those of others. Different parties will differently evaluate possible outcomes. Is *any* life worth living, or must a worthwhile life have a certain level of functional (physical/cognitive) capability? Both respect for persons and beneficence urge pursuing the patient's "best interests," but what counts as best interests is informed by other value commitments. To know what is really in a patient's best interests, one must grapple with issues such as whether life is sacred or has intrinsic value apart from its quality, and the nature of a meaningful life; and whether such a life requires a place in the community into which one is born (but which one has not autonomously chosen).

Put another way, we must consider *whose* definition of "a life worth living" should prevail. Even if we could achieve consensus—say, that the person living the life should determine its value—how would that consensus inform decision making for newborns who are unable to make such determinations? We cannot use personal autonomy as the standard because neonates have no self-reflective values. Parents' decisional authority typically extends to managing the affairs of their minor children, but the state can step in when parents fail to consider the welfare of their children. Then, too, we might look to evaluations made by persons (or their surrogates) whose lived experience incorporates disability, but here, too, evidence is ambiguous. While some surveys of even profoundly disabled children demonstrate that they rate their quality of life as very high,[7] those surveys are contested.[8]

What about decisional authority? Although Western medicine typically locates decisional authority in the individual patient, many communities subordinate the authority of the individual to the community.[9] What, if anything, morally justifies ignoring this alternative conception of decisional authority?

All parties in this case might autonomously agree to one moral obligation: do no harm. But, again, what will count as a harm? Surely pain and suffering to Anna should be minimized, but is saving her for a possible life of profound disability itself a harm, even if it is a harm outweighed by the benefit of life? Again, who should decide this question?

The personal and professional contexts out of which one comes—medicine, nursing, parenting, pastoral counseling, disability advocacy, (religious) community membership—profoundly influence one's definition not only of the good life, but also of appropriate decisional authority.[10] The team approach to caring for patients and families in NICUs, where information and decision making are shared and where sustained discussion generates better understanding, can ameliorate some of the distress surrounding treatment decisions. Misunderstanding, discomfort, a lack of trust, anger and resentment, feelings of isolation and confusion can be overcome by "taking care." But however caring they may be, a team whose members embrace disparate visions of the good life, of harms, or of appropriate decisional authority will have a hard row to hoe. Who, in the end, bears the moral responsibility for deciding what form Anna's care should take? The Amish community, accustomed to choosing with a view to group welfare? Society at large, concerned to protect *all* vulnerable persons and populations (as demonstrated by the Americans with Disabilities Act and the Baby Doe Regulations)? HCPs who suffer with babies like Anna and families like the Ns every single day? Helen Harrison argues that the parents, who will live most intimately with the outcomes, should decide. Jennifer Girod argues that the Amish community rightly informs the parents' decision. Eric Gampel worries that Anna's interests may be lost in the calculus and that, if this danger is real, HCPs should have the final word.

Rights Within the patient-professional relationship, Anna has a right to be aided by her HCPs. Do Anna's parents have this right? (Girod; Harrison) to the same degree? Anna and her parents both have a right to not be harmed, but what will count as harming her or them? (Harrison; Silvers) Anna has a right to self-determination, which is typically exercised for minors by their parents. (Gampel; Harrison)

Virtues Persons occupying various roles have role-related responsibilities. Parents have a role-related obligation of fidelity to promote their childrens' best interests. (Harrison; Silvers) HCPs have a role-related obligation of fidelity to promote their patients' best interests. (Catlin, Settle, and Thiel; Silvers) Members of communities have a role-related obligation of fidelity to factor in community interests when they conflict with their own. (Girod) Surely all parties should attend to Anna's needs with compassion. Does tolerance of or curiosity about the values of different communities or individuals require ceding decisional authority to those parties? What is the role of courage in this case?

Equality/Fairness (Justice) Is Anna being treated unfairly because if she lives she will be disabled? (Silvers) Are the parents being treated unfairly because of their community membership? Is the personal and financial burden Anna's parents and community will bear unfair? (Harrison) Would Anna's care unfairly deprive others of needed health care? (Gampel)

Even if we could agree on *who* has responsibility for decision making, we need to ask serious questions about the reasons people give for their decisions.[11]

Are specific justifications—for example, costs are too great—unfair to those who are, through no fault of their own, vulnerable? Are some visions of what we might want a child to "be"—or, more to the point, *not* "be"—morally impermissible? Are some projections of pain and suffering more than *any* child should have to "bear"? Is *any* decision that (apparently) disvalues disability inherently unjust?[12] As Harrison and as Catlin, Settle, and Thiel note, HCPs will not take home and raise the children they save. Is raising a child with some (unspecified) level of impairment unfair to the parents?

In a world of shared goals and values, some agreement on these issues is possible. But also, in a world of disparate perspectives, our moral reasoning and resources will sometimes seem impotent.[13] Each of the following commentators rules out various options for failing to respect some important value. If, as noted earlier, persons have radically differing definitions of a life worth living, how can consensus be achieved in particular cases? Tiny Anna demonstrates, in stark detail, how difficult moral dilemmas can be.

The Law   The following legal considerations are relevant to this case. (1) Are the parents, HCPs, or the hospital guilty of discrimination or of child abuse or endangerment if treatment and/or life support are discontinued in this case? (2) Is the decision to withdraw life-sustaining medical treatment from a child with this diagnosis and prognosis homicide?[14] Would cessation of treatment violate the Baby Doe Regulations? the Americans with Disabilities Act?

The following commentaries examine the application of various moral principles to this dilemma, thereby assisting the reader to undertake *Step 4: Analysis* and *Step 5: Justification*.

Recommended Readings

Paris, John J., Jeffrey Ferranti, and Frank Reardon. "From the Johns Hopkins Baby to Baby Miller: What Have We Learned from Four Decades of Reflection on Neonatal Cases? *The Journal of Clinical Ethics* 12, no. 3 (2001): 207–14.

Waltman, Gretchen H. "Amish Health Care Beliefs and Practices." In *Multicultural Awareness in the Health Care Professions*. Ed. Maria C. Juliá. Boston: Allyn and Bacon, 1996, 23–41.

Notes

1. For a poignant description of a family's struggle with a child like Anna, see Robert and Peggy Stinson, *The Long Dying of Baby Andrew* (New York: Atlantic–Little, Brown, 1983).
2. John Hardwig, "What About the Family?" *Hastings Center Report* 20, no. 2 (1990): 5–10; James Lindemann Nelson, "Taking Families Seriously," *Hastings Center Report* 22, no. 4 (1992): 6–12; Jeffrey Blustein, "The Family in Medical Decisionmaking," *Hastings Center Report* 23, no. 3 (1993): 6–13. But cf. Insoo Hyun, "Conceptions of Family-Centered Medical Decisionmaking and Their Difficulties," *Cambridge Quarterly of Healthcare Ethics* 12, no. 2 (2003): 196–200.

3. Anita Silvers, "Formal Justice," in *Disability, Difference, and Discrimination,* eds. Anita Silvers, David Wasserman, and Mary Mahowald (Lanham, MD: Rowman & Littlefield, 1998), 13–145; and Sara Goering, "Beyond the Medical Model? Disability, Formal Justice, and the Exception for the 'Profoundly Impaired,'" *Kennedy Institute of Ethics Journal* 12, no. 4 (2002): 373–88.

4. For a general discussion of issues facing HCPs in the NICU, see Hazel E. McHaffie and Peter W. Fowlie, "Impairments and Disabilities," and "Parental Involvement in Decision Making," in *Life, Death and Decisions: Doctors and Nurses Reflect on Neonatal Practice* (Manchester, England: Hochland & Hochland Limited, 1996), 94–107, 179–215.

5. Pam Hefferman and Steve Heilig, "Giving 'Moral Distress' a Voice": Ethical Concerns among Neonatal Intensive Care Unit Personnel," *Cambridge Quarterly of Healthcare Ethics* 8, no. 2 (1999): 173–78.

6. Ruth R. Faden and Tom L. Beauchamp, *A History and Theory of Informed Consent* (New York: Oxford University Press, 1986), 298–336; but see Berit Støre Brinchmann, Reidun Førde, and Per Nortvedt, "What Matters to the Parents? A Qualitative Study of Parents' Experiences with Life-and-Death Decisions Concerning Their Premature Infants," *Nursing Ethics* 9, no. 4 (2002): 388–404.

7. Saroj Saigal et al., "Self-perceived Health Status and Health-related Quality of Life of Extremely Low-birth-weight Infants at Adolescence," *JAMA: Journal of the American Medical Association* 276, no. 7 (1996): 453–59; Cedar Rapids Community School Dist. v. Garret F., 526 U.S. 66 (1999), 106 F.3d 822, affirmed.

8. Helen Harrison, "Making Lemonade: A Parent's View of 'Quality of Life' Studies," *The Journal of Clinical Ethics* 12, no. 3 (2001): 239–50; Karen Smith and Mary Ellen Uphoff, "Uncharted Terrain: Dilemmas Born in the NICU Grow Up in the PICU," *The Journal of Clinical Ethics* 12, no. 3 (2001): 231–38.

9. Leslie J. Blackhall et al., "Ethnicity and Attitudes toward Patient Autonomy," *JAMA: Journal of the American Medical Association* 274, no. 10 (1995): 820–25; Lawrence O. Gostin, "Informed Consent, Cultural Sensitivity, and Respect for Persons," *JAMA: Journal of the American Medical Association* 274 (1995): 844–45.

10. See Gostin, note 9, above.

11. Jonathan Muraskas et al., "Neonatal Viability in the 1990s: Held Hostage by Technology," *Cambridge Quarterly of Healthcare Ethics* 8, no. 2 (1999): 160–70.

12. See Silvers, note 3, above.

13. Enrico Chiavacci, "From Medical Deontology to Bioethics: The Problem of Social Consensus of Basic Ethical Issues Within Western Culture and Beyond It in the Human Family," in *Transcultural Dimensions in Medical Ethics,* eds. Edmund Pellegrino, Patricia Mazzarella, and Pietro Corsi (Frederick, MD: University Publishing Group, 1992), esp. 94–103.

14. For a number of recent legislative initiatives and federal regulations that have shaped the legal landscape in these sorts of cases, see Jerry Menikoff, *Law and Bioethics* (Washington, DC: Georgetown University Press, 2001), Chap. 12, "Futile Medical Care," 356–77. The Baby Doe Regulations (eventually subsumed under the 1984 Amendments to the Child Abuse Prevention and Treatment Act, 42 U.S.C.S. § 5102) stipulate the way in which best interest standards should inform treatment abatement decisions; the mandated treatment that should be provided to seriously ill/disabled newborns; and whether parents should be allowed to decide on the treatment provided to their seriously ill/disabled child. Additionally, the Americans with Disabilities Act of 1990 (42 U.S.C.S. § 12101) requires that individuals with disabilities be afforded equal opportunity in the areas of public life, including medical services. The ADA defines disabilities broadly and mandates significant efforts to provide reasonable accommodation and access to services. Though discussion of the

implications of this legislation for the treatment of severely ill/disabled newborns is sketchy, see American Medical Association, Council on Ethical and Judicial Affairs, *Code of Medical Ethics: Current Opinions with Annotations,* 2000–2001 Edition (Chicago: American Medical Association, 2000), § 2.17 "Quality of Life," 50–52; § 2.20 "Withholding or Withdrawing Life-Sustaining Medical Treatment," 55–71; and § 2.215 "Treatment Decisions for Seriously Ill Newborns," 79. Legal and ethical intersections, as well as issues related to decision-making authority and resource allocation are discussed by Pauline Challinor Mifflin, *Saving Very Premature Babies: Key Ethical Issues* (Edinburgh: Elsevier Science Limited, 2003), especially Chap. 6, "The Legal Framework," 59–77. Though more conceptual, Lainie Friedman Ross, *Children, Families, and Health Care Decision-Making* (Oxford, England: Clarendon Press, 1998), Chap. 7, "The Child as Patient," 131–51, and discussion of relevant court cases, 134–35, provides important insights.

A Parent's Analysis

Helen Harrison

By tradition and law, patients or their surrogates (parents in the case of infant patients) may refuse medical treatment, including life-sustaining care, if, in their reasonable judgment, the burdens of treatment outweigh the benefits.[1] However, health care providers, acting from personal beliefs or professional interests, vary in their willingness to honor the wishes of patients and surrogates.[2]

Ethical guidelines drafted by physicians,[3] by professional/lay collaborations,[4] and by experienced parents[5] describe situations in which the benefits of intensive care are doubtful, and life-sustaining care is, therefore, optional. Baby Anna, with her extremely low birth weight (539 grams), severe brain hemorrhage, poor response to treatment, and grave prognosis, is well within the "gray area" described in these documents in which parental decision making is appropriate.

Public opinion supports the parents' right to decide. Surveys show 70 percent to 86 percent of those polled would want the right to refuse life-sustaining care for a child with Anna's prognosis.[6] Eighty-nine percent of critically ill adult patients would also decline life-saving treatment for themselves if they risked an outcome similar to that predicted for Anna.[7] Family burden, in the view of 76 percent, is an important consideration in decision-making.[8] Roman Catholic ethicists cite excessive pain, risk, and expense, as well as patient or family "burden," as legitimate reasons to refuse life sustaining treatment.[9] The American Academy of Pediatrics has written: "Because the families bear the emotional and financial consequences of the birth of an extremely low-birth-weight infant, it is essential to inform [them] . . . regarding the expectations for infant outcome and the risks and benefits of various approaches to care."[10]

Anna's parents have been informed and, in close consultation with their community, have chosen comfort care for their daughter—pain relief, removal from life support, and a natural death.

The staff suggest that Anna's parents may be acting without cool-headed reflection and from selfish motives. However, staff members base their hopes for Anna's future on the false, but common, belief that infants are more resilient to trauma, especially trauma to the brain, than older patients.[11] And the staff may, themselves, have self-interested motives in continuing intensive care for a child with such a poor prognosis. Revenues from neonatal intensive care units (NICUs)—referred to as "profit centers"—provide crucial financial support for many hospitals.[12] Intensivists prosper[13] as they bask in personal and professional glory at the "miraculous" rescue of a marginally viable infant.[14]

Neonatal caregivers often indicate they would refuse the same treatments for their own marginally viable newborns that they routinely administer to other people's children.[15] But when parents in their units object to treatment, physicians may, as in this case, invoke the "Baby Doe" amendments to the Federal Child Abuse Act. These amendments mandate life-saving care in almost every case, a standard which conflicts with many state laws and with recent court decisions.[16] Ironically, the Baby Doe regulations, intended to protect the rights of handicapped infants, may actually discriminate against these infants by denying them the legal right granted to all other incompetent patients to refuse treatment through a surrogate.[17] Two-thirds of physicians polled believe that the regulations fail to consider the suffering of infants or the rights of parents.[18] It has been suggested that the regulations may actually become an instrument of child abuse ". . . prolonging dying under conditions of a brutal intensive care from which there is no escape."[19]

If the staff prevail, Anna will continue to endure arduous treatments that, like most of NICU care, have never been properly tested for safety or efficacy.[20] The acute and chronic pain of these treatments may be sufficiently stressful to worsen her brain damage or cause her death.[21] The costs of her immediate care may well exceed a million dollars.[22]

In the unlikely event that Anna survives, she may remain dependent on medical technology (ventilator, oxygen, tracheotomy, gastrostomy, ventriculo-perintoneal shunt). Her parents (without electricity or modern transportation) will almost certainly need to institutionalize their daughter or relinquish their Amish way of life to care for her.

Even urban affluent families find that providing lifelong care for such a child involves severe burdens: the anguish of coping with a constantly suffering child, the loss of health insurance and of health, bankruptcy, sibling neglect, the need to forgo future childbearing, divorce, mental and physical breakdown, suicide, mercy killing, or the abandonment of their child to institutional care.[23] Those who are eligible for government-funded services often find they are of extremely poor quality if they exist at all.[24] Parents feel isolated and ostracized by friends and family,[25] and by communities and school systems[26] that are unable or unwilling to help. Even parents who can obtain rigorous, costly rehabilitative therapies soon discover that they provide no proven benefit to disabled children.[27] Parents also feel abandoned by the medical profession, once eager to perform heroic care for their neonates, but now unenthusiastic about the unglamorous and less remunerative post-NICU care.[28] The difficult and mysterious ailments that afflict these children as they age are simply beyond the scope of most physicians, and good medical care may be unavailable at any price.[29]

At least Anna's parents have a supportive community willing to face the future and discuss life-and-death decisions with candor, realism, and compassion. By contrast, staff objections to the parents' decision are based on medical myth, a dismissive attitude toward the parents and their advisers, and on the Baby Doe regulations—selectively enforced rules of dubious legality,[30] which have been denounced as "abusive."[31] Although the staff may benefit financially and professionally from Anna's treatment and may chalk up another "save" for their statistics, they will not be around to witness the pain or bear the burdens of this child's life. The parents' decision is reasonable, ethically appropriate, moral, and, almost certainly, legal. It is time to begin Anna's comfort care.

Notes

1. President's Commission for the Study of Ethical Problems in Medicine and Biomedical and Behavioral Research, *Deciding to Forego Life-Sustaining Treatment: A Report on the Ethical, Medical, and Legal Issues in Treatment Decisions* (Washington, DC: US Government Printing Office, 1983), 195–229; Frank I. Clark, "Intensive Care Treatment Decisions: The Roots of Our Confusion," *Pediatrics* 94 (1994): 98–101.

2. John J. Paris, Jeffrey Ferranti, and Frank Reardon, "From the Johns Hopkins Baby to Baby Miller: What Have We Learned from Four Decades of Reflection on Neonatal Cases?" *The Journal of Clinical Ethics* 12 (2001): 207–14; SUPPORT (The Study to Understand Prognoses and Preferences for Outcomes and Risks of Treatments) Principle Investigators, "A Controlled Trial to Improve Care for Seriously Ill Hospitalized Patients," *JAMA: Journal of the American Medical Association* 274 (1995): 1591–98; Deborah J. Cook et al. for the Canadian Critical Care Trials Group, "Determinants in Canadian Healthcare Workers of the Decision to Withdraw Life Support from the Critically Ill," *JAMA: Journal of the American Medical Association* 273 (1995): 703–08; Thomas J. Simpson, "Response to 'Neonatal Viability in the 1990s: Held Hostage by Technology' by Jonathan Muraskas et al. and "Giving 'Moral Distress' a Voice: Ethical Concerns among Neonatal Intensive Care Unit Personnel" by Pam Hefferman and Steve Heilig (CQ vol. 8, no. 2): Navigating Turbulent and Uncharted Waters," *Cambridge Quarterly of Healthcare Ethics* 8 (1999): 524–26.

3. Jon Tyson, "Evidence-based Ethics and the Care of Premature Infants," *The Future of Children* 5 (1995): 197–213, http://www.futureofchildren.org (6 Apr. 2004); and California Association of Neonatologists, "Guidelines for Neonates at the Threshold of Viability," February 18, 1996, http://cansite.org (30 Mar. 2004).

4. Wisconsin Association for Perinatal Care (1010 Mound Street, Madison, WI 53715), "Position Statement: Guidelines for the Responsible Utilization of Neonatal Intensive Care," 1997, 1–8; CCMD (Colorado Collective for Medical Decision Making (777 Grant Street, Suite 206, Denver, CO 80203), "Guidelines for the Management of Low Birth Weight/Early Gestational Age Newborns: Revised Neonatal Guidelines," 20 March 1997.

5. Helen Harrison, "The Principles for Family-Centered Neonatal Care," *Pediatrics* 92 (1993): 643–50.

6. Humphrey Taylor, "Withholding and Withdrawal of Life Support from the Critically Ill," *New England Journal of Medicine* 322 (1990): 1891–92; Frederick R. Abrams et al.,

Colorado Speaks out on Health: The Final Report of a Two-year Educational Program and Study of Public Opinion on Critical Care Issues (Denver: Colorado Speaks Out on Health, 1988), 7–8.

7. Terri R. Fried et al., "Understanding the Treatment Preferences of Seriously Ill Patients," *New England Journal of Medicine* 346 (2002): 1061–66.

8. See Abrams, note 6, above.

9. *Declaration on Euthanasia,* adopted by the Sacred Congregation for the Doctrine of the Faith, approved by Pope John Paul II, released to the public 26 June 1980; Pope Pius XII, "The Prolongation of Life," in *Ethics in Medicine: Historical Perspectives and Contemporary Concerns,* eds. Stanley J. Reiser, Arthur J. Dyck, and William J. Curran (Cambridge: MIT Press, 1977), 393–96; David L. Oskandy, *Severely Defective Newborns: The Catholic Physician's Dilemma* (St. Louis: The Catholic Health Association of the United States, 1985), 9–11.

10. American Academy of Pediatrics, Committee on Fetus and Newborn, American College of Obstetricians and Gynecologists, Committee on Obstetric Practice, "Perinatal Care at the Threshold of Viability," *Pediatrics* 96 (1995): 974–76.

11. Jerome Y. Yager and Jim A. Thornhill, "The Effect of Age on Susceptibility to Hypoxic-ischemic Brain Damage," *Neuroscience & Biobehavioral Reviews* 21 (1997): 167–74; John D. Lantos, M. Corpus, and William Meadow, "Pediatric Academic Medical Centers' Increasing Dependence on NICUs: Joan of Arc or Thelma and Louise?" *Pediatric Research* 47 (2000): 316A.

12. Lagnado L. Deja, "In a Poor Baby's Fight to Survive, a Parable of a Medicaid HMO," *The Wall Street Journal,* 27 Dec. 2000, A1, A6; William A. Silverman, "Lifesavers," in *Where's The Evidence? Debates in Modern Medicine* (New York: Oxford University Press, 1998), 85–88; M.R. Sanders et al., "Perceptions of the Limit of Viability: Neonatologists' Attitudes Toward Extremely Preterm Infants," *Journal of Perinatology* 15 (1995): 494–502.

13. See Simpson, note 2, above.

14. Pam Hefferman and Steve Heilig, "Giving 'Moral Distress' a Voice: Ethical Concerns among Neonatal Intensive Care Personnel," *Cambridge Quarterly of Healthcare Ethics* 8, no. 2 (1996): 173–78.

15. Hazel E. McHaffie and Peter W. Fowlie, *Life, Death, and Decisions: Doctors and Nurses Reflect on Neonatal Practice* (Cheshire, England: Hoachland & Hoachland, 1995), 84; Helen Harrison, "Making Lemonade: A Parent's View of 'Quality of Life' Studies," *The Journal of Clinical Ethics* 12 (2001): 239–50; Marcia Angell, "The Baby Doe Rules," *New England Journal of Medicine* 314 (1986): 642–46; Loretta M. Kopelman, Thomas G. Irons, and Arthur E. Kopelman, "Neonatologists Judge the 'Baby Doe' Regulations," *New England Journal of Medicine* 318 (1988): 677–83.

16. See Clark, note 1, above.

17. Joy H. Penticuff, "The Impact of the Child Abuse Amendments on Nursing Staff and Their Care of Handicapped Newborns," in *Compelled Compassion,* eds. Arthur L. Caplan, Robert H. Blank, and Janna C. Merrick (Totowa, NJ: Humana Press, 1992), 267–84.

18. William A. Silverman, *Retrolental Fibroplasia: A Modern Parable* (New York: Grune & Stratton, 1980).

19. Helen Harrison, "Preemies on Steroids: A New Iatrogenic Disaster?" *Birth* 28 (2001): 57–59.

20. See note 5; eds. Bonnie Stevens and Ruth E. Grunau, "Pain in Vulnerable Infants," *Clinics in Perinatology* 29 (2002); Jeffrey J. Pomerance, L.J. Pomerance, and J.A. Gottlieb, "Cost of Caring for Infants Weighing 500–749g at Birth," *Pediatric Research* 33 (1993): 231A; U.S. Department of Health and Human Services, Agency for Healthcare Policy and Research, "High Costs of Caring for a Disabled Family Member May Negatively Affect Receipt of Needed Care for Other Family Members," *AHCPR Research Activities* 226 (1999): 8.

21. Gloria Culver et al., Informed Decisions for Extremely-Low-Birth-Weight Infants (letter), *JAMA: Journal of the American Medical Association.* 283 (2000): 3201–02.

22. Jimmy J. Barthel, "Should He Have Been Allowed to Live?" *McCalls,* Nov. 1985: 109–11, 156–61.

23. See Kopelman, note 15, above; S. Eikner, "Dealing with Long-term Problems: A Parent's Perspective," *Neonatal Network* 5 (1986): 45–49; Nancy Montalvo and Brian P. Vila, "Parent's Grand Rounds Speech on Neonatal Intensive Care Unit Experience," *Journal of Perinatology* 19 (1999): 525–27; Nancy Montalvo and Brian P. Vila, "Response to letter to editor by Charles Rait, RN, (*Journal of Perinatology* 20 (2000): 143–45)," *Journal of Perinatology* 20 (2000): 399–403; Canadian Press, "Mother Found Dead with Son Denied Funds," *Globe and Mail,* 7 Dec. 1994, A5; A. Jacobs, "Pennsylvania Couple Accused of Abandoning Their Disabled Son," *New York Times,* 30 Dec. 1999; C.U. Battle, "Beyond the Nursery Door: The Obligation to Survivors of Technology," *Clinical Perinatology* 14 (1987): 417–27; C. Trost, "Prisoners of Technology: Modern Science Has Rescued These Children, but for What Kind of Life?" *The Wall Street Journal,* 13 Nov. 1989, R25; J. Ryan, "Caught Between Exhaustion and Love," *San Francisco Chronicle,* 16 Jan. 2003, D-4; Anne Mitchell, "I Can't Hate the Kelsos," 4 Jan. 2000, http://www.dir.salon.com/mwt/feature/2000/01/05/kelsos/index.html (6 Apr. 2004); Helen Featherstone, *"A Difference in the Family: Living with a Disabled Child* (New York: Penguin Books, 1980).

24. Sam Allis, "The Struggle to Pay for Special Ed," *Time,* 4 Nov. 1996, 82–83; Cecilia M. McCarton et al. for the Infant Health and Development Program Research Group, "Results at Age 8 Years of Early Intervention for Low-Birth-Weight Premature Infants: The Infant Health and Development Program," *JAMA: Journal of the American Medical Association* 277 (1997): 126–32.

25. See Canadian Press, note 23, above; Alfred A. Baumeister and Verne R. Bachrach, "A Critical Analysis of the Infant Health and Development Program, *Intelligence* 23 (1996): 79–104.

26. Frederick B. Palmer et al., "The Effects of Physical Therapy on Cerebral Palsy: A Controlled Trial in Infants with Spastic Diplegia," *New England Journal of Medicine* 318 (1988): 803–8.

27. Alan D. Rothberg et al., "Six Year Follow-up of Early Physiotherapy Intervention in Very Low Birth Weight Infants," *Pediatrics* 88 (1991): 547–52; E. Tirosh and S. Rabino, "Physiotherapy for Children with Cerebral Palsy," *AJDC* 143 (1989): 552-55; Robert E. Arendt, William E. MacLean, and Alfred A. Baumeister, "Critique of Sensory Integration Therapy and Its Application in Mental Retardation," *American Journal on Mental Retardation* 92 (1988): 401-11; Theodore P. Hoehn and Alfred A. Baumeister, "A Critique of the Application of Sensory Integration Therapy to Children with Learning Disabilities," *Journal of Learning Disabilities* 27 (1994): 338–50; Jean-Paul Collet et al., "Hyperbaric Oxygen Therapy for Children with Cerebral Palsy: A Randomized Multicentre Trial," *The Lancet* 357 (2001): 582–86.

28. See Stevens, note 20, above; see Montalvo and Vila, both citations, note 23, above.

29. Ibid.

30. See Clark, note 1, above.

31. See notes 17–19, above.

A Nurse Ethicist's Analysis

Jennifer Girod, PhD, RN

Modern medicine is currently able to save the lives of many critically ill individuals, although many of those individuals are left with significant disabilities that require extremely expensive and time-consuming lifelong care. Anna N's case is a perfect illustration of this ambiguous success. Because her family is Amish, her case also dramatically illustrates the burdens such a life can impose on an entire community. In Anna's case, I believe her parents are making a responsible, considered decision in the context of a compassionate and supportive community and that the staff should respect their decision.

The Amish are committed to helping one another in all kinds of crises. This commitment is embodied in their tradition of Mutual Aid, which has been present in the Anabaptist community since its founding.[1] Help with medical expenses and caregiving has always been one feature of their Mutual Aid commitment.[2] When individual families can't afford to pay their medical bills, the deacon of the community collects funds within the community and from neighboring Amish communities. When these efforts fall short, he will secure funds through bank loans.[3]

In addition to financial support, practical help is offered by the community in many forms. Visitors at the hospital are common, even though the Amish must hire a car and driver to get there. While families are at the hospital, others take care of their businesses. When they are home, they receive help cooking, cleaning, and taking care of their homes. This often includes young children (nieces and nephews) who can provide an extra set of hands or save a few steps.[4] In the event of a death, nonfamily community members plan the funeral, prepare the grave, and bury the body. They then increase acts of fellowship and charity for a full year following death.[5]

Until very recently, Amish communities have been able to raise enough funds to care for their members' medical needs without sustaining any debt. The costs of some recent treatments such as Anna's, however, are so high that the ability to attend to other community needs—such as building schools and caring for the poor—is threatened.[6] One alternative is to begin accepting private or governmental insurance. However, the threat this brings to the community may be even more serious than the specter of debt. The acceptance of insurance would break down boundaries that keep the Amish community separate from the larger society, which may make the community less distinct. It may endanger some of the exemptions (such as not paying Social Security tax) the Amish have won precisely because they have not accepted Medicare and Medicaid.[7] In addition, the Amish worry that depending on outsiders would decrease the interdependence inside the community.

Individuals and families in an Amish community are expected to submit their will and interests to the good of the community. The harmony that results from this attitude of submission (*Gelassenheit*) is necessary because the Amish believe that community purity is necessary for individual salvation. That is, the Amish create a redemptive community (*Gemeinde*) when they practice the true principles of Christianity as they understand them (including separation from the non-Amish world).[8] Thus it is natural that a family like the Ns would consider how Anna's care would affect the whole community.

What might bother some staff members about the Ns' decision to discontinue treatment is that it is presented in a way that suggests it is based more on the burdens to the family and the community than on burdens to Anna herself. However, it is unlikely that the Ns fear caring for Anna. The Ns would be supported both financially and emotionally by their community if they chose to continue medically supporting Anna. However, the intimacy of that community also makes the Ns aware of the collective sacrifices that would be necessary to help their child. The time-consuming nature of Anna's care will decrease the amount of time her family can contribute to others in the community, and will most likely result in lifelong financial dependence on the community. Although there is no stigma placed on poor families by others within the community, many families will feel some shame at being in this position.[9]

In addition, the Ns' concerns will necessarily extend to others within the community. Not only do they care about other members of the church who might be burdened (family, friends, and neighbors); it is also necessary for them to put the survival and holiness of the church above their own needs. Although they are unlikely to be told not to pursue certain medical treatments for themselves or their children, their fundamental commitment to the well-being and survival of the community will make them consider their own interests from this perspective.

Although it is easier to understand the Ns' reasoning when we look at their religious tradition, it does not settle questions about whether or not they should be allowed to refuse care for their children because of high medical costs. In this case, however, any family would likely be given broad decision-making discretion due to the nature of Anna's condition and her bleak prognosis. Although it is impossible to predict outcomes precisely, her physicians anticipate many serious obstacles to a good quality of life if she survives. Anna's prognosis is sufficiently bleak that her parents could reasonably argue against further treatment based on her interests alone. The issue would be different if her care were expensive but her prognosis were better.

Is a family or community permitted to limit medical care for its members for financial reasons? I think the answer must be "yes" for the Amish. They have created and sustained an alternative religious community that embodies compassionate care for all its members in an extraordinary manner. If they decide that a financial burden associated with medical care threatens the viability of their community, we should respect that decision rather than encourage them to follow us down our path of providing extravagant and expensive medical care.

Notes

1. John A. Hostetler, *Amish Society,* 4th ed. (Baltimore: Johns Hopkins University Press, 1993).
2. Ibid.
3. Jennifer Girod, "A Sustainable Medicine: Lessons from the Old Order Amish," *Journal of Medical Humanities* 23, no. 1 (2002): 31–42.
4. Ibid.
5. Kathleen B. Bryer, "The Amish Way of Death: A Study of Family Support Systems," *American Psychologist* 34, no. 3 (1979): 255–61.
6. Ibid.
7. Donald B. Kraybill, ed., *The Amish and the State* (Baltimore: Johns Hopkins University Press, 1993).
8. See note 1, above.
9. See note 3, above.

A Neonatal Intensive Care Unit (NICU) Analysis

Elizabeth A. Catlin, MD, Margaret Doyle Settle, RNC, MS, and Mary Martha Thiel, MDiv

And now here is my secret, a very simple secret: It is only with the heart that one can see rightly; what is essential is invisible to the eye.

ANTOINE DE SAINT EXUPÈRY, *THE LITTLE PRINCE**

Anna's short life has been complicated and tragic. Physicians and nurses caring for this infant must consider three key areas as they struggle, together with her parents, to make medically appropriate, compassionate, and moral decisions. They must understand: (1) accurate, pertinent medical data, (2) sociocultural, ethical, legal, and religious principles, especially as they relate to this infant's Amish family, and (3) the substance and quality of the nurse-parent-physician relationships.[1]

A first step in this analysis is to review relevant medical data to build a foundation for subsequent decision making. The majority of neonates born at 29 weeks of gestation survive.[2] Anna developed multiple medical complications, including a severe intracranial hemorrhage. Catastrophic syndromes of intracranial hemorrhage are associated with high mortality or profound morbidity because effective treatment doesn't exist.[3] Anna is very growth restricted; a birth weight of 1 pound, 3 ounces indicates that prior to birth she was a very ill fetus. After one week of maximal support she is gravely ill, comatose, and ventilator dependent, with renal

---

*Antoine de Saint Exupèry, *The Little Prince*, trans. Katherine Woods (New York: Harcourt, Brace, and Company, 1943), 70.

insufficiency. This picture of extensive multi-organ system failure raises concerns that continued aggressive treatment might not confer clear benefit, except to sustain biological existence.

The burdens of aggressive treatment are many for the baby: pain, suffering, and discomfort caused by invasive tests, tubes, needles, and catheters entering her body, and the constant forced breaths of the mechanical ventilator. Considerations regarding appropriate treatment, limiting resuscitation, and withdrawing mechanical supports are complex, painful, and stressful for parents and health care providers (HCPs).[4] Nonetheless, in some circumstances, limiting or stopping life-sustaining medical treatment may be appropriate.[5]

Parents are assumed to be the most appropriate decision makers for their babies. This assumption differs from earlier paternalistic practice where life-and death-decisions were made by the physician.[6] Because neonates are unable to articulate decisions, neither the autonomy principle nor substituted judgment is applicable in decision making. Parents, as surrogate decision makers, and HCPs must rely on the best interest standard.[7] This approach, whereby parents, together with physicians and nurses, make reasoned decisions about care for their critically ill newborn, is supported in practice and policy.[8] Anna's parents have met with staff, consulted with Amish community members, and concluded that treatment should be stopped.

The next step is to use sociocultural, ethical, legal, and religious considerations to understand *why* her family has made this request. In this instance, a very unusual set of reasons is provided: predicted financial expense for the baby's current and future care.

The cultural context of parenting and decision making for Anna's family is the Amish tradition, a Protestant Christian denomination with distinct theological beliefs and strong community values. The Amish community embraces members with ongoing medical needs and are said not to consider children "troubling" in any way.[9] Amish child care needs are supported by the extended family or church community, groups which overlap in membership.[10] Amish parents commonly believe that every child is a gift from God. Amish communities often show an exemplary willingness to love and honor "special needs" children and to integrate them fully into daily life. The response of Anna's parents to this dilemma is atypical. We make this observation, not to rely on stereotypic interpretation of the Amish, but to highlight this unexpected response as a focal point to be explored in further communications.

The third focus is nurse-parent-physician relationships. Neonatologists and neonatal nurses have a fundamental moral obligation to care for and protect infant patients. However, our infant patients are not our children. We must be vigilant not to supercede parental authority, except in unusual cases. The health team for Anna (and each infant) must establish a mechanism to communicate with parents to convey data, caring, and compassion. HCPs must create an atmosphere of trust as they build relationships with parents; without trust, communication and mutual decision making are difficult.

In our practice, we use the team meeting followed by family meeting format[11] with an emphasis on pastoral resources.[12] All HCPs provide input during the broader team meeting. Once consensus is reached, the attending neonatologist, primary nurse, social worker, and, at times, clergy/chaplain join the parents for definitive family meeting(s).

The entire NICU care team plays a critical role in providing a consistent, supportive environment for parents who are frightened and distressed. In Anna's case, the team has not provided a consistent, supportive, setting. In fact, the staff is demonstrably fragmented. This case and the resulting lack of consensus likely represent a 'critical incident' for this NICU.[13] As such, nursing and medical leadership (the NICU nurse manager, the medical director of the NICU, and Anna's attending neonatologist) must respond by providing structure, support, debriefings, and clear communication avenues.

The ethical dilemmas that we encounter in caring for critically ill neonates change over time as technology advances and our culture evolves. Responses of caregivers change, as well.[14] Baby Doe regulations, enacted nearly 20 years ago, mandated best medical therapy for all newborns except those in chronic coma, or if treatment only prolonged dying or provided no possible benefit.[15] Institutional ethics committees (IECs) have emerged as important resources for consultation and for helping to resolve conflict surrounding treatment decisions.[16] In this case, an IEC consultation would be appropriate. Working closely with the team, the IEC can assist in creating a cooperative, informed, consensus-driven decision-making process.[17]

Anna's parents have requested withdrawal of life support based on the expense of her care. Limiting medical therapy based on considerations of cost in critically ill infants is not supported by the American Academy of Pediatrics (AAP),[18] and surveyed pediatricians reject restrictive fiscal policies when asked about decisions for critically ill infants.[19]

Nonetheless, as Anna is in a coma and her condition grave, treatment is likely prolonging her dying without providing benefit. Thus, an analysis of prospective burdens to *her* may mean that caregivers are not prevented from withdrawing support.[20] We could support reorganizing care to minimize Anna's suffering and discontinue virtually futile treatment; however we would not support withdrawal based on expense.

Further communication with Anna's parents is desperately needed prior to invoking child protective services or proposing foster care in the unlikely event that she survives. Finally, throughout this ordeal, Anna's parents must be treated with sincere respect, sensitivity, and compassion. Parents never "get over" the death of a child and the death of the dream for a healthy child is a profound loss.[21]

Notes

1. Avraham Steinberg, "Decision-making and the Role of Surrogacy in Withdrawal or Withholding of Therapy in Neonates," *Clinics in Perinatology* 25 (1998): 779–90; E. N. Kraybill, "Ethical Issues in the Care of Extremely Low Birth Weight Infants," *Seminars in Perinatology* 22, no. 3 (1998): 207–15.

2. James A. Lemons et al., "Very Low Birth Weight Outcomes of the National Institute of Child Health and Human Development Neonatal Research Network, January 1995–December 1996," *Pediatrics* 107, no. 1 (2001): E1; Rita G. Harper et al., "Neonatal Outcome of Infants Born at 500–800 Grams from 1990 through 1998 in a Tertiary Care Center," *Journal of Perinatology* 22, no. 7 (2002): 555–62.

3. Joseph J. Volpe, "Intracranial Hemorrhage: Germinal Matrix-intraventricular Hemorrhage of the Premature Neonate," in *Neurology of the Newborn,* 4th ed. (Philadelphia: W.B. Saunders, 2001), 448–53.

4. Michael S. Jellinek et al., "Facing Tragic Decisions with Parents in the Neonatal Intensive Care Unit: Clinical Perspectives," *Pediatrics* 89, no. 1 (1992): 119–22.

5. Christine Mitchell, "When Living Is a Fate Worse than Death—Doctors and Nurses at My Hospital Did 'Everything' to Keep a Child Alive. If Only Her Parents Had Let Her Go," *Newsweek,* 28 Aug. 2000, 9; American Academy of Pediatrics, Policy Statement: "Guidelines for Forgoing Life-sustaining Medical Treatment (RE9406)," *Pediatrics* 93 (1994): 532–36.

6. Raymond S. Duff and Alexander G. M. Campbell, "Moral and Ethical Dilemmas in the Special Care Nursery," *New England Journal of Medicine* 289 (1973): 890–94.

7. Raymond J. Devettere, "Neonatal Life," in *Practical Decision Making in Health Care Ethics,* 2nd ed. (Washington, DC: Georgetown University Press, 2000), 380–419.

8. American Academy of Pediatrics, Policy Statement: "Ethics and the Care of Critically Ill Infants and Children (RE9624)," *Pediatrics* 98, no. 1 (1996): 149–52.

9. John A. Hostetler, "The Life Ceremonies," in *Amish Society,* rev. ed. (Baltimore: Johns Hopkins Press, 1968), 172.

10. Mary J. Banks and Rosalie J. Benchot, "Unique Aspects of Nursing Care for Amish Children," *American Journal of Maternal/Child Nursing* 26 (2001): 192–96.

11. See note 4, above.

12. Elizabeth A. Catlin et al., "Spiritual and Religious Components of Patient Care in the Neonatal Intensive Care Unit: Sacred Themes in a Secular Setting," *Journal of Perinatology* 21, no. 7 (2001): 426–30; see also note 4, above, for a description of the NICU decision-making process.

13. Brad H. Reddick, Elizabeth Catlin, and Michael Jellinek, "Crisis Within Crisis: Recommendations for Defining, Preventing and Coping with Stressors in the NICU," *Journal of Clinical Ethics* 12 (2001): 254–65.

14. I. David Todres et al., "Moral and Ethical Dilemmas in Critically-ill Newborns: A 20 Year Follow-up Survey of Massachusetts Pediatricians," *Journal of Perinatology* 20, no. 1 (2000): 6–12.

15. "Child Abuse Neglect and Prevention Program: Final Rule," 50 *Federal Register* (1985): 14878–901.

16. American Academy of Pediatrics, Committee on Bioethics, "Institutional Ethics Committees," *Pediatrics* 107, no. 1 (2001): 205–9.

17. Avery B. Gordon, "Futility Considerations in the Neonatal Intensive Care Unit," *Seminars in Perinatology* 22, no. 3 (1998): 216–22.

18. See note 8, above.

19. See note 14, above.

20. See note 15, above.
21. See note 4, above; Bernadette Reilly-Smorawski, Anne V. Armstrong, and Elizabeth A. Catlin, "Bereavement Support for Couples Following the Death of a Baby: Program Development and Fourteen-year Exit Analysis," *Death Studies* 26, no. 1 (2002): 21–37.

An Ethicist's Analysis

Eric H. Gampel, PhD

This case raises the sad possibility that a baby could be left to die because her family cannot afford the medical care she needs. We have to assume this is not a simple case of medical futility:[1] Anna has a chance to live, and even some chance of a rewarding life. If the parents had medical insurance, there would be no serious doubt that treatment should continue. In other words, beneficence toward Anna would lead us to try to save her, despite the low odds and the burdens and risks (to Anna) of treatment. So the hospital has to decide whether to go along with the request of the parents. Of course, the hospital must consider the legality of ceasing Anna's treatment and the financial risk of being sued, whether by the parents or by an outside group. But assuming the legal and risk assessment calculations do not force their hand, physicians have to consider the moral question: should they accede to the parents' request? To do so would conflict with beneficence toward Anna, an important value; but to treat Anna against her parents' wishes would conflict with principles of rights (parental decisional authority) and autonomy (respect for parents' decision regarding their own family). So a moral dilemma exists, with hazards regardless of which horn is chosen.

The first thing to say here is that some creative strategies are worth trying. The case does not indicate that anyone has pressed the parents to consider accepting Medicaid, despite the general opposition of the Amish to doing so. Perhaps these parents, more educated than most Amish, would in this extreme crisis consider an exception to their rule. Another possibility is a compromise in which some treatment is continued for the short-term, until physicians have a better sense of the prognosis. It has been only a week—albeit an expensive one—and a few more days, or another week, could allow a more reliable estimate of Anna's chances for living a more rewarding life. The parents seem to have in mind an all-or-nothing decision; perhaps they would delay if physicians think that could help gain important information. Of course, a delay may lead to worse scenarios: the parents (and their community) lose tens of thousands more dollars and Anna's treatment is withdrawn in any case a week or two later; or even worse, Anna lives only for a short period with enormous pain and suffering, minimal cognitive function, and exorbitant financial costs. But these may be gambles they would be willing to take, so the possibilities should be explored.

But suppose these strategies fail; the parents continue to reject Medicaid and refuse to delay the decision, or the physicians think it would take months or years to have a better estimate of Anna's prospects. Now the moral dilemma becomes immediate. Continued treatment is not medically futile, but Anna's parents are rejecting it. Their main concern does not seem to be Anna's death or potential disabilities, but the financial burden of the treatment. Framed this way, I do not think the parents' request has much merit. While the parents' religious and social beliefs require rejecting Medicaid, at this point Anna's interests must take center stage. The hospital should seek *temporary* legal custody in the hopes that Anna's prospects will improve. The parents should not be allowed to impose their religious or cultural strictures on their daughter. This strategy risks harming the parents and splitting them from Anna, perhaps even in the long term, but those risks are less important than giving Anna a chance to have a life which, we are assuming, would be worth living.

The parents might be thinking that further efforts to save Anna would be a misuse of medical resources, that beneficence toward Anna must give way to social utility. Perhaps that is, in part, their reason for refusing to allow Medicaid to pay for Anna's care. But in a modern democracy, it is not for parents to make this social utility calculation. Moreover, it seems highly unlikely that not using Medicaid in this situation will allow the funds to be used for some other important medical purpose. More likely, the cost of Anna's care would disappear as a tiny figure in a much larger budget battle at state or national levels.

Notice that the reasoning thus far assumes that Anna's continued treatment is medically recommended—that is, that she has a reasonable chance of having a life worth living, even if that life involves some serious disabilities. But suppose the physicians are themselves unsure: They do not consider treatment medically futile, but they worry that with such low odds, it may be best for Anna that she be allowed to die now rather than go through months, years, or decades of burdensome medical care for an uncertain result.[2] This means a difficult risk/burden/benefit judgment must be made for Anna, one that would ordinarily be left in the hands of well-intentioned parents. The problem is that Mr. and Mrs. N, though trying to do what is best *for all concerned*, are being driven partly by financial concerns, rather than strictly by reference to what is best for Anna. Nevertheless, if the physicians are genuinely uncertain of what would be medically best for Anna, I would recommend going along with the parents' request to withdraw treatment, because there is insufficient ground to question the parents' reasoning. But if the physicians are convinced the potential benefits to Anna would be worth the burdens and risks, they should seek legal guardianship and continue to treat. The parents' strictures should not be respected at the cost of Anna's welfare; beneficence toward the patient must override respect for parental rights and autonomy when childrens' lives are at stake.

Notes

1. Simple, because if physicians judge a treatment to be futile and the family agrees, there is little moral controversy over ceasing treatment. Futility cases only generate dilemmas when family and HCPs differ about the merits of treatment. For discussion of such dilemmas, see

Robert D. Truog, A. S. Brett, and Joel Frader, "The Problem with Futility," *New England Journal of Medicine* 326 (1992): 1560–64; B. E. Wilson, "Futility and the Obligations of Physicians," *Bioethics* 10 (1996): 43–55; and William Harper, "Judging Who Should Live: Schneiderman and Jecker on the Duty Not to Treat," *Journal of Medicine and Philosophy* 23 (1998): 500–15.
2. For a discussion of the difficulty of making such risk/benefit judgments, see John Lantos et al., "The Illusion of Futility in Clinical Practice," *The American Journal of Medicine* 87 (1989): 81–84.

A Philosopher and Disability Advocate's Analysis

Anita Silvers, PhD

As is often the case when disability enters the picture, conversation about this case is dominated by generalizations that may be exaggerations or may not even apply to Anna or her situation. The sad history of stereotyping disabled people as being burdensome to themselves, their families, and the general public has been a pretext for exclusionary and brutal treatment.[1] The wrongs this history evidences create a special obligation to exercise careful scrutiny when considering the life prospects of any person who may be more limited, physically or mentally, than is typical for our species. In thinking about them, we must focus on facts, not fears.

Are the Ns, and their community, deciding on the basis of the facts about Anna? Or are they swayed by fears fed by suspect generalizations? If so, from whence have these overwrought claims come?

The Ns themselves are hardly likely to have originated the claim that "the average cost of subsequent care for premature infants like Anna is roughly $100,000 per year—for each year of her life." Further, the claim is not true. Even a study published by the Lucille and David Packard Foundation—one that emphasizes the costliness of low birth weight as an argument for increased prevention—estimates the first-year medical costs for babies born at less than 1000 grams and with respiratory distress at $33,000.[2] Incremental health care costs after the first year are estimated at $470 annually for low birth weight children. In fact, 75 percent of the additional costs associated with the health care and education of these children occur in their infancy.[3]

Why have Anna's parents come to believe that she will require special schooling that is unavailable in her community? We are told physicians imparted this information. Possibly physicians overestimate the need for special expertise in educating children with disabilities and discount the resources of traditional rural settings. Until the middle of the nineteenth century, cognitively and visually impaired children commonly remained in and grew up to contribute their labor to their communities. The belief that they needed "special" care developed as part of an economic revolution that moved families from farm to factory and, at the same time, drove disabled people out of their communities and institutionalized them.[4] But it is exactly this social change that the Amish way of life escaped.

Amish lifestyle makes family caregiving available and offers an environment in which disabled people may contribute and flourish. Very-low-birth-weight children are less likely to achieve in reading, spelling, and mathematics than full-term children are, and they are more likely to be shy and unassertive.[5] These propensities—disadvantages in an urbanized lifestyle—are not so for the Amish way of life.

If Anna is disabled and needs special equipment to learn or move, she will receive assistive technology under the federal Individuals with Disabilities Education Act through the K-12 schooling in which Amish children are allowed to participate. Asthma and related respiratory infections are the health problems for which very-low-birth-weight children most commonly need extra medical care.[6] However, recent studies show that children raised around animals, as the Amish are, seem much less prone to asthma than their city peers.

The realities about very-low-birth-weight children seem quite different from what Anna's parents have been told. Nor is it clear why the hospital staff believes her future is so limited. Only 20 percent of less than 1000 gram neonates develop spastic motor problems, and only 5 percent–6 percent are blind.[7] In Anna's case, we are told, hypoxia led to intracranial hemorrhage, which progressed to coma. But we are not told, and therefore Anna's parents presumably have not been told, that sonography reveals a dimmer prognosis based on the extent or location of the hemorrhage, and perhaps an exacerbating hydroencephaly is present.[8]

What the hospital staff has told Anna's parents is important because, from a moral point of view, we must know whether they believe themselves to be acting in the interests of a child who probably will not survive, and for whom aggressive measures most likely will do no more than prolong suffering, or for a child who probably will survive, but with an increased risk of neurological limitations and respiratory problems. We cannot assess the parents' decision from a moral point of view without knowing what they believe about the child for whose interests they stand surrogate, and whether their beliefs about the child are fair and true. The presumption is that families act in the best interests of their members. Only with persuasive evidence to the contrary may we discard this premise to conclude that the state is more likely than her family to act in a child's real interests.

This brings us to the Baby Doe Regulations about which some hospital staff are concerned. Initially issued in 1984 as an application of the antidiscrimination provisions of the 1973 Rehabilitation Act, these federal regulations threatened hospitals with loss of federal funds if they withheld treatment from handicapped infants. The Supreme Court ruled that the Rehabilitation Act did not apply to medical care, so Congress passed the Child Abuse and Treatment Act, which defined withdrawal of medically indicated treatment as child abuse. This Act permits withholding treatment if it is virtually futile or the infant is chronically comatose; a footnote to the regulations declares that they were not developed with premature infants in mind.[9] Nor does the Americans with Disabilities Act "forbid denying treatment solely on the basis of disability." The Supreme Court's ADA rulings require only that public medical services offered to nondisabled people in community settings be made available to disabled people in the same settings so they need not accept institutionalization as the price of obtaining treatment.[10] As neither the Baby Doe Regulations nor the ADA protect individuals who are chronically comatose or in persistent vegetative conditions, their moral and legal status remains a troubled issue, but to place Anna firmly within this category demands more information about her individual condition than we have been told.

In sum, Anna's autonomy (as represented by her parents, her surrogate decision makers), and the autonomy of all people with actual or potential disabilities, is compromised by judgments based on inaccurate or incomplete information about their potential and by incorrect claims about the legal protection that exists for them. From a moral point of view, the hospital staff should focus on providing full and accurate information. Further, in discussing Anna's prognosis, staff should be especially alert to the resources and strengths of community ways of life.

Notes

1. Leslie Francis and Anita Silvers, eds., introduction to *Americans with Disabilities: Exploring Implications of the Law for Individuals and Institutions* (New York: Routledge, 2000), xiii–xxix.

2. Eugene M. Lewit et al., "The Direct Cost of Low Birth Weight," *The Future of Children: Low Birth Weight* 5, no. 1 (1995), http://www.futureofchildren.org/information2826/information_show.htm?doc_id=79879 (31 Mar. 2004).

3. Maureen Hack, Nancy K. Klein, and H. Gerry Taylor, "Long-Term Developmental Outcomes of Low Birth Weight Infants," *The Future of Children: Low Birth Weight* 5, no. 1 (1995), http://www.futureofchildren.org/information2826/information_show.htm?doc_id=79895 (31 Mar. 2004).

4. Anita Silvers, "People with Disabilities," in ed. Hugh LaFollette, *The Oxford Handbook of Practical Ethics* (New York: Oxford University Press, 2003), 300–327.

5. See note 3, above.

6. Ibid.

7. See note 2, above.

8. David Annibale and Jeanne Hill, "Periventricular Hemorrhage-Intraventricular Hemorrhage," *eMedicine Journal* 2, no. 10, 30 Oct. 2001, http://author.emedicine.com/ped/topic2595.htm#section~test_questions (31 Mar. 2004).

9. Ascension Health, Inc., "Baby Doe, Baby Jane Doe, Baby Doe Regulations, and the 1983 Amendment to the Child Abuse Law," n.d., http://www.ascensionhealth.org/our_essence/ethics/affiliates/cases/all_cases.asp (3 Aug. 2003); Dana Wechsler Linden and Mia Wechsler Doron, "Eyes of Texas Fasten on Life, Death and the Premature Infant," *New York Times*, 20 Apr. 2002, http://www.tripletconnection.org/texas.html (26 Mar. 2004).

10. Leslie Francis and Anita Silvers, eds., *Americans with Disabilities: Exploring Implications of the Law for Individuals and Institutions* (New York: Routledge, 2000), Introduction, xiii–xxix; "Foundations," 1–85; and "Health," 223–68.

Further Reflections

Consequences

1. Compare the analysis of outcomes given by Catlin, Settle, and Thiel with that given by Silvers. On what *factual* assumptions and *presumed* consequences does each depend?

2. The moral principle of beneficence is central to the practice of good neonatal intensive care unit (NICU) care. Compare the discussions by Gampel, Silvers, and Harrison about what beneficence requires concerning treatment and treatment abatement.

Autonomy

3. Many people believe that we cannot determine whether and how to treat a patient without knowing whether the patient will have a "life worth living," which hinges in part on how we define a "life worth living." Compare the *value* assumptions about a life worth living that are advanced by Catlin and her colleagues, by Gampel, and by Silvers. Is consensus among these analysts possible? What might such a consensus look like?

4. At least three commentators (Catlin et al., Silvers, and Harrison) are critical of the decision-making process in or absent from this case. What does each commentator feel is most wrong with the way the resolution of this dilemma is proceeding? What limitations, blind spots, missed or misinterpreted moral commitments and erroneous presumptions are at work in this NICU? Are these significant enough to compromise parental autonomy?

Rights

5. The right of parents to make decisions for their minor children is well established ethically and legally. What conditions, if any, can *morally* override this right?

6. What obligations, if any, do HCPs have in regard to the parents' right to not be harmed?

Virtues

7. If the government makes available funds to provide health care for children like Anna through the Medicaid program, does the role-related virtue of fidelity morally obligate the Ns (in their role as parents) and their community (in its role of protecting its members) to accept those funds and the care they provide? What arguments are advanced by Girod in this regard? Compare her analysis to the observation by Gampel that the family's "main concern does not seem to be Anna's death or potential disabilities, but the financial burdens of

treatment. Framed in this way, I do not think the parents' request has much merit." Is the observation by Catlin, Settle, and Thiel that "Limiting medical therapy based on considerations of cost in critically ill infants is not supported by the [American Association of Pediatrics]" based on professional integrity (role of physicians)?

8. Why does making health care decisions based on "costs" cause so much consternation among HCPs and others? Why, for example, are nearly all commentators opposed to factoring in costs and financial burdens on the family and Amish community as the decisive reason to abate or discontinue Anna's treatment?

Justice

9. In response to public concerns about failure to treat disabled infants, the U. S. Department of Health and Human Services published the so-called "Baby Doe Regulations" that require treatment unless: (1) The infant is irreversibly comatose; (2) Treatment would be futile in terms of survival; or (3) Treatment would be virtually futile in terms of survival and would also be inhumane. How might the principle of justice support or denounce these regulations? Are the restrictions they place on treatment for seriously ill neonates unfair? If not, why are so many HCPs who work in NICUs—as well as our commentators— so critical of these regulations?

10. If Anna's care is likely to have implications for future and further discrimination against persons with disabilities, should her parents or HCPs factor that information into choices about her care?

Chapter 12

Patients We Love to Hate: The Obese

Mr. P is a 42-year-old, self-employed architect who works out of his home; he has severe rheumatoid arthritis. His hands, knees, and ankles are chronically swollen and inflamed. Despite aggressive medical treatment, his disease has progressively limited his mobility. Chronic anemia (a low red blood cell count) leaves him with fatigue and subsequent limitation of his ability to work. He weighs 370 pounds. A recent fall left him with a fracture and dislocation of two thoracic (chest) vertebrae (bones in his spine), requiring surgery to remove bone chips from his spinal column and to repair and stabilize the fractures. He will be confined to bed rest in his small community hospital for several weeks until the fractures heal.

Mr. P poses a number of challenges to the nursing staff. In addition to his fractures, Mr. P has multiple skin folds, most of which are raw and oozing. He has severe perianal excoriation and scrotal ulcerations, and yeast infections in both these regions. His feet and legs are weeping from cellulitis.

Mr. P's obesity, wounds, and immobility make frequent skin care and repositioning essential, yet his weight makes these interventions impossible with fewer than four staff members—three to establish and maintain correct alignment (so his spine will heal properly) and one to provide skin and wound care. The staff try to reposition him at least hourly (especially as Mr. P gets so uncomfortable if he lies in the same position even that long), but finding four people who can spare 10–15 minutes every hour is always difficult and often impossible.

The fact is that virtually every staff member is assigned to care for Mr. P, always at some cost to other patients and to unit morale. Nurses as-

226

signed as Mr. P's primary caregivers dislike being unable to provide his care without intruding on their colleagues' schedules. Their colleagues dislike being unavailable to their own patients frequently and for extended periods of time. Some of the staff have tried to get the job done with fewer than four people, resulting in three nurses with acute low back strains, one severe enough to require treatment. In less than a week, Mr. P has seen the time between repositionings lengthen from 60- to 90- or even 120-minute intervals. The staff no longer answer his light as promptly, and the receptionist no longer even asks what he wants, saying only, "Be patient, Mr. P; it will take time to round up enough people."

Mr. P's dietary habits are a source of constant friction. His physician put him on a 1200-calorie diet developed by the American Diabetic Association, about which he grumbles constantly: The food is uninteresting and the portions too small; he is always hungry; denying him food is denying him the only source of enjoyment and comfort left to him. The staff grumble too: He should see that losing weight would improve his health; they can't change the doctor's order; he should quit complaining. When Mr. P's visitors were discovered smuggling in "junk" food, several staff overtly chastised Mr. P for his behavior, for his obesity, for the extra burden his extra weight places on his caregivers. The nurse who discovered potato chips in Mr. P's skin folds was especially harsh in her criticism.

In addition, pain control has been challenging. Both the surgical repair and the rheumatoid arthritis cause him pain. The staff recognize this but are reluctant to medicate Mr. P because he requires narcotics for pain control and the doses required for full relief make him lethargic, raising worries about pneumonia. In addition, sufficient pain medication makes him flaccid and, thus, even more difficult to position, to clean, etc.

In short, no one wants to take care of Mr. P. Given the frustrations of providing his care, the staff prefer to rotate the responsibility. But given the challenges, a better approach for Mr. P is a stable team who could establish and provide efficient, effective routines with minimal confusion and fumbling. Further, the staff are increasingly resentful of the additional time and personnel needed to get even the simplest tasks done. And Mr. P's ongoing complaints of pain and food deprivation are as wearing on the staff as they are on him. Finally, usurping four staffers for 15 minutes each hour slights other patients. As Mr. P will be hospitalized for several more weeks, the problems must be solved.

After much soul-searching the nurse manager, Ms. Y, informs Mr. P that the hospital simply cannot provide adequate staffing to meet his *needs. She cites two reasons: (1) As this is a small community hospital with limited professional resources, providing additional personnel each shift is impossible (cost concerns aside); and (2) Compromised care to the other patients on the unit is unfair. Since Mr. P has rejected transfer to a larger, distant facility (if he is hospitalized locally, he can continue to meet with clients), Ms. Y gives him an ultimatum: The hospital will continue to assign a licensed nurse to coordinate his care and give his medications; however, Mr. P will have to hire two (preferably three) full-time private duty nursing assistants for each shift to assist with his physical care (bathing, turning, etc.). This approach will ensure that he receives the physical and professional care he needs without compromising care to other patients. It will also make the staff more willing to medicate him adequately.*

Mr. P protests that he cannot afford to hire private duty personnel. The ongoing costs of his illness are a significant financial burden. Because he is self-employed, he must purchase his own health insurance (approximately $1600/month), as well as assume full financial responsibility for all his medications. His insurance policy does not cover private duty staff and he cannot afford to pay for personnel out of his own pocket. He adds that the hospital should not assume that every patient will be "perfect" because many will require greater-than-normal resources, and that a well-run hospital should plan for such contingencies. He feels he should not be penalized for administrative inefficiency or shortsightedness.

What is Ms. Y's moral obligation at this point?

Introduction

This case raises three significant moral issues:

1. Do appeals to autonomy justify holding persons responsible for the effects—including restricted health care services—of health-risking behavior?

2. Do considerations of fidelity obligate health care professionals (HCPs) and/or health care institutions (HCIs) to particular patients, patient populations, or both?

3. What is the morally appropriate criterion for just allocation of scarce health care resources?

The AJ Method

Step 1: Information Gathering   How likely is Mr. P's care to burden staff? other patients? Can Mr. P's pain be controlled without making his physical care more difficult? What motivates the staff dislike of Mr. P? Is Mr. P's obesity—in and of itself—a source of staff rejection? Are the hospital staffing levels appropriate, or are too few nurses assigned to Mr. P's unit? Can Mr. P afford private duty nurses? Can Ms. Y increase the staffing on the unit?

Step 2: Creative Problem Solving   A creative solution would have to meet Mr. P's needs without *unduly* burdening staff and other patients. (Brown; Silvers)

Step 3: Pros and Cons   Survey CARVE principles to identify important moral reasons that support conflicting options for resolving this case.

   Consequences   Who will be harmed if Mr. P is required to hire private staff? if he is not so required? (Silvers) Who will be benefited? What does the principle of utility advise? (Brown; Resnik)

   Autonomy   Recall that autonomy, most broadly understood, applies to choosing the values in terms of which to live one's life, as well as the means to achieve those values. Does autonomy confer a responsibility to suffer the ill effects of one's lifestyle choices? (Silvers) Whose autonomy is relevant here?

   The moral principle of autonomy requires respect of persons' choices about how to live their lives, even—perhaps especially—those choices of which others disapprove.[1] Further, persons are—and are presumed willing to be—held responsible for choices they autonomously make. Since many people make lifestyle choices that are likely to have effects on their health (e.g., over-eating, lack of exercise, high-risk hobbies), are HCPs or HCIs morally justified in holding such persons responsible for negative outcomes that result from these choices? Or can one make a case that such choices were not (fully) autonomous?[2] If so, is responsibility attenuated? But perhaps one could argue that virtually every person engages in some health-risking behavior. Why should those who are unlucky enough to actually realize the risks be penalized?

   An appeal to autonomy might also raise the question of whether or to what extent persons choosing health-risking behavior have, by extension, made an autonomous choice to forgo easy access to a full range of health care opportunities (especially those living in small communities with limited access to health care services). Are residents of small or geographically isolated towns morally responsible for—and thus required to suffer through—less than optimal care?[3] Or do they fail to appreciate this particular burden (i.e., are not fully informed of the risks of their choices) until they need health care that is too extensive, too expensive, or too sophisticated?

Rights   Mr. P has rights of privacy and confidentiality that may be violated if external staff are employed. Mr. P, within the context of the patient-professional relationship, has a right to be aided. Mr. P and the staff have a right to not be harmed. Mr. P has a right of self-determination.

Virtues   The virtues of integrity, fidelity, and compassion can inform the discussion. (Brown; Resnik; Silvers)

The virtues of integrity and fidelity speak to the question of to whom HCPs and HCIs are morally responsible. Does nursing's Code of Ethics require nurses to do whatever is necessary to meet the needs of every particular patient?[4] Or should they weigh the needs of the one against the needs of the population? Does the Code give assistance to nurses who, like Ms. Y, are functioning in a supervisory rather than a patient-care mode? Who, or what, has first claim on the nurse? Similarly, the American Hospital Association's "Bill of Rights" specifies that "The patient has the right to expect that, within its capacity and policies, a hospital will make reasonable response to the request of a patient for appropriate and medically indicated care and services." What counts as a "reasonable response"?[5] Do reasonable responses fluctuate, depending on the needs of patient populations or staffing levels? on other resources?

Justice   Is anyone treated unfairly (and, if so, who) if Mr. P is required to purchase private staff? if he is not? (Brown; Resnik; Silvers) Is Mr. P being discriminated against because of his obesity? (Silvers) his lifestyle?

Justice in allocation arises whenever demand exceeds supply, and requires specifying some standard(s) for distributing these scarce resources. Criteria for just distribution of health care goods and services are contested.[6] Some scholars argue that service-oriented institutions should distribute goods based on a criterion of need.[7] Others argue that in a market-based economy goods and services should be distributed on ability to pay.[8] Still others argue that distribution of any resource should maximize the welfare of the group, rather than of particular persons.[9] To date little agreement has been reached on which criterion is apt.

The moral principle of utility raises further questions about the nature and extent of institutional obligations: How should we interpret the American Hospital Association's mandate that "The patient has the right to considerate and respectful care"?[10] Does *every* patient have this right? Again, what of the claim (above) regarding a "reasonable response" to the patients' appropriate requests for "medically indicated care and services"? Is "reasonable response" defined in terms of the welfare of the individual patient or of populations? If the two conflict, which is more "reasonable"? These questions are particularly pressing for small hospitals serving small communities whose citizens—especially those with greater than average needs—may lack access to alternative providers and who may feel professional staffing shortages more keenly than their urban counterparts.[11] All institutions have budgetary constraints. Should income be spent on one or a few patients if that means reducing access to or quality of services for (many) more patients, present and future? Similarly, all HCPs have limited personal resources—time, energy, stamina, patience.

The Law   In conclusion, the following legal considerations are relevant to this case: (1) Would insisting on private nursing staff legally constitute a violation of privacy or a breach of an implicit contractual agreement with Mr. P or his insurance carrier? (2) To whom is the nursing supervisor legally obligated in such a situation—the patient, unit employees, other patients, or the institution? (3) What course of action (premised on risk assessment) should be taken to adjudicate competing obligations? (4) Are there legal limits to the obligations that the various parties involved in this case have to Mr. P?[12]

The following commentaries examine the application of various moral principles to this dilemma, thereby assisting the reader to undertake *Step 4: Analysis* and *Step 5: Justification.*

Notes

1. H. Tristram Engelhardt, Jr., *The Foundation of Bioethics,* 2nd ed. (New York: Oxford University Press, 1996), 288–330.
2. Obesity is an especially vexing problem. The extent to which persons *can* control their caloric intake is currently under scrutiny. What is known is that even persons with serious food-related illnesses find controlling what they eat difficult. For example, nearly 100 percent of diabetics fail to strictly follow dietary recommendations, and 98 percent of obese dieters gain back lost weight within two years. See, for example, Norman B. Levy, MD, "A Psychiatrist Answers Questions About Noncompliance," *E-NEPH Archive: Dialysis & Transplantation* 24 (April 1995), http://www.eneph.com/feature_archive/Compliance/v24n4p187.html (27 Mar. 2004).
3. For a related discussion, see "Are We Our Patients' Keepers?" (Chap. 14, this volume).
4. American Nurses Association, *Code of Ethics for Nurses with Interpretive Statements* (Washington, DC: ANA, 2001), 2001, http://nursingworld.org/ethics/code/ethicscode150.htm (27 Mar. 2004), §§ 1, 2.
5. American Hospital Association, "A Patient's Bill of Rights" (Chicago: American Hospital Association, 1998), #8, adopted 1973, revised 21 Oct. 1992, http://www.hospitalconnect.com/aha/about/pbillofrights.html (27 Mar. 2004).
6. For a fine overview of distributive justice, see Tom L. Beauchamp and James F. Childress, *Principles of Biomedical Ethics,* 5th ed. (New York: Oxford University Press, 2001), 225–82.
7. John Rawls, *A Theory of Justice* (Cambridge: Harvard University Press, 1971).
8. Robert Nozick, *Anarchy, State, and Utopia* (New York: Basic Books, 1974).
9. John Stuart Mill, *Utilitarianism,* ed. Oskar Piest (Indianapolis: Bobbs-Merrill, 1975), Chap. 5.
10. See note 5, above, #1.
11. Gladys B. White, "Ethical Implications of the Nursing Manpower Crisis, Shortage and Staffing," *American Nurses Association Ethics & Human Rights Issues Update* 1, no. 2 (2001), http://www.nursingworld.org/ethics/update/vol1no2b.htm#reflect (27 Mar. 2004).
12. The Americans with Disabilities Act of 1990 (42 U.S.C.S. 12101) requires that individuals with disabilities be afforded equal opportunity in the areas of public life, including medical services. The ADA defines disabilities broadly and mandates significant efforts to provide reasonable accommodation and access to services. American Medical Association, Council

on Ethical and Judicial Affairs, *Code of Medical Ethics: Current Opinions with Annotations*, 2000–2001 Edition (Chicago: American Medical Association, 2000), § 10.02 "Patient Responsibilities," 234–35, provides some general guidelines, although the issue of who is legally and morally responsible to assure quality care in such situations and the extent of that obligation is unclear.

A Nurse's Analysis

Janet Brown, RN, MSN, CNS

Caring for an unpleasant, noncompliant, demanding patient with a complex illness is difficult and time-consuming. Nonetheless because respect and caring are the moral imperatives that drive nursing, patients are entitled to their nurses' individualized care and respect, regardless of the nature and cause of their illnesses.

Obesity is a serious health condition. *Bariatrics* (the branch of medicine focusing on prevention, control, and treatment of obesity) identifies excess weight as a medical and/or health condition. Thus obese patients have genuine medical and nursing needs and are entitled to respectful care in meeting those needs.

Further, the American Hospital Association's "Patients' Bill of Rights," which specifies patients' rights and the responsibilities of hospitals and health care providers (HCPs), acknowledges a right to receive medically needed care and services.[1] In recognizing this right, the hospital assumes responsibility for providing whatever care a patient needs. An institution may be excused from this responsibility if it literally cannot provide the care, but not merely because doing so is difficult.

But resource limits are real. As the shortage of licensed, professional nurses increases, hospitals face this type of challenge more frequently.[2] The nursing shortage will likely result in less care for all, rather than limited care for some and adequate care for others. Still, one might argue that the greater good of the nursing staff and other patients on the unit support using private duty aides for Mr. P's care. Ms. Y's intent when she appraises the resources on the unit and determines that Mr. P's care should be limited is at least partly a question of whether scarce resources should be used to promote the welfare of one patient or of all. The intent is to protect all patients. However, denying appropriate care to Mr. P could ultimately slow his recovery and contribute to additional health problems. On the other hand, consequences for other patients for whom less nursing time and skill may be available must be considered.

The American Nurses Association's (ANA) Code of Ethics' first standard states: "The nurse . . . practices with compassion and respect for the inherent dignity, worth and uniqueness of every individual, unrestricted by considerations of social or economic status, personal attributes, or the nature of health problems."[3] Further, nurses have a fiduciary relationship with clients. Clients, vulnerable as the result of their illnesses, are dependent on the integrity of the professional who literally promises to help. Deciding that because Mr. P's care is too difficult he will be required to provide his own attendants violates the Code's first standard and the fiduciary relationship; thus, this decision is morally wrong.

In addition, nonprofessional health care workers have limited knowledge and skills. Mr. P could be at increased risk because his complex needs require ongoing professional assessment. Less knowledgeable personnel would be less able to identify significant changes and make sound judgments about necessary changes to his care plan.

One solution may address many of these concerns: renting equipment designed for obese patients. If Mr. P had a bed that turned him mechanically then, despite an increased cost in equipment initially, costs in human resources (and related injuries) would decrease. More effective repositioning would also promote wound healing and help prevent lung problems. A mechanical bed could promote his independence (turning when he chose) and his well-being (beneficence) and that of his caregivers (utility).

Withholding Mr. P's pain medication cannot be defended ethically. The moral principle of nonmaleficence requires a nurse to do no harm. While one could argue that his sedation from pain medication may contribute to complications, data indicating the therapeutic value of adequate pain relief are so compelling that the Joint Commission on Accreditation of Healthcare Organizations has adopted standards for hospitals related to the assessing and managing of pain.[4] Pain relief is expected to be a primary organizational priority. By conferring with a knowledgeable pharmacist, the nursing staff could identify analgesics with fewer sedative effects.

Finally, while we may believe in a holistic basis for nursing (addressing the individual client's total experience), patients whose pathology is the result of personal lifestyle choices raise two common responses: disgust and the suspicion that they are "wasting" resources. Nurses shouldn't be judgmental, but they may be unable to avoid feeling resentful. It may seem as if Mr. P's choices intentionally harm his nurses, but this is unlikely to be what Mr. P intends. The challenge is to move beyond negative reactions to patients with conditions, such as obesity, which seem to result from their own choices and which tax the resources of institutions and providers.

Even as his nurses acknowledge Mr. P's right to respectful and appropriate care, they recognize the drain on resources, especially the physical and psychological resources of his caregivers. As a result, HCPs wonder if distributive justice, which addresses proper use of scarce resources, applies to these patients. Distributive justice requires that each individual be given the care to which he is entitled. But who determines what a person deserves, either independently of or compared to others? Does Mr. P truly deserve only the same level of care as the "average" patient, given his additional need? Every acute-care hospital is required to have a patient classification system for determining nursing care needs, or acuity, of individual patients based on an assessment by a registered nurse on a shift-by-shift basis. So staffing requirements for each day and shift vary with the varied and varying acuity of patients. In addition, nurses providing patient care make decisions about how to allocate their time during any one shift. As such they can choose, to some degree, the amount of care provided to each patient. However, the controversy of which patient is more or less deserving of resources is a problem that cannot be answered by policies about allocation of resources relative to patient acuity.

As patient advocates the nursing staff must work collaboratively with Mr. P to effectively address his needs. As a member of a profession committed to welfare of individual patients, Ms. Y must address—not shift responsibility for—the problem of inadequate available resources.

RECOMMENDED READING

Hahler, Barbara. "Morbid Obesity: A Nursing Care Challenge." *MEDSURG Nursing* 11:2 (2002); 85–90.

Notes

1. American Hospital Association, *A Patient's Bill of Rights* (Chicago: American Hospital Association, 1998), adopted 1973, revised 21 Oct. 1992, http://www.hospitalconnect.com/aha/about/pbillofrights.html (27 Mar. 2004).
2. Judith Erlen, "The Nursing Shortage, Patient Care, and Ethics," *Orthopaedic Nursing* 20, no. 6 (2001): 61–65.
3. American Nurses Association, *Code of Ethics for Nurses with Interpretive Statements* (Washington, DC: American Nurses Association, 2001), http://www.ana.org/ethics/ (27 Mar. 2004).
4. The Joint Commission on Accreditation of Healthcare Organizations, *Accreditation Manual for Hospitals* (Oakbrook Terrace, IL: The Joint Commission on Accreditation of Healthcare Organizations, 2000).

A Philosopher and Disability Advocate's Analysis

Anita Silvers, PhD

The quandary that pits nurse manager Y against patient P is a common one. Do providers of health care services owe more than the usual care to atypical patients who do not fit our standard expectations of patients' needs? Similar problems about the treatment of atypical patients include:

1. If the typical psychiatric patient can choose to receive mental health care services in the community, does the provider owe the same opportunity to mentally retarded individuals with similar psychiatric problems?
2. Must medical facilities give wheelchair users equal access to examination rooms, treatment rooms, bathrooms, and recreation rooms, as is required of schools, airports, stores, and restaurants?

In all such cases, the answer is Yes!

In its famous *Olmstead* decision, the Supreme Court decreed that states which provide psychiatric services in the community to the general run of patient may not require mentally retarded people to accept institutionalization in order to receive the same psychiatric services.[1] More generally, federal law requires that hospitals offer disabled people access equivalent to that afforded the nondisabled (but hospitals need not offer medical services to disabled people that other people neither are offered nor need).[2]

In this case a patient's atypically corpulent body increases the difficulties of his care. Who bears responsibility for rising to these difficulties—the patient or the professional caregiver?[3] On principle, healthcare professionals (HCPs) should not turn away from patients who present unusual challenges. How can we rely on caregivers who withdraw their help when people's situations make their care troublesome? Permitting such abandonment subverts the regulative principle of rescue, which nourishes the trust we place in the health care professions.

Nevertheless, the rule of rescue may be defeasible if patients, intentionally and with full foresight, cause certain kinds of difficulties for themselves. Patients who patently act contrary to their own interests sometimes are perceived as signaling their permission, freely given, for others to disregard their welfare. Has patient P done so?

Mr. P's behavior is described in language designed to defeat hospital responsibility by establishing Mr. P as the cause of the problems with his care. His obesity is blamed on his noncompliance with dietary proscriptions, and the extra care he needs in turn is attributed to his obesity. Notice, however, that even Mr. P's transfiguration into a model dieter would not afford the hospital staff relief, for months will pass before he is appreciably lighter. Thus, reference to this matter seems based on the staff's distaste of his character, rather than on any principle delineating patients' obligations to make their care easier for their caregivers.

Allocating health care resources with reference to patients' characters and personal traits is morally suspect. Few of us agree that our own access to health care should be diminished if HCPs (dis)approve of us as persons, or take a dim view of our quality of life. To illustrate: transplantable organs initially were allocated on this basis, but when the public learned of this rationing procedure an ethical outcry against such preferences ensued.

Let's summarize the discussion so far. Despite what some staff members view as irresponsible or self-destructive behavior on his part, nothing Mr. P has done defeats the professional responsibility to care for him. Further, it is morally suspect to deprive him of an effective level of care by arguing that there are patients whose attractive characters or situations make them more deserving.

Looking at the case from a different perspective, however, may compromise Mr. P's claim. HCPs have duties to themselves and to each other as well as to their patients. One's duty to one's self recommends against risking injury. Nurses thus have a prima facie obligation to avoid injuring themselves in the course of caring for others.[4]

From this wider perspective on duties, nurses must care for themselves by avoiding back injuries. Musculoskeletal injuries are much more common among nurses and nurses aides than among workers generally.[5] Developing a workplace safety culture, which includes providing mechanical devices such as lifting and rolling aids, greatly reduces the incidence of back injuries in nurses. Indeed, though patient P is heavy, his weight falls within what some ordinary hospital lifting devices can handle, and is well within the specifications of heavy-duty devices.[6]

Now we are closer to understanding nurse manager Y's obligations. By improving the conditions under which nurses work, which also are the conditions under which patients are cared for, health care managers facilitate ethical conduct by reducing the potential for conflicts between the interests of caregivers and care-receivers. Rather than insisting that Mr. P pay for a squad of extra nurses to lift him, Ms. Y should be insisting that the hospital meet OSHA (Occupational Safety and Health Act) standards by adopting ergonomic approaches to safe lifting. Acquiring ergonomic equipment often pays for itself over time by reducing employee sick leave use and increasing retention, surely a plus for a community hospital with nurses in short supply.[7]

Nurses are professionally obligated not only to their patients individually but also to the population collectively. They have professional duties to enlarge the public's access to health care and to ensure that this access is equitable for everyone. Broadly, nurses have professional responsibilities to shape the institutions that affect their patients.[8]

Nurses have a crucial role to play in developing adequate institutional responses to the challenge of achieving equitable health care for the atypical patient. Nurses, especially those with managerial duties, also are obligated to protect the professional capabilities of other caregiving personnel, and they have a professional obligation to improve the organizations in which they work.[9] Their organizational role positions nurse managers to promote institutional responsibility, which in this case may mean exercising leadership to develop a hazard-free lifting program for the hospital.

Notes

1. Olmstead v. L. C., 527 U. S. 581 (1999).
2. Alexander v. Choate, 469 U.S. 287 (1985).
3. Mary Crossley, "Impairment and Embodiment," in *Americans With Disabilities,* eds. Leslie Francis and Anita Silvers (New York: Routledge, 2000), 111–23.
4. American Nurses Association, *Code of Ethics for Nurses with Interpretive Statements* (Washington, DC: Author, 2001), http://nursingworld.org/ethics/ecode.htm (27 Mar. 2004).
5. U.S. Department of Labor, Bureau of Labor Statistics, "1999 Annual Survey of Nonfatal Injuries & Illnesses," 12 Dec. 2000, http://www.bls.gov/iif/home.htm (27 Mar. 2004).
6. Craig Shepard, OTR/L, "Dimensions of Care: Ergonomics for the Hospital Setting," *Health Tracker* 4, no. 2 (2001), http://www.systoc.com/Tracker/Summer01/ErgonHosp.asp (14 Aug. 2003).

7. Ibid.
8. Edward M. Spencer et al., eds., *Organization Ethics in Health Care* (New York: Oxford University Press, 2000).
9. Remarks of Beth Piknick, RN, for the American Nurses Association, 22 Nov. 1999, http://www.nursingworld.org/pressrel/1999/st1122.htm (27 Mar. 2004); see ANA, note 4, above.

An Ethicist's Analysis

David B. Resnik, PhD, JD

The fundamental moral challenge that Mr. P poses is allocation of scarce resources on the unit—specifically, staff time. As a result of problems related to his fractures and co-morbidities associated with his obesity, Mr. P requires more attention and nursing care than do other patients on the unit. Time spent taking care of Mr. P's many needs takes away time from the other patients. As a consequence, Mr. P is having a negative impact on the unit's overall morale.

Although Mr. P is obese, the challenge he poses is not unique to obesity. Patients with other complex medical problems—such as hepatitis, tuberculosis, advanced HIV/AIDS, multiple bedsores, dementia, schizophrenia, and quadriplegia—may also require more nursing care than the average patient. While one might be tempted to focus on Mr. P's obesity as the source of the moral dilemma and scold him for causing his own problems through his unhealthy lifestyle, the most important issue here concerns the allocation of nursing care. This commentary will not explore ethical issues related to holding patients responsible for the consequences of their unhealthy behavior; it will focus only on the allocation issues.

Ms. Y has told Mr. P that the hospital cannot provide adequate staffing to meet his needs and that he must hire his own private nursing assistants to help with his care, if he plans to remain a patient in this particular hospital. Is this fair to Mr. P? To answer this question, one must determine what constitutes a just (or fair) allocation of health care.

The four basic approaches to allocating health care are based on equality, medical needs, utility, or ability to pay.[1] If Ms. Y follows a principle of equality, she should ensure that all patients receive equal nursing care. Under this approach, Mr. P would receive less care than he is receiving now because all patients would receive the same amount of care, and Mr. P needs more care than the average patient. Other patients might receive more care than they are currently receiving because they *need* less care than the average patient. Since different patients have different medical needs, one might argue that equality is not a very fair or effective way of allocating nursing care.

Perhaps Ms. Y should follow a principle of medical need and allocate more resources to patients who require more care and fewer resources to patients who require less care. Under this approach, Mr. P would get as much nursing care as he needs. The problem with this approach is that some patients may require so much attention that taking care of their needs will take care away from the other patients and reduce the overall health of patients on the unit. By attending to medical needs, one may fail to promote utility. If ten patients are on the unit, completely attending to Mr. P's needs may result in substandard care to five of the remaining nine patients. Thus, only five of the ten patients would receive the full standard of care.

To promote utility, Ms. Y could decide to provide substandard care to Mr. P and the full standard of care to the other patients. Thus, nine of ten patients would receive the standard of care, as opposed to five of ten. This approach to allocation would maximize the overall health care of all the patients on the unit at Mr. P's expense. Something like a principle of utility plays an important role in triage procedures in medicine, which are used in the emergency department setting, on the battlefield, and during natural disasters. The problem with the principle of utility, however, is that it implies that one could ignore the medical needs of one (or a few) patients in order to promote the needs of other patients, which would result in a highly unequal and (possibly) ineffective distribution of health care.

Ms. Y appears to be allocating health care based on the ability to pay, since she has told Mr. P that he can get the nursing care that he needs only if he pays for it. The problem with using this principle to allocate resources is that many patients cannot afford care that they need. In this case, Mr. P cannot afford to hire extra private nurses. Thus, allocation based on ability to pay, like allocation based on utility, may also ignore medical needs.

So how should Ms. Y approach this allocation problem? Most solutions to resource allocation problems should involve some complex weighing and balancing of different principles for distributing resources. In this case, Ms. Y first attempted to take care of Mr. P's medical needs, but she had to deviate from that plan to attend to the health care needs of all patients on the unit. To avoid ignoring Mr. P's needs, she offered him the option of paying for his own nurses.

The approach Ms. Y took is justifiable. Since this is a small community hospital with limited resources, it is not able to meet all of the medical needs of every patient. The hospital must also consider utilitarian and economic factors. Ms. Y made a fair choice that carefully balanced the principles of need, utility, and ability to pay.

Furthermore, her decision will probably avoid some of problems with morale on the unit, since it will shift some of the burden of caring for Mr. P to private nurses. Good morale among the nursing staff enhances the health care of all the patients on the unit.

Making Mr. P pay for extra care makes a great deal of sense as a general rule for community hospitals, since a community hospital that responded to every patient demand for additional resources would soon go bankrupt. For example, if a patient needs an MRI to determine whether he has a brain tumor, he has no right to require a community hospital to purchase an expensive MRI machine to meet his medical needs. If he wants an MRI, he must seek treatment at a facility that can afford one. Likewise, if Mr. P wants the full standard of care, he must either help to pay for it or seek treatment elsewhere. To do otherwise would be unfair to the other patients, to whom the unit also has moral obligations.

Note

1. For a useful review of these different approaches, see Tom L. Beauchamp and James F. Childress, *Principles of Biomedical Ethics*, 5th ed. (New York: Oxford University Press, 2001), 225–82.

Further Reflections

General

1. Reflect on the fact that one's medical needs are shaped by the way one was raised by family, or socially conditioned, as well as one's genetic predispositions and tendencies about which one has no knowledge or control, everyday limitations of human willpower, and ignorance about the outcomes of choices we all make and the lifestyles we all fall into. Is it possible that individuals are not nearly as free in the choices they make as we think, and therefore not morally responsible for the results of their choices? Might not an attitude of "forgive and forget" or "recognize the fallibility in all persons" be a better attitude to have for individuals like Mr. P (and all of us)? If so, how might this new agnosticism about human responsibility alter the way in which we think about resolving this case?

2. How does our society factor freely chosen lifestyle choices into a determination of the obligations of health care professionals (HCPs) to those who require medical help? What sorts of diseases and illnesses are most likely to generate a feeling of "they had this coming" among HCPs and society; and which (though also a result of lifestyle choice) are less likely to generate this feeling? Compare attitudes toward infant and juvenile obesity, schizophrenia, obsessive-compulsive disorder, HIV disease, late-onset diabetes, manic-depression, injuries due to sports accidents, lung cancer, cardiovascular disease, skin cancer, infections and viruses acquired from living overseas, and acute traumatic injuries acquired in falling from a step ladder vs. bungee jumping.

3. How does the location of a small town and community hospital complicate the facts of this case and the nature of what is owed to patients?

Consequences

4. Brown suggests that employing private duty nurses could slow Mr. P's recuperation. How can we determine if this is true and, if it is, how should the consequences for Mr. P be adjudicated in light of the needs of other patients?

Autonomy

5. Review the criteria for the moral concept of respect for autonomy. To what degree does *respect* for autonomy require active support (as opposed to mere noninterference) of other persons? What might it require? To what degree does autonomy require something of persons demanding respect for their own autonomy? What might it require? Does allowing people the freedom to make whatever choices they want require holding them responsible for the results of the choices they make (and forgo)—even if those results are toxic?

6. If lifestyles *are freely chosen,* how should those choices figure in the assessment of an individual's responsibility for his or her medical problems? In other words, should personal responsibility determine, at least in part, what a patient is due, with respect to medical access and treatment?

Rights

7. What would need to change in this case in order for Mr. P to argue that he has greater rights to care than other patients? than those affirmed by the HCPs?

Virtues

8. What are the obligations of the *health care system* and hospital to Mr. P? What moral principles and professional commitments shape the nature and content of these obligations? Be specific.

9. What moral principles and professional promises are relevant for understanding the professional commitments of nurses to patients in situations like this? What does the American Nurses Association Code of Ethics specify? Can these specifications ever be set aside? If so, under what conditions? If not, why not?

Equality/Fairness (Justice)

10. Resnick suggests that, in allocating the scarce resources of health care, four different approaches might be used. Which, in your opinion, is most justified? How would your preferred theory of justice resolve the case of Mr. P?

11. Silvers argues that patients with extra needs may not justly be denied the resources to meet those needs. To what theory of justice might she be implicitly appealing?

12. To what degree is this a problem case because the patient is obese? Do discrimination and negative attitudes toward obese persons figure in any significant way in the issues that surface in this case? Would a similar dilemma arise if we were dealing with a patient who suffered from some other ailment/physical problem?

Chapter 13

Professional Promises in the "Real" World: Skilled Nursing Facilities (SNFs)

Ms. E still remembers the sense of pride she felt when she received her results from the State Board of Nursing. It had been quite an accomplishment to balance work, education, and responsibilities as a single mother of two. She was excited to begin her career as a registered nurse and confident she could do the job.

Ms. E's first job was at a home health agency, where she worked for four years. During her employment, she was recognized as employee of the month three times and employee of the year once. Colleagues enjoyed working with Ms. E and she was happy with her own performance; she felt she was a good nurse and others agreed. Sadly, Ms. E's agency closed. Employees were given the option of relocating to another city 120 miles away. Ms. E considered moving, but decided that her children, both in high school, would be better off staying in their current environment. After an extensive job search Ms. E accepted a position as charge nurse for the evening shift at a local SNF. She counted herself fortunate to find a job in her small community of 7000.

After a brief orientation Ms. E became the only licensed staff member on site between 4 PM and midnight. Ms. E was unaccustomed to such professional isolation and was concerned about the lack of a resource person to whom she could turn when facing unfamiliar problems. She also worried that she would not be able to attend to all her patients within the time

241

limits of her shift. She discussed her concerns with the director of nursing, Mr. T. Mr. T reviewed good time management practices, such as prioritizing tasks and effectively utilizing ancillary staff. He assured Ms. E that a period of adjustment was both normal and expected, ending their conversation by advising Ms. E to "do the best you can; you'll be fine."

Weeks of frustration followed. Ms. E tried to fulfill her more critical responsibilities—medications, tube feedings, glucose testing of diabetic patients—at the beginning of her shift. On a good day she could accomplish the most crucial tasks. The problem was that there were so many bad days—days with new doctor's orders to implement, new admissions to assess, patients who needed catheters inserted, bowel care, wound care. On these days Ms. E found herself staying one to two hours after shift to complete her responsibilities. She believes she is giving her patients pretty good care, but she cannot seem to do so in the time allotted.

One evening Ms. E asked some of her staff if they shared her concerns. Everyone agreed additional staff was needed, but the experienced nursing assistants let Ms. E know that patients and their needs may change but staffing levels do not. They also let her know she was one of many nurses who had rotated through her position. Most nurses who left did so out of frustration, citing the inability to meet their professional obligation to ensure patients' welfare. Nonetheless, the experienced staff felt they had no choice but to live with the current conditions, especially since the last nurse to leave had been fired when she threatened to go public with the problem.

One evening Ms. E opened a chart to note a doctor's order and, to save time, charted a dressing change she had not yet completed. The next day she realized, to her horror, that she had never changed the dressing. As Ms. E thought about the omission, she recalled several occasions where procedures charted for the preceding shift seemed not to have been done—soiled dressings charted as having been changed, patients with bloated abdomens and complaints of constipation who had supposedly had enemas. Maybe other employees had similar problems organizing or completing patient care.

Ms. E summoned her courage and discussed her mistake with Ms. F, the nurse in charge of the preceding shift. Ms. F replied, in strictest confidence, that all the nurses chart treatments and medications at the beginning of the shift. "After all," Ms. F bemoaned, "we may never get another chance." When Ms. E confessed her charted, but undone, dressing change, Ms. F replied, "Well, sometimes you just can't get everything done. The important thing is, we're doing the best we can. You should see how bad things are in other places!"

Ms. E talked to Mr. T again, thinking perhaps he was unaware of the real situation. Mr. T listened patiently, then informed Ms. E that the facility had to comply with corporate staffing patterns and that "this is as good as it gets."

After ten weeks Ms. E's situation is out of control. After her conversations with Ms. F and Mr. T, she began routinely charting at the beginning of the shift. Not surprisingly, more omissions followed; more than once a charted treatment didn't get done. No one commented on it, but Ms. E was plagued by the memories of so many errors.

What bothered Ms. E most was what she did not remember. How had one event snowballed so quickly? How had she advanced from a single, unintended error to a pattern of deliberate deception? One omitted dressing change had grown into a bad habit. And this approach seemed to work so well. The on-coming staff did not want to know if treatments had really been done; they were satisfied if they had just been charted. Doctors rarely came to see the patients. Families were usually unaware if treatments were missed. Patients' complaints could be ignored or deferred. Besides, if these patients were at home in the care of their families, such omissions of basic care would occur as well. It's one thing to talk about what one would ideally hope for in-patient care, but reality forces all of us to compromise in life. The facility was in compliance with corporate staffing levels. On paper everything looked fine, but in reality patients were not getting the care they needed.

And what about Ms. E's moral responsibility? She had promised when she entered the profession to put her patients' welfare first, to always protect their interests over all others. What had happened to that promise? She could report her concerns to the state oversight board, but she fears losing her job. And she still feels the care she does give is good care, in spite of the fact that she cannot give all the care that is needed.

What, from a moral point of view, should Ms. E do now?

Introduction

This case prompts two important moral questions:

1. What is the *moral* justification for particular staffing levels, and what professional and institutional obligations follow from this?
2. To whom does Nurse E have primary moral obligation: patients, colleagues, or her employer (or the corporate office)?

The AJ Method

Step 1: Information Gathering   What is the nature of the tension between the welfare of patients and of other stakeholders? *Is* Ms. E a good nurse? Can Ms. E take additional steps to improve the efficiency of her own performance? of the performance of her staff? to meet patients' needs through nontraditional approaches (for example, enlisting family volunteers)? If Ms. E reports conditions in her facility, how likely is she to be fired or otherwise punished? How likely is it that her report will change conditions for patients? What motivates corporate staffing patterns?

Presently approximately 1.6 million Americans reside in Skilled Nursing Facilities (SNFs).[1] According to a 1999 survey, 75 percent of SNF residents required assistance with at least three activities of daily living (ADL): 94 percent required assistance with bathing, 87 percent with dressing, 56 percent with toileting, and 47 percent with eating.[2] By any measure, caring for SNF residents is labor intensive.

Step 2: Creative Problem Solving   A creative solution would have to meet patients' needs without jeopardizing Ms. E.

Step 3: Pros and Cons   Survey CARVE principles to identify important moral reasons that support conflicting options for resolving this case.

Consequences   What are the likely consequences for the patients if Ms. E reports the conditions in the facility? (Mills; Peter) if she does not? (Hill) Are patients likely to be better or worse off? (Peter) What about other staff? Ms. E?

SNF residents are vulnerable and dependent. Those who cannot bathe, dress, feed, or toilet themselves must depend on the kindness of strangers. Any moral obligation to advance patients' interests surely implies an environment in which at least residents' basic needs can be met. Derivatively, this environment must incorporate the staffing adequate to those needs.

This analysis of moral obligations is complicated by two facts. First, unlike physicians or nurses, SNFs are responsible—under the moral principles of beneficence *and* utility—to advance the well-being of *all* patients in their facility. Beneficence obliges protecting residents as *individuals*.[3] But SNF administrators might argue that limited resources (financial or—in a small town—staffing), give utility priority over beneficence. Utility mandates distributing benefits and burdens so as to minimize harms/burdens and maximize benefits/interests/welfare of the group or community, to achieve the best *general* outcome. The commitment to utility requires hard choices about who gets what, when. Its proponents argue that utilitarian decisions maximize welfare, all things considered. Perhaps; but a utilitarian approach may result in compromised care for particular individuals. In an ideal world healthcare professionals (HCPs) would provide highest quality of care to every patient at all times; staffing would be sufficient to meet all needs. In our world, utility will almost certainly support suboptimal attention to some patients; staffing will be sufficient to maximize group welfare.

A utilitarian analysis becomes even more complex when one realizes that patients are not the only stakeholders. Caregivers, families, and communities also have a stake in SNFs' success. In the current fiscal environment, both for-profit and not-for-profit SNFs face budget restrictions increasingly strained by suboptimal reimbursement. In addition, investors in for-profit SNFs expect returns on their investments.

Some might argue that any SNF that is unable to provide good care should be closed. But families and communities face tremendous costs when a SNF closes. Families must become primary caregivers for the frail elderly. This burden falls disproportionately on women, who subsequently experience diminished personal and professional opportunities. Job loss forces HCPs to search for employment elsewhere; the community loses HCPs' income if they leave the area.

In sum, a SNF's survival depends on efficient use of resources that demands balancing patient needs and *limited* resources. SNFs are forced to ration care; by definition, "rationed" care implies (at least some) suboptimal care. A utilitarian calculation that takes account of the burdens and benefits to all patients *and* other stakeholders *can* (at least in theory) justify less-than-optimal staffing patterns.

Autonomy Whose autonomy is relevant here? (Mills)

Rights Within the context of the patient-professional relationship, patients have a right to be aided. All parties have a right to not be harmed. Is the right of self-determination relevant here? privacy? confidentiality?

Virtues What does the virtue of fidelity require? (Hill; Mills; Peter) Does courage play a role? Does compassion? Honesty?

Should Nurse E accept a utilitarian calculation? HCPs, as well as administrators of SNFs, must be especially cognizant of their moral obligations to their incapacitated residents. Indeed, their codes of ethics speak to these obligations.[4]

For most HCPs professional identity and integrity are intimately related to advancing the interests of *particular* patients. In particular, the American Nurses Association Code of Ethics specifies: "A fundamental principle that underlies all nursing practice is respect for the inherent worth, dignity, and human rights of *every* individual."[5] The Code further notes: "The nurse's primary commitment is to the health, well-being, and safety of *the* patient. . . ." (§ 3.5, *emphases added*). So it would seem that clinical nurses should focus on each patient rather than on a patient population.

Nurses expect—perhaps naïvely—that their professional communities and institutions will affirm and enable this commitment. When nurses perceive that an institution or its caregivers are failing to live up to the standards of quality care, due consideration of patient well-being, and conformity to ethical and legal standards, moral condemnation (and, quite possibly, guilt) follows. Nurse E experiences this moral dilemma as violation of her professional obligations and her silence as complicity with wrong-doing.

But if a utilitarian calculation supports suboptimal staffing in Nurse E's institution, how should she adjudicate between the SNF's consequence-based obligations and her own professional integrity? As an employee, must Nurse E affirm the full range of institutional commitments? We can agree that SNFs have obligations to various stakeholders (of which patients are but one group), and that SNF investors expect a "return on investment." But do *nurses* have an obligation to stockholders? If so, how are these measured against other obligations? If not, to what action(s) does the virtue of professional integrity (and possibly the virtue of courage) commit Nurse E?

Equality/Fairness (Justice) Are patients being unfairly burdened by current conditions? Is Ms. E? Are other staff members? Are patients being discriminated against because of their age?

The Law In conclusion, the following legal considerations are relevant to this case. (1) Is legal negligence an issue in this case? Does professional "underperformance" count as elder abuse in such a situation? Or is the problem simply a misfit between internal institutional standards and professional ideals? (2) Who is legally liable for the poor care administered in this institution: individual nurses, nursing supervisors, SNF administration, or the corporation (profit or not-for-profit) that owns the SNF? (3) Do HCPs have a legal obligation to report negligence or elder abuse? To whom? (4) What legal requirements and protections cover whistle blowers in such a situation?[6]

The following commentaries examine the application of various moral principles to this dilemma, thereby assisting the reader to undertake *Step 4: Analysis* and *Step 5: Justification*.

RECOMMENDED READINGS

Fletcher, James J., Jeanne M. Sorrell, and Mary Cipriano Silva, "Whistleblowing as a Failure of Organizational Ethics." *Online Journal of Issues in Nursing,* 31 Dec. 1998, http://www.nursingworld.org/ojin/topic8/topic8_3.htm (27 Mar. 2004).

Mills, Ann E. and Edward M. Spencer. "The Healthcare Organization: New Efficiency Endeavors and the Organization Ethics Program." *The Journal of Clinical Ethics* 13, no. 1: 29–39.

Notes

1. National Center for Health Statistics, "Fast Stats A to Z: Nursing Home Care," 14 Apr. 2003, http://www.cdc.gov/nchs/fastats/nursingh.htm (27 Mar. 2004).
2. National Center for Health Statistics, "The National Nursing Home Survey: 1999 Summary," 27 Sep. 2002, http://www.cdc.gov/nchs/about/major/nnhsd/nnhsd.htm (27 Mar. 2004).

3. Centers for Medicare and Medicaid Services, Department of Health and Human Services, "Nursing Homes: Residents' Rights," n.d., http://www.medicare.gov/Nursing/ResidentRights.asp? (27 Mar. 2004).

4. American College of Healthcare Executives, "Code of Ethics," 2000, http://www.ache.org/abt_ache/code.cfm (27 Mar. 2004), § II; American Nurses Association [ANA], *Code of Ethics for Nurses with Interpretive Statements* (Washington, DC: ANA, 2001), http://www.ana.org/ethics/ (27 Mar. 2004), §§ 3.4, 3.5; see also Public Affairs, Parliamentary and Access Branch, Commonwealth Department of Health and Aged Care, Canberra, Australia, "Codes and Declarations: Guide to Ethical Conduct for Providers of Residential Aged Care: Code of Ethics for Residential Aged Care," *Nursing Ethics* 10, no. 1 (2003): 89–94.

5. See ANA, Note 4, above, § 1.1 (emphasis added).

6. George P. Smith, II, *Legal and Healthcare Ethics for the Elderly* (Washington, DC: Taylor and Francis, 1996), 91–106, provides an overview of the Patient's Bill of Rights, long-term care ombudsman representation, the use of physical and chemical restraints, forced psychotropic medication, and elder abuse issues. From the perspective of the medical director of such an institution, see American Medical Association, Council on Ethical and Judicial Affairs, *Code of Medical Ethics: Current Opinions with Annotations*, 2000–2001 ed. (Chicago: American Medical Association, 2000), § 8.02, "Ethical Guidelines for Physicians in Management and Other Non-Clinical Roles," 141–42; and § 2.095, "The Provision of Adequate Health Care," 28–30. Peter J. Buttaro and Emily L. H. Buttaro, *Legal Guide for Long-Term Care Administrators* (Sudbury, MA: Jones and Bartlett, 1999) provides an overview of issues related to torts, negligence, administrative liability, and protective arrangements for person and property.

A Nurse's Analysis

Elizabeth Peter, PhD, RN

Nurse E's primary moral obligation is to ensure a high-quality health care environment.[1] The Canadian Nurses Association (CNA) Code of Ethics states, "Nurses value and advocate for practice environments that have the organizational structures and resources necessary to ensure safety, support and respect for all persons in the work setting."[2]

The poor care in this skilled nursing facility (SNF) is unlikely to result from Nurse E's incompetence or an idiosyncratic perception. Despite her recent history of errors, her former peers and employer have recognized her as an outstanding nurse. Moreover her staff agrees additional nurses are needed to provide good care and have witnessed other nurses who were in Nurse E's position leave because they felt incapable of meeting their professional obligations to patients. The firing of Nurse E's predecessor, who threatened to go public with the problem, is a sign that the organization does not support or respect its employees or its patients. Therefore we can reasonably conclude that this SNF is not a quality health care environment.

Nurse E has no ethically justified option but to take action. The American Nurses Association (ANA) code states, "Acquiescing and accepting unsafe or inappropriate practices, even if the individual does not participate in the specific practice, is equivalent to condoning unsafe practice."[3] Acting to ensure a quality health care environment, however, can be politically and ethically challenging. Both the CNA and ANA codes, and a CNA document entitled "I See and Am Silent/I See and Speak Out: The Ethical Dilemma of Whistleblowing," provide direction to nurses that can facilitate this process.[4]

First, Nurse E must report her errors to Mr. T and must ensure that these errors are responsibly disclosed to her patients.[5] In the disclosure of errors nurses promote, advocate for, and strive to protect the health, safety, and rights of patients. Second, as an advocate for her patients she must address her concerns regarding staffing through the appropriate channels.[6] She has already spoken with the director of nursing twice and with Ms. F, another charge nurse. Nevertheless, Nurse E must persistently continue to advocate for change, likely through collective action also.[7] She should inform Mr. T that she will report the problem further if he does not act. Although the SNF is small and may not have many channels through which Nurse E can expand her efforts, she must take this issue as far as she can—perhaps to the SNF administrator or board of directors. Third, if these efforts fail, partnering with other nurses and a professional organization to report the problem of understaffing could strengthen Nurse E's efforts. Through this process these nurses should be open with their managers about their activities and should fully document all steps taken. If these actions also fail Nurse E must consider reporting the SNF's patient care problems outside of the organization—whistleblowing—either on her own or in conjunction with others. Possibilities include reporting the problem to the state oversight board or the media. Actions such as whistleblowing are ethically justified because nurses must "value and advocate for quality practice environments that have the organizational structures and resources necessary to ensure safety, support and respect for all persons in the work setting."[8]

Whistleblowing, however, should be considered a last resort because it can create chaos and suspicion in an organization. Individuals, if falsely accused, could lose their employment and their reputations.[9] Although patients are the nurse's primary moral responsibility, nurses also have a moral obligation to maintain "compassionate and caring relationships with colleagues and others."[10] In addition, the whistleblower herself can experience harassment, a tarnished reputation, or job loss. Thus, the actual or potential harm must be serious and the nurse must have reported concerns through the hierarchy without satisfactory explanation or action.[11]

In small communities some unique features must be taken into account when whistleblowing is considered. Potential harms can be magnified. If the community is close-knit, a loss of reputation could have a profound impact on a community member's public and private life. In addition, because employment opportunities are likely less plentiful than in a large city, the loss of employment, along with reputation, could make finding new work nearly impossible for someone like Nurse E. Outside supports, such as one's professional association, may also be less accessible.

On the other hand, the character of a small community could lead those threatened with public exposure to act more quickly to protect their reputations. It also may be easier for Nurse E to garner the support of her colleagues and members of the community in collective action because SNF patients are likely well known to family members, neighbors, friends, former coworkers, and so forth.

In conclusion, Nurse E has the moral obligation to continue to act until she has reported the problem through all reasonable channels. Unfortunately she may suffer personal loss as a result, but in the end her moral integrity as a person and as a nursing professional is preserved.

RECOMMENDED READINGS

Wilmot, S. "Nurses and Whistleblowing: The Ethical Issues." *Journal of Advanced Nursing* 32, no. 5 (2000): 1051–57.

Notes

1. American Nurses Association [ANA], *Code of Ethics for Nurses with Interpretive Statements* (Washington, DC: ANA, 2001), http://www.ana.org/ethics/ (27 Mar. 2004); Canadian Nurses Association [CNA], *Code of Ethics for Registered Nurses,* 2002, www.cna.aiic.ca (14 Jan. 2003), http://www.cna-nurses.ca/_frames/search/searchframe.htm (30 Mar. 2004).
2. See CNA, note 1, above, 8.
3. See ANA, note 1, above, § 6.3.
4. See ANA, note 1, above; see note 1, CNA, above; Canadian Nurses Association, "I See and Am Silent/I See and Speak Out: The Ethical Dilemma of Whistleblowing," (Ethics in Practice), 1999, http://www.cna-nurses.ca/.
5. See ANA and CNA, note 1, above.
6. See ANA, note 1, above.
7. See ANA and CNA, note 1, above.
8. See CNA, note 1, above, 17.
9. See "I See," note 4, above.
10. See ANA, note 1, above, § 1.5.
11. See "I See," note 4, above.

A Medical Director's Analysis

Terry Hill, MD

Nurse E is right to question how she could have gone so far so fast, from a one-time shortcut to "a pattern of deliberate deception." Contributing factors include the stress and isolation of a new job in a new clinical setting. She apparently has no training and no previous experience in nursing facilities, and she has no professional colleagues on her shift. She has yet to consult the Code of Ethics for nurses[1] or colleagues outside the facility. Nurse E needs to awaken and begin to extricate herself from this nightmare, relying on and restoring her integrity and professionalism.

The threat of sanctions provides a very real frame for the day-to-day temptations that clinicians face. It is true that state surveyors on their annual or episodic visits may not detect her charting deceptions. Even if they do, they will most likely punish the facility, which may or may not discipline Nurse E. The advent of quality indicators and quality measures increases the likelihood that the facility will face regulatory or corporate scrutiny for its pressure sores and other conditions. But Nurse E and the other nurses in the facility correctly perceive that these threats are *indirect*. The *direct* threat of sanctions comes from the state's board of nursing. "Precharting" is considered falsification of records that could cost Nurse E her license.[2] If a colleague were to bring this point home, it could serve as a wake-up call and Nurse E might find her next steps much easier to make.

Nurse E should stop precharting treatments and medications. She also needs to think through how to respond to the fact that other nurses are precharting. Consistent with other health professional codes, the Code of Ethics for Nurses articulates nurses' responsibilities to advocate for patients and to improve healthcare environments. The Code's interpretive statements call for addressing directly the person engaged in questionable practice. Depending on the "detrimental effects" of the practice on patients and the integrity of nursing practice, Nurse E should proceed up the reporting hierarchies. "Reporting unethical, illegal, incompetent, or impaired practices, even when done appropriately, may present substantial risks to the nurse; nevertheless, such risks do not eliminate the obligation to address serious threats to patient safety."[3] While it is appropriate for Nurse E to think through the gravity of the situation and the consequences of her decisions, taking into account other factors such as her obligation to provide for her children, the fact remains that her failure to report illegal and unethical practices violates her *professional*, if not her *personal*, code of ethics.

Should Nurse E leave the facility? "Nurses should not remain employed in facilities that routinely violate patient rights or require nurses to severely and repeatedly compromise standards of practice or personal morality."[4] If the facility and corporate leadership continue to stonewall her, she will probably have to leave.

On the other hand, she might be able to find an ally within the corporate structure, especially if the facility's pressure sore prevalence, posted on the federal Medicare website, has already raised concerns.* Many corporations hire nurse con-

---

*Since 1999, facilities and surveyors have been getting "quality indicator" data derived from the Minimum Data Set submitted to the state on each skilled nursing facility resident. Each SNF sends data to the state, which analyzes it and submits a "quality assessment" for each patient. Since 2002 similar data have been posted on the Nursing Home Compare Web site: http://medicare.gov/nhcompare/home.asp (27 Mar. 2004). These data are nationwide.

sultants who routinely visit their facilities and occasionally can help transform a facility's practices and culture. Multiple intermediate situations between these two responses will require Nurse E to weigh her obligations and choices. Her deliberations will be vastly less frightening once she develops exit options to use as needed.

The narrative does not describe others within the facility or corporation who are interested in improving the facility's practices, outcomes, staff retention, or moral climate. Mr. T's first conversation with Nurse E, in which he gave her time management advice and encouragement, may have been appropriate for a new employee struggling to learn the routines in a new practice setting. Their next conversation, in which he apparently condones the precharting practice, reflects profound moral and professional deficits. If the director of nursing cannot uphold practice standards, the facility is likely to face serious trouble soon, either from regulatory sanctions or lawsuits or both. His comment about "how bad things are in other places" is manipulative and incorrect. There is consensus that almost all nursing facilities are understaffed.[5] Even so, most facilities staff higher than the minimum cut-off below which substandard care is inevitable.[6] Nurses do not commonly collude in charting their treatments and medications at the beginning of the shift. Facilities with such widespread, egregious violations tend to be recognized as "chronically poor performers" by regulatory agencies.

Corporations, state agencies, and state professional organizations have an obligation to provide appropriate reporting processes which could support Nurse E's moral and professional recovery and minimize her risk. While these are a good start, a moral environment depends on much more than reporting procedures. This facility has fallen far short of facilitating an "open forum for moral discourse" with supportive working conditions, policies, ethically informed education, and grievance mechanisms.[7]

As individuals within the facility and corporate leadership become aware of the facility's poor practices, they need to weigh factors and options that are quite similar to those Nurse E had to weigh. They should begin by making the needs of the residents their highest priority. They will need to argue that a commitment to quality improvement, professional standards, and caring relationships can reduce the facility's risk. Transforming an organization's practices requires knowledge, skills, resources, leadership commitment, and persistence. Our codes of professional ethics require that we continually take small steps in the right direction.[8]

Notes

1. American Nurses Association [ANA], *Code of Ethics for Nurses With Interpretive Statements* July 2001, http://nursingworld.org/ethics/code/ethicscode150.htm (27 Mar. 2004).
2. Mississippi Board of Nursing, *Board Notes* 17, no. 3, (2000), http://www.msbn.state.ms.us (27 Mar. 2004).
3. See ANA, note 1, above.
4. Ibid.

5. Institute of Medicine, *Report: Improving the Quality of Long-term Care* (Washington, DC: National Academy Press, 2001).

6. *Report to Congress: Appropriateness of Minimum Nurse Staffing Ratios In Nursing Homes Phase II Final Report* (Washington, DC: Centers for Medicare and Medicaid Services, 19 Mar. 2002), http://www.cms.hhs.gov/medicaid/reports/rp1201home.asp (27 Mar. 2004).

7. See ANA, note 1, above.

8. American College of Physicians, *Ethics Manual*, 1998, http://www.acponline.org/ethics/ethics_man.htm (27 Mar. 2004); American Medical Association, *AMA Code of Medical Ethics*, 18 Jul. 2003, http://www.ama-assn.org/ama/pub/category/8600.html (27 Mar. 2004); National Association of Social Workers, "Code of Ethics," 1999, n.d., http://www.naswdc.org/pubs/code/code.asp (27 Mar. 2004); see ANA, note 1, above.

An Organizational Ethicist's Analysis

Ann E. Mills, MSc (Econ), MBA

Approaching a case from an organizational ethics viewpoint means asking, "Is there a role for an organization ethics program to play in this dilemma?" In this instance an organization ethics program certainly *could* play a role. Ms. E could approach members of the program confidentially; she could state her dilemma and ask for help. The program could then follow whatever consultation steps have been outlined in its charter—gathering facts, approaching stakeholders, making recommendations. In this instance, as I explain below, it is doubtful that an organization ethics program would ever be established, let alone have the authority and moral prestige to play an effective role.

The ethical climate of an organization results from an organization's culture which depends, in large part, on the beliefs and behaviors of its stakeholders. The ethical climate of any organization can be positive or negative and—from a moral point of view—good or bad. A negative ethical climate results from the gap between what the organization *says* are its mission and values and what its stakeholders *perceive* about its daily operations and goals.

Since all health care organizations deliver health care, they should all endorse the delivery of quality care. Since there is a consensus in this country that health care is not solely a market commodity and that effective interventions may require the trust of patients and the compassion of providers, all health care organizations should endorse other (nonmarket) values (like trust or compassion). Most health care organizations do subscribe to these kinds of values. In all probability, this organization has some kind of mission and values statement that says that it endorses them. They may be part of the organization's marketing or advertising programs. However, "subscribing" to particular values doesn't mean much unless the organization lives up to them.

Organization leaders in authority set the examples and supply the policies—either explicitly stated or not—for others to follow. To establish a fully functioning organization ethics program, organizational leaders must embrace this goal; this implies that organization leaders believe in the goals of the program: to articulate and enhance the ethical climate of the organization by helping to align the organization's mission and values with its daily operations and goals.

In this example, organization leaders obviously value something other than the delivery of quality care—perhaps return on investment—and there is no evidence of any other value that society generally associates with the delivery of care. Organization leaders seem to be satisfied with the state of affairs that currently exists and my guess is that they would not see the necessity for such a program. If it were established, perhaps for accreditation reasons, the program would be ineffective as its role and function would at best be meaningless to organization leaders. At worst, organization leaders would see it as a threat to the *actual* (as opposed to its espoused) values and goals of the organization.

The ethical climate of any organization, driven by the actual values of the organization, forms the basis for stakeholder roles and relationships. In this case stakeholder roles are confused and relationships are poisoned. Ms. E is confused about her role as a nurse; she cannot trust her supervisor; and her relationships with her coworkers and her patients and their families are deteriorating. She has been told to "do the best she can" and she perceives a policy of silence surrounding the delivery of chronically indifferent and sloppy care. She knows it is wrong and probably illegal, but feels powerless to do anything about it. Her choices are bleak: Ms. E can do nothing, she can quit, or she can become a whistleblower.

Ms. E knows in the short term that if she does nothing the values that propelled her to nursing school and which she thinks are important will be slowly eroded, and that her conduct and beliefs will shortly resemble those of her coworkers. Ms. E is an intelligent woman, however, and probably knows that in the long term, this situation will result in an incident that neither the families of the residents, the organization leaders, nor the regulators can ignore. In that event, most probably, some degree of culpability will be laid at the feet of the health care professionals associated with the organization, and Ms. E's reputation and career prospects will be severely damaged: she could quite possibly be charged with criminal behavior. Doing nothing is not a long-term option Ms. E can afford to consider, and it is a dangerous short-term option.

Quitting is not a short-term option. Ms. E has two children that she must support and employment prospects are not abundant in her community. In the long term, however, finding employment elsewhere is a viable option and one that confronts many Americans every day. Given Ms. E's qualifications, she could likely find reasonable employment in a good community with a good school system. This choice however, begs the question of Ms. E's moral responsibility to her patients.

Most states regulate the conditions under which care is delivered to residents in nursing homes and unacceptable conditions in long-term care facilities can be confidentially reported to a dedicated agency. If Ms. E chooses this option, it would probably mean the end of her career in the facility. The community is small; since Ms. E has already complained to her supervisor, organization leaders would have an idea of who was responsible for contacting the regulators. Organization leaders have already shown their willingness to terminate employees who do not follow the policies endorsed by the organization. But even if she is not fired, and even if regulators allow the facility to remain open, she would be inviting investigation of her own role in the facility that she herself views as unacceptable. In reality, she would probably be sanctioned—or even blamed for some of the conditions in the facility.

The only option that Ms. E has to safeguard her future and the future of her children is to find employment in another locality. The only option that Ms. E has to ensure the safety and well-being of her patients without inviting harm to herself is to contact regulators anonymously after she has moved.

Further Reflections

General

1. Mills notes that "the ethical climate of an organization results from an organization's culture, which depends, in large part, on the beliefs and behaviors of its stakeholders." Develop a short list of what might reasonably be included in the skilled nursing facility's (SNF's) mission and values statements. Develop a short list of the major stakeholders in this case. Discuss the relationship between the values and the stakeholders, noting areas of divergence and convergence.
2. Compare and contrast the recommendations of Hill, Mills, and Peter. Given your work in question #1 (above), which of these is most likely to succeed?
3. Does the fact that this is the only SNF in this small town inform your moral analysis of this case? If so, how and why?

Consequences

4. What are the outcome-based arguments for whistleblowing in this case? against whistleblowing?
5. What role do the following stakeholders play in guaranteeing that the SNF functions optimally? What does optimum functioning mean for each of them?
   a. SNF administration
   b. Oversight committees for nursing practice
   c. State and federal SNF regulatory boards
   d. Shareholders in the private company

    e. Nurses
    f. Physicians
    g. Patients
    h. Patients' families

Autonomy

6. According to Hill, precharting is a species of falsification of records. Why might SNF regulators see it as such a serious problem?

Rights

7. Medicare has determined that SNF residents have a "right to be treated with dignity and respect." What does this right imply for staffing levels?

Virtues

8. The ANA Code of Ethics seems to require beneficence to individual patients; Ms. E's colleagues and the administration of the SNF seem to advocate beneficence to the corporation. Assuming Nurse E wishes to perform with integrity, which of these obligations is most/more demanding?

Equality/Fairness (Justice)

9. One often hears complaints that the needs of elders are shorted in U.S. society. In your estimation, is inadequate staffing in SNFs due to the fact that most residents are over 65 years of age? In any case, is the staffing—even if substandard when compared to, for example, staffing in hospitals that care for patients who are acutely, rather than chronically ill—morally permissible?

Are We Our Patients' Keepers?

Pleasantville is a geographically remote town of 40,000, situated in north-ern California in the foothills of the Sierra Nevada mountains. The near-est town of comparable size is 110 miles away. Because the area enjoys moderate weather, a relatively low cost of living, and lovely scenery, it has attracted large numbers of retirees. The major sources of employment in the region are agriculture, a cannery, a mobile-home manufacturer, a hos-pital, and a regional community college, all of which (excepting agricul-ture) provide health insurance for employees and their families. Six years ago insurance options for these employers included fee-for-service and preferred provider options and six health maintenance organizations (HMOs).

Most local physicians are members of an independent professional as-sociation (IPA) that negotiates covered services and fees with all insurance providers. The last six years have seen a loss of five HMOs when they could not reach mutually agreeable contracts with the IPA. Eighty-five percent of the town's residents are now insured by the single remaining HMO. Recently the IPA announced its intention to not renew its contract with the HMO. At a town hall meeting the administrators of the IPA and several member physicians discussed their reasons for this decision. These included, first, a reluctance to be in a position of having to balance the needs of particular patients against the needs of patients collectively. Most physicians felt uncomfortable with the inevitable conflict that continu-ously arose between their commitments to advance individual patients' in-terests and their obligations to keep costs under control as players in the health financing game. The physicians noted that they had taken an oath to put the interests of each individual patient first. The HMO policies make keeping this professional promise always difficult and sometimes impossible.

Second, most physicians speaking that night felt that under managed care they had also lost much of their professional freedom and autonomy. They noted that HMO policies constrain management of patient care. Generally, the HMO was not willing nor able to take account of the nec-essarily individual nature of therapy. Although patients with the same di-agnosis do not necessarily benefit from a single therapeutic approach, the HMO demanded identical treatment of diagnoses (not of patients). In complying with one-size-fits-all therapies, some patients' best interests have not been served. Further, the HMO drug formulary limits the drugs physicians can prescribe, even though different patients with the same di-agnosis respond differently to different drugs. The result, according to the physicians, has been a deterioration of the quality of care afforded their patients. Further, this loss of professional autonomy has contributed to patients' perceptions that they were not receiving the care they needed. When the HMO refused to pay for certain treatments or drugs, physi-cians often found themselves trying to convince patients that particular drugs, diagnostic procedures, interventions, or referrals to specialists were inadvisable. Efforts to persuade patients to accept different (cov-ered) approaches were both time-consuming and increasingly adversar-ial, especially if patients believed the physician's motivation was financial rather than beneficent, or if patients had requested a specific medicine or treatment.

Finally, the physicians have become concerned about their own finan-cial interests in the face of HMO reimbursement policies and financial arrangements with the IPA. They have been forced under the present HMO arrangement to accept appreciably lower personal incomes. Many physicians have found themselves forced to spend increasingly larger amounts of (unreimbursed) time in convincing their patients that the quality of their care was not being sacrificed for profits. Nor is time the only resource for which physicians have been (in their estimation) poorly paid. Increasing uncompensated care (care needed by patients and given by physicians but not reimbursed by the HMO) has lowered the local av-erage annual physician income from $140,000 to $90,000. To preserve their income, physicians have needed to see more patients (35–40 instead of 20–25 patients each day). As a result, quality of care and patient and *physician satisfaction have suffered, though not necessarily because physicians were prescribing inferior (or no) treatment. Rather, the very resource—physician time—that is crucial to ensuring patient trust and satisfaction has been in shorter and shorter supply. The doctors are worried that they may have been subconsciously making treatment decisions based on their own financial interests, though they feel they have not done so intentionally.*

The physicians spoke eloquently about their concerns, emphasizing that the most pressing issue is increasing strain on patient-professional relationships. How, they worried, could they help people who might not perceive them as honorable or trust them as professionals? Their solution is to abandon their relationship with the HMO which, they believe, has been the source of these negative effects.

The patients and a few health care advocacy workers present at the meeting were sympathetic to some of these arguments, but by and large they remained unpersuaded by them. They feel that the HMO represents the most (in many cases, the only) affordable insurance option for literally thousands of persons in the community. The town's rural nature generates salaries that are lower than those of their urban counterparts. Senior citizens noted that they retired to Pleasantville in large part because of its lower cost of living, and that their fixed incomes give them little fiscal flexibility. For all citizens, but especially seniors, the HMO's pharmacy benefit is critical to their welfare. Many would be unable to afford their numerous prescription drugs if they had to purchase them outside the HMO—that is, at full price. Many residents claimed they would have to forgo physician visits as well. The much larger monthly premiums, co-payments, and annual deductibles required by the remaining insurance options are beyond the means of well over half of the citizens, especially those with chronic conditions that require frequent physician visits. These individuals also face the problem of being unable to get any new health insurance at an affordable rate, given their preexisting conditions. While urban dwellers might be able to "vote with their feet" (i.e., establish relationships with physicians who have not severed relationships with the HMO), the town's geographic isolation makes this practically impossible.

As to the loss of physician autonomy, the patients argued that most HMOs permit exceptions in treatment modalities if a physician can make a persuasive case for the exception. Many patients had anecdotes suggesting that such exceptions had been granted fairly regularly by the HMOs in the past. Most patients saw such requests by physicians as an effective method for addressing worries about individualizing therapy. The physi-

cians replied that the paperwork needed to get exceptions approved is burdensome, adding not only to their workload, but further reducing their income (because they had to hire personnel to submit the paperwork and were not compensated for the resources—time, personnel—needed to process these requests). Thus, this approach has aggravated many of their concerns.

Nor were most residents sympathetic to the loss of physician income. At the meeting they noted that physicians, like other citizens, enjoy the lower costs of living associated with the rural environment. In fact, very few other residents' income even approximates $90,000, although most enjoy a comfortable (albeit simple) life. The physicians replied that they have made—and are now stuck with—financial commitments (e.g., student loans, mortgages) based on anticipated incomes greater than $90,000/year; reneging on these commitments would have negative ripple effects throughout the community. A few farmers in the audience reported that on more than one occasion they have had to renegotiate loans when crops garnered less income than anticipated; that's just life. The physicians were less sanguine about this approach; some said that continued affiliation with the HMO would force them to relocate, depriving the community of their services. And replacing them would be difficult, as new physicians would be reluctant to come to a community with so low an average income. One or two citizens suggested that maybe the physicians have been making individualized care decisions based on their own financial interests; at the very least they certainly seem to be making career decisions on that basis.

Most citizens at the town meeting, however, affirmed trust in their physicians' professional abilities and judgments, fiscal and therapeutic. They realized the physicians—as they themselves—have been under pressure from the HMOs. Knowing that, they have had to become more proactive; to assume that their physicians are thinking only of patients' interests would be foolish. Most think they have become responsible consumers seeking to protect the welfare of their families and communities; they don't really want to be antagonistic toward the doctors themselves, many of whom have become family friends over the years.

The meeting concluded with the citizens reiterating that their best interests generally would be served by having this more affordable insurance option; they implored the representatives of the IPA to reconsider its position.

Are the physicians morally obligated to renew their contract with the remaining HMO?

Introduction

At least three moral issues are raised by this case:

1. What are the *consequences* of failing to insure individuals/populations?
2. Is failing to insure individuals/populations *(un)just?*
3. Does failing to participate in some/any insurance program violate physicians' *professional integrity?*

The AJ Method

Step 1: Information Gathering   What is the nature of the tension between patients and physicians? What harms will patients suffer if physicians refuse to renew the contract? Will many (how many?) be genuinely unable to afford health care? What harms will physicians suffer if they renew the contract? Is the HMO obstinate about reimbursement rates? What motivates the physicians' decision to abandon the contract?

The burdens of failing to insure U.S. citizens are well documented: the uninsured "live sicker and die earlier."[1] Inadequate insurance and, derivatively, access to health care typically afflict rural residents more harshly than urban dwellers: rural Americans have a 20 percent higher rate of uninsurance than urban dwellers, partly because so many are self-employed.[2] Nor has managed care improved rural insurance coverage; less than 8 percent of rural Americans receive health care from a health maintenance organization (HMO).[3] Further, rural areas are more likely to experience a shortage of physicians.[4] The causes and causal relationships of these deficiencies is unclear, but all contribute to reduced health care access for rural residents.

Step 2: Creative Problem Solving   A creative solution would have to meet patients' needs and physicians' needs simultaneously. (All commentators)

Step 3: Pros and Cons   Survey CARVE principles to identify important moral reasons that support conflicting options for resolving this case.

Consequences   Who will be harmed if the contract is not renewed? What will be the nature of those harms? (Campbell; Magnus and Goold) What, specifically, will be the effects on the trust relationship between patients and physicians? (Campbell; Magnus and Goold) Who will benefit if the contract is renewed? What will be the nature of those benefits? What might an appeal to the principle of utility advise? (Gannett)

The current problems in Pleasantville would be ameliorated by national or state universal health insurance coverage.[5] Absent that, citizens and physicians might begin by examining their dilemma in consequential terms.

Consequential discussions examine results to all affected and seek to maximize benefits while minimizing burdens. Complex dilemmas incorporate burdens *and* benefits, and consequentialist analysis involves trade-offs *in principle*—that is, benefits to some typically entail burdens to others. The dilemma at hand involves consequences to both the community and individuals. If the morally justifiable (as opposed to merely self-interested) benefits to physicians of eschewing HMO affiliation are sufficiently great, burdens to patients are morally justified—even if this entails onerous burdens to particular individuals. Similarly, if the consequences of denying insurance to some maximize benefits to the citizens considered collectively (including physicians), such denials are morally permissible.

Autonomy Whose autonomy is relevant here? (Campbell) What option best preserves or promotes autonomy?

Rights Within the context of the patient-professional relationship, patients have a right to be aided. (Gannett) All parties have a right to not be harmed. Do all parties have a right of self-determination?

Virtues What do professional integrity and fidelity to patients advise? (Campbell; Gannett) Is honesty relevant? compassion?

Assuming small-town citizens ought to be guaranteed reasonable access to health insurance and providers, the question remains: who is responsible for providing these benefits?

Appeals to professional integrity and fidelity are often made to assert an obligation of faithfulness to patients who have come to be dependent on professional assistance. The American Medical Association (AMA) explicitly endorses priority of patient needs over preservation of an insurance company's resources.[6] Yet is fidelity to one's patients inescapable? Or are physicians allowed to opt out of relationships for some (if not just any) reasons? Is reimbursement ever one such reason? If so, how "poor" must a physician be to call it quits?

Perhaps one might appeal to fidelity to the profession, if not one's patients. The AMA's *Principles of Medical Ethics* states that physicians should "recognize a responsibility to participate in activities contributing to the improvement of the community and the betterment of public health" (principle VII), and "support access to medical care for all people" (principle IX).[7] Such statements suggest physicians have some obligations to establish social contracts with communities and, given the current methods of financing health care, contracts with insurance companies. But then, what of Principle VI: "A physician shall, in the provision of appropriate patient care, except in emergencies, be free to choose whom to serve . . ."?[8] What the profession morally requires is unclear.[9]

Two conflicts of interests bear on this dilemma (which can also be analyzed from a consequential perspective): a primarily financial conflict between physicians and the HMO over reimbursement rates; and the conflicts that arise within managed care itself. Bernard Lo explains: "A conflict of interest exists when a person entrusted with the interests of a client, dependent, or the public violates that trust by promoting his own self-interest or the interests of third parties, such as hospitals or insurance plans."[10] If physicians, first and foremost, should be ". . . dedicated to providing competent medical care, with compassion and respect for human dignity and rights,"[11] to what extent can they be required, in compliance with professional integrity, to sacrifice their own (in this case, financial) interests?[12]

Managed care arrangements also generate conflicts between the interests of individual patients and patient populations (e.g., reducing care to one so that all may be better served), as well as between the interests of patients and providers (e.g., a subsequent loss of trust by patients who suspect their physicians may be rationing their care).[13]

Equality/Fairness (Justice)   If the contract is not renewed, are patients unjustly burdened? (Campbell) If the contract is renewed, are physicians unjustly burdened? (Gannett) What role does equality—for example, equal access, equal earning power—play here? (Magnus and Goold)

One must ask whether abandoning the HMO affiliation is (un)just. Justice—getting what one deserves—may be incompatible with maximizing good out-comes.[14] Are the disproportionate health care burdens faced by rural and small-town Americans unjust?[15] Perhaps less-than-optimal health care access, higher cost for desired care, or lower salaries for health care professionals (HCPs) are fair trade-offs for the benefits of living in a small community.

Denying health insurance/care merely on the basis of geography *seems* unjust. Perhaps, but people choose their addresses for many reasons, and rural conditions that generate burdens also generate benefits. Persons may decide to reside in small towns because they find this environment attractive. Urban emigrants report moving to escape the chaos, crime, and crowding of urban centers; to reconnect on a personal level with neighbors and family; to simplify expensive or complicated lifestyles; to have more time to do things they value. People move to small towns to "live" their values. Many Pleasantville residents chose the community for lifestyle reasons. The choice to join a particular community—as a retiree, urban refugee, or new physician—is typically freely made. However, once ensconced in the Pleasantville ethos, an implicit social contract may require residents to relinquish some freedom in order to nurture and perpetuate that lifestyle.[16]

Have Pleasantville citizens (tacitly) consented to forgo certain conveniences? Might the easier access to insurance and physicians found in urban settings be *justly* denied in small towns? Or is reliable access to insurance and physicians independent of context—even if improved access damages the context itself?

The Law   In conclusion, the following legal considerations are relevant to this case: (1) Does this situation constitute patient abandonment, and what are the legal issues surrounding such actions? (2) Does a patient-professional relationship constitute a legal contract, even if only implicit? If so, under what conditions may it be legally breached or rendered void? (3) What legal responsibilities, if any, are binding on the HMO in this case?[17]

What guidance can consequences, justice, and integrity provide for adjudicating between health interests of individual patients and patient populations, and for determining what economic arrangement will—in the long run—provide a sustainable balance between the competing commitments to health care access, quality, and cost containment?[18] This dilemma requires us to determine what might count as a legitimate reason to terminate a patient-physician relationship; the consequences of doing so; whether doing so is (un)just; and the extent to which *personal* interests can inform *professional* decisions.

The following commentaries examine the application of various moral principles to this dilemma, thereby assisting the reader to undertake *Step 4: Analysis* and *Step 5: Justification*.

Notes

1. American College of Physicians–American Society of Internal Medicine, "No Health Insurance? It's Enough to Make You Sick—Scientific Research Linking the Lack of Health Coverage to Poor Health," n.d., http://www.acponline.org/uninsured/lack-contents.htm, p. 4 (13 July 2003); Board on Health Care Services (HCS), Institute of Medicine, *Hidden Costs, Value Lost: Uninsurance in America*, 2003, www.amcp.org/press/release/weekly/index_weekly.asp (13 July 2003).

2. National Rural Health Association, "Access to Health Care for the Uninsured in Rural and Frontier America," 1999, http://www.nrharural.org/dc/issuepapers/ipaper15.html (22 June 2003).

3. American Academy of Physicians Assistants, "Managed Health Care and Rural America," 1997, http://www.aapa.org/policy/managed-health-care.html (22 June 2003).

4. National Rural Health Association, "What's Different about Rural Health Care," n.d., http://www.nrharural.org/pagefile/different.html (13 July 2003); Health Resources and Services Administration, "Selected Statistics on Health Professional Shortages Areas, Division of the Shortage Designation Bureau of Primary Healthcare," n.d., http://ruralhealth.hrsa.gov/links (22 June 2003).

5. See, however, Charlene A. Galarneau, "Health Care as a Community Good: Many Dimensions, Many Communities, Many Views of Justice," *Hastings Center Report* 32, no. 5 (2002): 33–40, for an argument that locating health care control in local communities is more likely to be effective.

6. Council on Ethical and Judicial Affairs (CEJA), American Medical Association, "Ethical Issues in Managed Care," *JAMA: Journal of the American Medical Association* 273 (1995): 332.

7. American Medical Association, "E-Principles of Medical Ethics," 15 July 2002, http://www.ama-assn.org/ama/pub/category/8292.html (22 June 2003).

8. Ibid.

9. Susan M. Wolf, "Health Care Reform and the Future of Physician Ethics," *Hastings Center Report* 24, no. 2 (1994): 28–41.

10. Bernard Lo, "Overview of Conflicts of Interest," in *Resolving Ethical Dilemmas: A Guide for Clinicians* (Baltimore: Williams & Wilkins, 1995), 267.

11. AMA, see note 7, above, Principle 1.

12. Ezekiel Emanuel and Nancy N. Dubler, "Preserving the Physician-Patient Relationship in the Era of Managed Care," *JAMA: Journal of the American Medical Association* 273 (1995): 323–29; see CEJA, note 6, above.

13. Allen Buchanan, "Trust in Managed Care Organizations," *Kennedy Institute of Ethics Journal* 10 (2000): 189–212; CEJA, note 6, above, 330–35; Mark A. Hall et al., "Trust in Physicians and Medical Institutions: What Is It, Can It Be Measured, and Does It Matter?" *The Milbank Quarterly* 79, no. 4 (2001): 613–39; Patricia Illingworth, "Trust: The Scarcest of Medical Resources," *The Journal of Medicine and Philosophy* 27, no. 1 (2002): 31–46; John H. McArthur and Francis D. Moore, "The Two Cultures and the Healthcare Revolution: Commerce and Professionalism in Medical Care," *JAMA: Journal of the American Medical Association* 277 (1997): 985–89; Laurence B. McCullough, "Moral Authority, Power and Trust in Clinical Ethics," *The Journal of Medicine and Philosophy* 24, no. 1 (1999): 1–10; Laurence B. McCullough, "A Basic Concept in the Clinical Ethics of Managed Care: Physicians and Institutions as Economically Disciplined Moral Co-fiduciaries of Populations of Patients," *The Journal of Medicine and Philosophy* 24, no. 1 (1999): 77–97; David Orentlicher, "Managed Care and the Threat to the Patient-Physician Relationship," *Trends in Healthcare, Law & Ethics* 10, no. 1/2 (1995): 19–24; Steven D. Pearson, James E. Sabin, and Tracey Hyams, "Caring for Patients within a Budget: Physicians' Tales from the Front Lines of Managed Care," *The Journal of Clinical Ethics* 13, no. 2 (2002): 115–23.

14. Norman Daniels, *Am I My Parents' Keeper? An Essay on Justice Between the Young and the Old* (New York: Oxford University Press, 1988).

15. For an excellent discussion of the injustice of employment-based insurance, see John D. Banja, "The Improbable Future of Employment-Based Insurance, *Hastings Center Report* 30, no. 3 (2000): 17–25.

16. Eugene Borowitz, "The Autonomous Self and the Commanding Community," *Theological Studies* 45 (March 1984): 34–56; H. Tristram Engelhardt, Jr., *The Foundations of Bioethics*, 2nd ed. (New York: Oxford University Press, 1996), 74–83; Howard K. Rabinowitz and Nina P. Paynter, "The Rural vs. Urban Practice Decision," *JAMA: Journal of the American Medical Association* 287 (2002): 113.

17. Peter D. Jacobson, *Strangers in the Night: Law and Medicine in the Managed Care Era* (New York: Oxford University Press, 2002) provides a sociological and economic analysis of the often contentious relationship between law and medicine in the context of recent managed care arrangements. Broader social policy, and legal and economic issues related to physicians and the care of their patients in managed care settings are discussed by E. Haavi Morreim, *Balancing Act: The New Medical Ethics of Medicine's New Economics* (Washington, DC: Georgetown University Press, 1995), especially chap. 4, "Fiscal Scarcity: Challenging Fidelity," 45–70; and chap. 6, "The Obligations and Limits of Fidelity: Physicians' Professional Services," 105–32. See also Mark Hall, *Making Medical Spending Decisions: The Law, Ethics, and Economics of Rationing Mechanisms* (New York: Oxford University Press, 1997), esp. chap. 5, "Motivating Physicians with Financial Incentives," 171–92. Of particular interest with respect to physician and health plan tort liability issues is E. Haavi Morreim, *Holding Health Care Accountable: Law and the New Medical Marketplace* (New York: Oxford University Press, 2001). A review of recent court decisions and legislation regarding these issues and their implications for the practice of medicine appear in American Medical Association, Council on Ethical and Judicial Affairs, *Code of Medical Ethics: Current Opinions with Annotations*, 2000–2001 ed. (Chicago: American Medical Association, 2000), § 8.05, "Contractual Relationships," 154–55; § 8.051, "Conflicts of Interest Under Capitation," 155–56; § 8.13, "Managed Care," 175–81; and § 9.12, "Patient-Physician Relationship: Respect for Law and Human Rights," 218–20.

18. Hilda R. Heady, "A Delicate Balance: The Economics of Rural Healthcare Delivery," *JAMA: Journal of the American Medical Association* 287 (2002): 110.

A Physician's and a Philosopher's Analysis

Stephen A. Magnus, PhD, MAE, MS,
and Susan Dorr Goold, MD, MHSA, MA

Do the physicians of Pleasantville have a moral obligation to renew their contract with the one health maintenance organization (HMO) remaining in the area? If pressed to deliver a single answer, we would have to say "no." No codes of professional ethics obligate physicians to maintain a contractual, legal relationship with the HMO, or even to continue practicing medicine in Pleasantville. There are, however, morally weighty considerations that should be factored into such a decision. Canceling the HMO contract is likely to impair the affordability of health insurance for Pleasantville's citizens—a problem compounded by the town's geographic isolation—and harm patients' access to health care and, in turn, their health.

It is important to distinguish practical, even self-interested, concerns from ethical ones. The physicians are understandably worried about lower personal incomes, reduced professional autonomy, and increased bureaucratic hassles from participation in the HMO. They are also worried about their patients' access to affordable, high-quality health care. A useful way to frame the physicians' dilemma is in terms of trust and trustworthiness, a core professional value.

Many citizens of Pleasantville have entrusted their health care to physicians under contract with the HMO. These citizens have also entrusted the HMO to pay for health care that meets medical needs, while exercising stewardship over pooled financial resources. Physicians *and* health care organizations face an ethical obligation to deserve the trust placed in them. Although little is said in the case about the health plan, it is a central moral actor.

If the physicians cancel their contract with the HMO, there are likely to be significant, deleterious effects on patient trust. First, many doctor-patient relationships will end; patients will either seek care from new physicians or lack a personal physician. Either consequence displaces an established, trust-based relationship. Second, canceling the contract could lessen trust in physicians because of perceptions that they are more concerned about incomes than about patients. Despite declining incomes, Pleasantville's physicians still earn more than most other town residents. It behooves the physicians to remember that their salaries are not strictly a practical matter, but also raise questions of social justice, social obligation, and equity*

Agreeing to the proposed HMO contract, however, could also adversely affect trust. If physicians believe that patients are likely to be harmed by restrictions on medical practice (e.g., overly stringent prescription formularies or limitations on

---

*Note, however, that there is a tension between patient/community perceptions of physician greed and the desire to attract and retain good physicians by offering "decent" incomes.

referrals and tests), it would be untrustworthy for them to accept those conditions. Even when physicians can overcome restrictions through appeals, all appeal processes require time. In combination with declining reimbursements for patient visits, the need to request many exceptions to HMO guidelines may pressure physicians to see more patients per day in order to maintain desired income levels. Physician time—critical to patient trust and satisfaction—diminishes.

Is there no "middle path" that could accommodate the diverse interests and constituencies represented at the town meeting? The community wants and needs an affordable health plan; the health plan needs to control costs in order to stay in business; and the physicians want to practice high-quality medicine and earn a fair wage. Pleasantville's physicians should not underestimate their power and prestige, which may enable them to advocate effectively on behalf of patients and the community.

For instance, physician meetings with HMO administrators and community or political leaders could focus on the need to keep the HMO in town and maintain affordable premiums. Other topics for discussion include patients' waiting times for medical appointments, bureaucratic hassles for physicians, and the amount of time physicians can spend with their patients. Finally, physicians can illustrate the importance of flexibility in medical treatment by providing anonymous examples from their practices. They can suggest physician involvement in the development of practice guidelines and stipulate streamlined appeals processes.

Like physicians, the HMO needs to seek and deserve the trust of its enrollees— a trust that, according to the case, is profoundly lacking. Working with physicians toward patient and community goals of affordable, individualized, high-quality health care could strengthen trust in this insurer.

In negotiations, the issue of uncompensated care for enrollees poses a particular challenge.* According to the physicians, the volume of uncompensated care delivered to HMO enrollees has increased; the physicians find it difficult to refuse patient requests for services that are not covered by the insurer. Again, physicians (and HMOs) enhance trust when they focus on access to medically necessary or prudent care. In addition to negotiating which services are covered, the physicians and HMO could work together to educate community leaders, and patients, that some frequently requested services (e.g., yearly Pap smears for low-risk women, or COX-2 inhibitors for patients with arthritis but no history of ulcers) are not medically necessary. Trusted physicians and health plans are less likely to encounter perceptions that refusals of medical treatment are motivated by greed.

If a mutually agreeable contract cannot be reached with the HMO, what other options could enhance trust in physicians? Perhaps the physicians could help to or-

---

*Of course, there is also an urgent need to provide uncompensated medical care for the uninsured (i.e., non-HMO enrollees), but that topic is beyond the scope of the case study.

ganize a community shuttle service to the town 110 miles away, thereby easing the travel burden for patients who wish or need to change physicians due to the end of the HMO contract. They could also try to negotiate an urgent-care contract for patients who require more timely access to a physician, or for whom traveling is an excessive burden. In all of these matters, physicians who campaign on behalf of their patients, and not merely themselves, enhance the trust placed in them.

In order to both strengthen and justify trust, Pleasantville's independent physician association (IPA) needs to present moral, rather than financial, arguments for changing the HMO's proposed contractual arrangements. In doing so, the physicians must balance their legitimate practical interests with concern for patients and the community. Negotiations should strive to improve quality and access to care, and to nurture the patient-physician relationship by permitting physicians to spend adequate time with all of their patients. The HMO faces similar obligations to strengthen and justify the trust placed in it.

A Philosopher's Analysis

Lisa Gannett, PhD

With 85 percent of Pleasantville's 40,000 residents insured by the town's only remaining health maintenance organization (HMO), the decision by the physicians independent association (IPA) not to renew the existing contract with the HMO risks adding thousands from Pleasantville to the 41 million Americans who lack health care coverage.[1] Is this morally permissible? Or are the IPA physicians morally obligated to renew the HMO contract in order to ensure continued coverage for their patients?

As self-employed professionals, the Pleasantville physicians are entrepreneurs as well as health care providers; they are forced to juggle their finances alongside their patient caseloads. When physicians become members of an IPA in order to share income, expenses, facilities, and equipment, they do so as physicians—not accountants—and joint responsibility for the provision of quality medical care for their patients therefore ensues. Should conflicts between these competing demands arise, the American Medical Association's (AMA's) *Principles of Medical Ethics*[2] and *Opinions and Reports of the Council on Ethical and Judicial Affairs*[3] provide standards of conduct to aid in their resolution.

Except in emergencies, a physician is "free to choose whom to serve, with whom to associate, and the environment in which to provide medical care."[4] The freedom of physicians to choose their associates and work environments entitles the IPA to decide not to renew the HMO contract. However, this freedom does not annul all existing responsibilities of IPA physicians to provide care for their HMO patients once the contract between the IPA and HMO expires. Physicians are permitted to exercise their freedom "to choose whom to serve" only with respect to *potential* patients. Where physician-patient relationships already exist, patients have "the right to continuity of health care," and physicians are not permitted to discontinue medically indicated treatment "without giving the patient reasonable assistance and sufficient opportunity to make alternative arrangements for care."[5]

Realistically, "alternative arrangements for care" are unlikely to be forthcoming for many of the Pleasantville patients who would be affected by this course of action, regardless of "reasonable assistance and sufficient opportunity" on the part of physicians. Even if the town's employers were to continue to offer HMO coverage, most of the town's physicians are members of the IPA. With the nearest town of comparable size 110 miles away, Pleasantville residents, unlike their urban counterparts, cannot simply enroll in another HMO. And fee-for-service (FFS) and preferred provider options (PPOs) are beyond the financial means of well over half of those residents now covered by the HMO. As a result, should the IPA physicians proceed with their plan not to renew the HMO contract, they are morally obligated to continue to provide care for those among their existing patients who find themselves unable to make "alternative arrangements for care." This includes existing patients who, upon the loss of their HMO coverage, may be unable to bear the full financial burden of medical services they need.

This leaves the IPA physicians with a financial decision to make. If the HMO contract is not renewed, income gains that accompany FFS and PPO billing will be offset by uncertainties about receiving compensation for medical services that the physicians are obliged to continue to provide for their existing patients who become uninsured. Physician salaries will not be restored overnight from $90,000 to $140,000.

But the decision about whether or not to renew the HMO contract cannot just be a financial one. In making decisions about their practices, physicians have "ethical obligations to place patients' welfare above their own self-interest."[6] The IPA physicians must consider the impact that the loss of HMO coverage will have on the welfare of their patients, not just those who join the ranks of the uninsured but those who cannot afford the co-pays, annual deductibles, or higher costs of prescription drugs associated with the other insurance options. The decision not to renew the HMO contract is morally justified if these negative impacts on patient welfare are mitigated by benefits associated with practicing outside the HMO, such as the ability to put the interests of each individual patient first, improved quality of care, and heightened patient satisfaction.

It would be inadequate to analyze this case only from the perspective of the physician-patient relationship and fail to consider the community and societal levels. The physicians' preference for FFS and PPO clientele represents a desire to return to traditional models of health care delivery. In a sense, this is a retreat from the changes that have taken place in health care delivery over the past several decades, specifically, attempts by third parties to use HMOs to contain spiraling health care costs, followed by the conversion of many not-for-profit HMOs and insurance companies to for-profit corporations. These developments may not have served physicians well, but they certainly have not served patients well either. A "system" of health care delivery that threatens to leave a large proportion of a rural town's residents without coverage is too dysfunctional to be called a system. The responsibility of physicians to help build a genuine system of health care delivery is recognized in the AMA's Code of Ethics: "Because society has an obligation to make access to an adequate level of healthcare available to all of its members regardless of ability to pay, physicians should contribute their expertise at a policy-making level to help achieve this goal."[7]

It may be possible to make changes at the community level in the case of Pleasantville. The town hall meeting is evidence of a cohesive community structure and recognition on the part of the IPA physicians that their decision not to renew the HMO contract has an impact on the community as a whole, and not just their current patients. The physicians' willingness to participate in the town hall meeting is consistent with the ethical responsibilities of physicians "to participate in activities contributing to the improvement of the community"[8] and to "advocate for patients in dealing with third parties when appropriate."[9] Third parties need also to be part of any community-based resolution of this crisis; after all, the managed care revolution in the United States was an attempt on the part of employers and governments to contain health care costs and their share of these costs. It may be possible for the town's employers to join together to attract a different HMO and for a period of time provide that organization with a contract adequate for controlling health care spending while protecting and improving the health of patients. Without shareholders and the pressure to make profits over the short term, a not-for-profit HMO may also agree to terms of practice more amenable to the physicians.

Notes

1. Kaiser Commission on Medicaid and the Uninsured, "The Uninsured and Their Access to Health Care: Key Facts," Jan. 2003, http://www.kff.org/content/2003/142004/142004.pdf (12 June 2003).

2. American Medical Association, *Principles of Medical Ethics*, June 2001, http://www.ama-assn.org/ama/pub/category/2512.html (12 June 2003).

3. American Medical Association, *Code of Medical Ethics: Current Opinions of the Council on Ethical and Judicial Affairs*, 1995–1998, http://www.ama-assn.org/ama/pub/category/2503.html (12 June 2003).

4. See note 2, above, Principle VI.

5. See note 3, above, § 10.01(5).

6. See note 3, above, § 10.015.

7. See note 3, above, § 2.095.

8. See note 2, above, Principle VII.

9. See note 3, above, § 10.01(6).

An Ethicist's Analysis

Courtney Campbell, PhD

The facts that five health maintenance organizations (HMOs) have stopped providing coverage to Pleasantville residents in the past six years, and that 85 percent of the population are insured through the one remaining HMO, leaves the independent physicians association (IPA) dealing with a virtual monopoly in health care delivery. Ironically, however, should the existing HMO contract be terminated, the circumstances of Pleasantville's rural locale and its elderly population demographic mean the IPA will itself assume essentially a monopoly position. Pleasantville's healthy population is unlikely to travel excessive distances (perhaps up to 110 miles) to receive primary care; its elderly population on fixed incomes will not be able to go elsewhere to obtain comparable coverage and pharmacy benefits; and a good portion of its general population, especially those who are chronically ill, may find themselves priced out of health care options altogether as healing and caring are displaced by cold economic reality and even abandonment.

Thus, the IPA has good reason to be worried about the "increasingly strained"— and in some circumstances, "adversarial"—quality of the evolving professional-patient relationship. It is not the role of the IPA or of organized medicine generally to solve the social justice question of inadequate or nonexistent access to basic and necessary health care services. But the IPA does have a moral responsibility to prevent current inequities in the cost, accessibility, and quality of health care from becoming worse. Moreover, the IPA must work to meet the requirements of the moral principle of fairness, that disparities in resource allocation work to benefit society's least advantaged members. These responsibilities are generated by the inner demands of medicine as a vocation oriented to healing and caring, and by the social duties assumed by medicine in its public role as a "profession." As it stands, however, the burdens of a decision to terminate the contract with the remaining HMO appear to fall most heavily on those citizens, such as those with fixed incomes and chronic ailments, who are least able to carry them.

The IPA does have a legitimate interest in maintaining both its identity and its integrity as an association of health care providers. It cannot maintain either identity or integrity if its role is reduced to merely a gatekeeping function for the HMO or, for that matter, solely to an advocacy role for health care consumers. Medicine is a distinctive profession owing to its defining commitments to healing and caring of the ill, which is possible only when mutual trust and respect exist between caregivers and patients. The IPA is thereby on solid professional grounds to resist the encroachments of the HMO on provider freedom and autonomy.

Various regulatory and economic provisions of a bureaucratic organization can undoubtedly inhibit physician freedom. However, the freedom of a professional provider is neither unbounded nor self-serving; it is always a freedom to serve those to whom the professional—individually and/or as a member of a collective body—has made a vow or promise to promote their welfare. Physician autonomy is an instrumental good because it enables caregivers to direct their knowledge and skills to the healing and caring of patients. Thus, the moral issue related to provider autonomy is whether the contractual provisions with the HMO impede the quality, accessibility, or reasonable cost of health care delivery to patients, and to the Pleasantville community generally. The IPA argues that restrictions on physician autonomy (a matter of professional identity) lead to depersonalized and less efficacious provision of care (a matter of professional integrity). Bureaucratic accountability and economics, the providers claim, have displaced professional knowledge and practical wisdom in the care of patients.

The IPA argument about inadequate compensation for professional services also brings together issues of identity and integrity. Capitation requirements can either inhibit a physician's earning capacity or enable this to be achieved only by compromising quality patient care. A fair level of compensation is an appropriate professional expectation and a sign of the value society places on the accumulation and application of professional skills.

Yet, society has also made a substantial investment to ensure the acquisition of these skills and their basis in theoretical knowledge. Society provides educational resources for aspiring physicians, and supports hospitals and other teaching institutions in which mentoring and training occur. Moreover, the physician's "practice"—which has the dual meaning of learning what will be effective care for a particular patient and the kind of work that advances a professional career—requires patients and research subjects to entrust their bodies and their well-being to the physician's growing, but always incomplete, knowledge and skills. Thus, as with the question of physician autonomy, the level of physician compensation has a broader communal dimension.

Society has a legitimate interest in physicians not exercising their professional autonomy in order to transform medicine from a practice defined by moral commitments into an entrepreneurial career. That transformation cannot but help erode the nature and quality of the physician-patient relationship. Indeed, since some Pleasantville citizens express suspicion that physician treatment decisions are rooted in the financial self-interest and career interests of physicians, the vital fabric of trust between physician and patient is already beginning to unravel.

If financial interests rather than trust and respect become the medium of exchange in the provider-patient relationship, that relationship will be irreparably damaged. The physicians clearly indicate they do not want to be under a cloud of ethical suspicion and do not want to have to choose between quality patient care and HMO capitation. However, the decision to terminate the HMO contract cannot help but be seen by the community as physician capitulation to entrepreneurial careerism.

The physician as autonomous entrepreneur also implies a construct of health care as a private commodity. As with other commodities, the means by which consumers gain access turns on their ability to pay. But access to health care is precisely what a good share of the residents of Pleasantville say will not be possible should the contract be terminated. Their inability to pay will mean exacerbating the economic stratification of health care delivery. An alternative understanding, which seems to have been the basis for the caring partnership between the IPA and the community to this point, is that health care is a *communal* good. This builds into the notion of health care provision both mutual accountability and mutual sharing of benefits. It may be the case that the disagreement between the IPA and the community over the disposition of the HMO contract may reflect implicit differences in beliefs about the kind of good health care is. An ethical resolution of the controversy may require that the substantive question of whether health care is a private commodity or a communal good be part of the professional and professional-community conversation.

To its credit, in keeping with the value of procedural justice, the IPA has given the Pleasantville community a voice in the decision-making process. The IPA's public justification of its decision to break ties with the HMO and its openness to the concerns of the community can be an opportunity to affirm those moral commitments that define medicine as a distinctive profession.

Still, the Pleasantville community is in a very vulnerable position vis-à-vis the IPA due to its rural location and aging population. It has few alternatives for reasonable and affordable quality care. The IPA, by contrast, has a position of relative power and choice. The IPA can choose to not renew the contract with the HMO; or it could use its position of influence to negotiate a better contract, one that is more accommodating of the providers' concerns, but also ensures continuity of care for the community. The IPA can, and ethically should, negotiate for contractual provisions that assure professional identity and integrity and enable healing and caring in a trusting relationship with patients. A contract premised on cooperative partnership rather than monopolistic dominance may be a hard-won achievement, but morally the IPA has an obligation to do no less.

Further Reflections

General

1. This case takes place in a small community where experienced physicians and insurance companies are in short supply. What role should this fact play in determining if the physicians have a moral duty to renew their contract with the health maintenance organization (HMO)? Would the morally appropriate response differ in an urban center with easier access to qualified physicians who had contracted with one's HMO?

2. Several years ago, former Surgeon General C. Everett Koop, in discussing (a) high quality, (b) low cost, and (c) universal access regarding health care, claimed societies could optimize any two of these three characteristics; but that no society could optimize all three. What moral principles support a social

commitment to these three criteria? Which two criteria are most important—practically and morally—to a society? Which of these criteria are most fully realized in our society, and which are sacrificed to the other(s)?

3. The commentators suggest that Pleasantville's physicians, community members, and representatives of the HMO might be able to work out an acceptable solution to this problem. Can these three parties *alone* solve Pleasantville's problem? Why (not)? If not, what else would have to occur or who else would need to be involved to resolve the problem?

Consequences

4. What important goods/benefits are sacrificed if the physicians break the contract with the HMO? Alternately, what important goods/benefits are lost by remaining in the HMO arrangement?

Autonomy

5. Do persons who move to small or rural communities to achieve the benefits of such settings agree to forgo the benefits—such as greater access to physicians or to multiple health care plans—that they would have in urban areas?

Rights

6. Do persons have a moral right to health care? If so, what is the basis of that right? What does the right consist of (in other words, what is it a right to)? Who is the right against (that is, who has the responsibility to meet the right)? In what circumstances (if any) does a person—or community—lose or relinquish that right?

Virtues

7. Discuss the physician's dilemma of patient- vs. self-interest. How strong is the professional promise to promote the welfare of one's patients first and foremost? What conditions, if any, excuse physicians from this promise? What morally justifies these conditions?

Equality/Fairness (Justice)

8. What particular problems with health care quality, cost, and access are experienced by small communities? What would it take to reverse these problems or deficiencies for small communities? Would such solutions themselves be just?

9. All commentators claim that the commitment to core professional values of trust and fidelity can help resolve the challenge faced by small communities. In attempting to solve other financially challenging dilemmas, society rarely appeals to these values. Why is health care different from so many other "goods" that societies allocate?

Chapter 15

You're Just His Doctor; I'm His Boss!

Mr. F is a 43-year-old employee of a local lumber supply company. He is responsible for overseeing five other employees in the lumber yard. His tasks include coordinating orders from contractors as well as supervising the loading of supplies onto 18-wheel and other trucks. Often his responsibilities involve operating the forklifts and tractors used to load rafters, drywall, lumber, conduit, and siding for shipment.

Recently a minor accident occurred at the lumber yard during some early evening overtime. A stack of lumber collapsed while Mr. F was loading rafters; in the accident he suffered a deep laceration of his thigh. A colleague drove him to the local emergency room (ER). The open bay structure (one large room with individual gurneys separated only by curtains) of the ER provided privacy for the physical examination, but several other patients and family members, including another lumber company employee, heard the physician, Dr. W, order a blood alcohol level and drug screen on Mr. F. The other employee hastily called the lumber yard owner, Mr. G.

While Dr. W was suturing the wound in Mr. F's thigh, the blood alcohol level was reported as 0.07 percent. (The state level for intoxication for driving is 0.08 percent.) The preliminary results of the drug screen were negative. As Mr. F was preparing to leave the ER, Mr. G arrived and demanded to know the results of both tests. Mr. F heatedly informed his boss that his medical records were confidential and that he had no intention of sharing the results. Mrs. F, who had arrived to take her husband home, echoed his sentiments. After their departure, Mr. G demanded the test re-sults from Dr. W.

Dr. W initially seconded Mr. F's claim of confidentiality, insisting that without the patient's permission, he was both legally and morally obli-gated to not reveal the test results. But Mr. G pressed Dr. W, indicating that he had legitimate business needs for this information. First, it was im-portant for future liability and insurance issues that he know Mr. F's con-dition when the accident occurred. If Mr. F was incapacitated, Mr. G wanted to seek release from liability for the accident and thus avoid in-creasing insurance premiums. But he stated his more serious concern was that if Mr. F had been intoxicated or under the influence of substances that affected his cognitive or motor acuity, Mr. G would need to restructure Mr. F's work requirements so his alcohol or drug use would not put other employees at risk. Providing a safe working environment is his obligation, and one he takes seriously. (There is also the possibility, not discussed by Mr. G, that he will terminate Mr. F's employment, based on an obvious breach of the employment rules at the lumber yard.)

After hearing Mr. G's discussion of the potential fallout from the situa-tion, especially the potential risk of Mr. F's behavior for many other people, Dr. W is less certain that Mr. F's test results should be kept confidential.

What is Dr. W morally obligated to tell Mr. F's employer?

Introduction

At least two important moral issues are present in this case:

1. What is the moral justification for respecting confidentiality? What moral justification, if any, could support health care *professionals* (HCPs) suspending respect for a patient's confidentiality?
2. Are *hospitals* also morally obligated to respect patient confidentiality? If so, what sorts of institutional policies or protocols should be embraced by hos-pitals to protect patient confidentiality?

The AJ Method

Step 1: Information Gathering   What facts are necessary for resolving this case? Was Mr. F functionally impaired? What is the hospital's policy regarding breach of confidentiality? (Spencer) Is Mr. F currently capable of autonomous decision making? Why did Dr. W order drug screening? (Lindberg and Iserson) What will Mr. G do with information about Mr. F? Are Mr. F's coworkers at risk if Dr. W withholds the information?

Rules for respecting and revealing secrets are present in all human cultures. In our society, we hold secrecy in high regard and, absent strong reasons to the contrary, consider persons morally obligated to protect information known to them to be confidential.[1]

Several moral principles justify keeping secrets. The principle of nonmaleficence precludes revealing secrets if doing so could cause harm; indeed, concerns about negative outcomes often justify keeping secrets, regardless of context. Respect for autonomy counsels keeping secrets as a means to respecting decisional authority of persons about what personal information to share with others. The virtue of fidelity deems persons to be virtuous when, in their personal or professional relations, they protect sensitive information acquired in the context of those relationships. These same moral principles support keeping secrets in medical contexts, where "keeping secrets" is recast as a "right of patient confidentiality" and is considered one of the most stringent principles in modern health care.[2]

Step 2: Creative Problem Solving   Any creative solution would have to provide information to Mr. G without violating Mr. F's right to confidentiality and Dr. W's integrity.

Step 3: Pros and Cons   Survey CARVE principles to identify important moral reasons that support conflicting options for resolving this case.

Consequences   Identify the effects on all parties concerned—Mr. F, his coworkers, Mr. G, Dr. W, the hospital—if Dr. W does, *and* if he does not, give Mr. G the information he is requesting. Are the effects on Mr. F likely to be better or worse if his medical information remains confidential? What effects will a breach have on patient-professional relationships? (Jollimore)

Numerous harms that can follow from disseminating sensitive medical information—ostracizing or condemning persons with conditions that taint their reputations, soured relationships with friends and family, loss of or inability to acquire health insurance, loss of trust in particular practitioners and of the profession generally—bring confidentiality under the umbrella of nonmaleficence.[3] Conversely, might beneficence argue against confidentiality if it undercuts a patient's own best medical interests?[4]

Concerns about confidentiality are especially pressing in small communities, where the relative anonymity of the urban health setting is absent. A slip of the tongue in a large city is usually only an interesting observation about human nature, considered abstractly. That same breach in a small town often provides listeners with information about an identifiable friend, neighbor, or colleague. Such intimate knowledge can change the nature of personal interactions—and not necessarily for the better.

Nonetheless, even if confidentiality should almost always be protected, few theorists or HCPs argue that *all* confidences need be kept.[5] In certain circumstances commitment to confidentiality may legitimately be overridden, for example, if breaching confidentiality can prevent some genuine catastrophe.[6]

Autonomy   Control over access to one's personal information is an important aspect of autonomy. To carry out one's life in a satisfactory fashion often depends on others having only limited information about one's values, habits, and behaviors. This principle is, however, less powerful if one's secrets place others at significant risk of harm.

Rights   The rights of confidentiality and privacy are central in this dilemma. (Lindberg and Iserson)

The rights of confidentiality and of self-determination require that the subject of the secret controls whether to divulge it.[7] These rights are derivative from respect for autonomy and the belief that the patient is best placed to identify and assess anticipated burdens and benefits of revealing sensitive information, and to determine whether he wants to assume the burdens he identifies. Occasionally a patient will consent to disclosure of his own medical information.

Virtues   Fidelity to the patient requires protecting confidential information. (Jollimore; Lindberg and Iserson)

Keeping patients' secrets is cast as a necessary means to nurturing patient-professional relationships. Without a stringent commitment to confidentiality, patients may not seek health care or, if they do, may lie to protect their "dirty little secrets." Unshared information can impede the therapeutic project, undercut patients' interests, and imperil public health.

If, however, one's HCPs are and will likely continue to be strangers (as is the case with HCPs in emergency settings), does the commitment to confidentiality, understood within a fiduciary relationship, still hold? What of the consequentialist argument against protecting confidentiality in the face of foreseeable, significant (even if not catastrophic) threats to other patients, individuals, or society as a whole? Perhaps a commitment to confidentiality, *all things considered*, is more sensible.

In fact, one might ask whether contemporary professionals should persist in considering confidentiality among their moral obligations. Interestingly, many patients in the age of managed care indicate that they have little, if any, trust in HCPs; they often suspect that HCPs make decisions solely based on economics.[8] If that belief (warranted or not) is widespread, the fidelity (or integrity)-based argument for confidentiality may be of historical interest only.

Even those who are not so cynical about HCPs' motives often suspect that the value of confidentiality, at the heart of the traditional, individual patient-centered conception of health care, may have less relevance in the context of contemporary health care. Physicians increasingly function in settings where their obligations extend beyond *individual* patients to institutions with fiduciary responsibilities to patient *populations*. Further, failure to release important information that affects public safety or welfare may place one—and one's institution—at risk of litigation.

Finally, we might ask about institutional integrity: what role should hospitals (and other institutions) play in defining the scope of confidentiality? The extent of respect owed to some moral values at the expense of others can be affected by institutional policies and protocols, with derivative obligations on professional employees. The American Hospital Association's *Patient's Bill of Rights* articulates only a *qualified* commitment to *individual* confidentiality:

> *The patient has the right to expect that all communications and records pertaining to his/her care will be treated as confidential by the hospital, except in cases such as suspected abuse and public health hazards when reporting is permitted or required by law. The patient has the right to expect that the hospital will emphasize the confidentiality of this information when it releases it to any other parties entitled to review information in these records.*[9]

Should hospitals—especially in small communities where guaranteeing patient confidentiality may be both particularly difficult and particularly important—more precisely define the extent of this commitment? Might institutions be morally obligated to construct policies and procedures that explicitly specify what constitutes a public health hazard, or what parties might be "entitled to review information"? Further, as Lindberg and Iserson note, the structural particulars of hospital architecture can enhance or diminish confidentiality. Might emergency rooms, for example, substitute glass walls for curtains, retaining visibility while decreasing intrusions on conversations?

In sum, preserving the confidentiality of individual patients by individual providers faces challenges from other individuals, patients themselves, providers, and institutions. Rethinking this cornerstone of the patient-professional relationship is increasingly important.

Equality/Fairness (Justice) Assuming Mr. F was functionally impaired, does protecting this fact pose an unfair burden to his employer or coworkers?

The Law   The following legal considerations are relevant to this case: (1) What federal and state legislation governs issues of confidentiality and privacy in health care? (2) Did the drawing of blood for alcohol and other drug screens constitute a legal violation of the patient's right to privacy? (3) Is the physician legally obligated to follow (and legally protected by) institutional policies (re: blood drawing or breach of confidentiality), assuming such policies exist? (4) What legal obligations to protect other workers exist? Might such obligations override presumptive obligations to protect privacy and confidentiality?[10]

The following commentaries examine the application of various moral principles to this dilemma, thereby assisting the reader to undertake *Step 4: Analysis* and *Step 5: Justification*.

Notes

1. Bok, Sissela, *Secrets: On the Ethics of Concealment and Revelation* (New York: Vintage, 1984), xv and chaps. 9 and 14.
2. Michael H. Kottow, "Medical Confidentiality: An Intransigent and Absolute Obligation," *Journal of Medical Ethics* 12, no. 3 (1986): 117–22.
3. Paul S. Appelbaum et al., "Confidentiality: An Empirical Test of the Utilitarian Perspective," *Bulletin of the American Academy of Psychiatry and the Law* 12, no. 2 (1984): 109–16.
4. Ibid.
5. American College of Emergency Physicians, "ACEP Policy Statements: Patient Confidentiality" (approved Jan. 1994, reapproved Oct. 2002), n.d., http://www.acep.org/1,629,0.html (31 July 2003).
6. Tarasoff v. Regents of the University of California, California Supreme Court, 17 California Reports, 3d series (1976).
7. J. O'Brien and C. Chantler, "Confidentiality and the Duties of Care," *Journal of Medical Ethics* 29, no. 1 (2003): 36–40.
8. Allen Buchanan, "Trust in Managed Care Organizations," *Kennedy Institute of Ethics Journal* 10 (2000): 189–212; Patricia Illingworth, "Trust: The Scarcest of Medical Resources," *The Journal of Medicine and Philosophy* 27, no. 1 (2002): 31–46; John H. McArthur and Francis D. Moore, "The Two Cultures and the Healthcare Revolution: Commerce and Professionalism in Medical Care," *JAMA: Journal of the American Medical Association* 277 (1997): 985–89; Laurence B. McCullough, "Moral Authority, Power and Trust in Clinical Ethics," *The Journal of Medicine and Philosophy* 24, no. 1 (1999): 1–10; David Orentlicher, "Managed Care and the Threat to the Patient-Physician Relationship," *Trends in Healthcare, Law & Ethics* 10, no. 1/2 (1995): 19–24.
9. American Hospital Association, *A Patient's Bill of Rights* (Adopted 1973; revised 21 Oct. 1992), n.d., http://www.hospitalconnect.com/aha/about/pbillofrights.html (30 July 2003), #6.
10. Important federal legislation relevant to this case includes the Health Insurance Portability and Accountability Act of 1996 (HIPAA, Public Law 104-191) which, among other things, regulates and restricts the management of health care information. Title II, §§ 261-264, of HIPAA (also known as Administrative Simplification) includes strict requirements for ensuring the security and privacy of individuals' medical information. For the text of the law and its implications for privacy, confidentiality, and its relationship to "individually identifiable health information," see http://www.hhs.gov/ocr/hipaa. Discussion of the conflict between physicians' duty of confidentiality to patients and obligations to warn third parties for foreseeable injuries under a Tarasoff-type scenario (Tarasoff v. Regents of the University of California, Supreme Court of California 551 P.2d 334 (Cal. 1976)), as well as related issues of tort liability for "failure to warn" are discussed in the context of HIV testing in American Medical Association, Council on Ethical and Judicial Affairs, *Code of Medical Ethics: Current Opinions with Annotations,* 2000–2001 ed. (Chicago: American Medical Association, 2000), § 2.23, "HIV Testing," 84–85.

    State and federal court decisions relevant to this case are reviewed in American Medical Association, Council on Ethical and Judicial Affairs, *Code of Medical Ethics: Current Opinions with Annotations,* 2000–2001 ed. (Chicago: American Medical Association, 2000), § 5.05, "Confidentiality," 105–17, and § 5.09, "Confidentiality: Industry-Employed Physicians and Independent Medical Examiners," 125–26.

An Ethicist's Analysis

Troy Jollimore, PhD

According to the American Medical Association's (AMA's) current *Code of Medical Ethics*, "Information disclosed to a physician during the course of the patient-physician relationship is confidential to the utmost degree."[1] The AMA also lists the right to patient confidentiality as one of the "fundamental elements of the patient-physician relationship."[2] Why place so much importance on confidentiality? One justification is the idea that physicians have special obligations to their patients, based in trust.[3] A second justification is consequentialist: patients will be less likely to seek medical attention, or less forthcoming when doing so, if they believe their medical information may be shared without their consent. Thus, a strict and general commitment to confidentiality is seen as a necessary condition for successful medical practice and a contributing factor to public health.[4]

Nevertheless, there are understood to be circumstances in which a physician may disclose medical information without the patient's consent. The justification of such exceptions usually appeals to public interest.[5] Particularly relevant are cases where "a patient threatens bodily harm to himself or to another person."[6] Thus, as stated in the AMA's *Fundamental Elements of the Patient-Physician Relationship*, "The physician should not reveal confidential communications or information without the consent of the patient, unless provided for by law or by the need to protect the welfare of the individual or the public interest."[7]

Perhaps, then, Dr. W is both permitted and required to disclose the results of Mr. F's drug test to his employer. Of course, Mr. G's desire to avoid raised insurance premiums hardly constitutes the sort of compelling public interest that can override the confidentiality requirement. But his other basis for demanding the test results—that Mr. F might have a drug problem that places himself and his fellow employees in danger of bodily harm—might be stronger.

But is it strong enough? If Mr. G possessed evidence that Mr. F had a potentially dangerous drug problem, he would perhaps be obliged to take steps to protect his other workers. But Mr. G has no such evidence. Due to an unfortunate coincidence, exacerbated by the lack of privacy in the local emergency room, Mr. G is aware that Mr. F's physician ordered a drug test. And he may conclude from this that the physician had reason to suspect Mr. F of having been incapacitated by drugs. But this is pure speculation. The mere fact that a person undergoes a drug test during treatment does not indicate that he is using drugs, nor even that the physician who orders the test believes that he is using drugs. Such tests might simply be part of standard procedure. Thus Mr. G has no more basis for concluding now that Mr. F might have a problem than he did when Mr. F first went in for treatment.

Of course, if Mr. G had some other reason, based on Mr. F's work performance, for suspecting him of having a potentially dangerous problem, then he might well be justified in taking precautions to protect his employees. The point, though, is that such precautions would need to be justified by evidence independent of the drug tests (whose occurrence, again, ought not to have been revealed to Mr. G in the first place). The test results themselves are and must be treated as irrelevant, and Mr. G should not have access to them.

This conclusion is supported by the fact that Dr. W apparently did not even consider that Mr. F might pose any sort of danger before being confronted with Mr. G's demands. If Dr. W did not originally think that the test results indicated a serious and immediate problem, why should the fact that Mr. G might interpret them otherwise compel him to violate confidentiality? Mr. G is no physician; moreover, he has a personal interest in the situation. It is therefore quite unlikely that his interpretation of the results would be either informed or objective. Had Dr. W himself judged, on seeing the results, that Mr. F posed a danger to those around him, his obligations would perhaps have been different.

As this example illustrates, physician-patient confidentiality can be especially difficult to maintain in small-town and rural settings, where the anonymity typical of urban environments is generally absent.[8] As Paul Ullom-Minnich and Ken Kallail write: "The increased visibility and social interconnectedness of rural life may confound personal privacy . . . . The challenge of confidentiality may therefore be more formidable in the rural environment."[9]

By the time Dr. W is confronted with Mr. G's demands, Mr. F's confidentiality has already been violated. As a result he may undergo increased scrutiny at work and be subject to other inconveniences. For Dr. W to compound this violation of privacy with a further breach of confidentiality would be ethically indefensible.

While public interest can sometimes override confidentiality, not just any public interest can do so; only in extreme cases can confidentiality be overridden. (The concept of a "clear and present danger," which has its origins in another context, is perhaps useful here, at least as a rough intuitive guide.) Given the value of confidentiality in securing patients' participation and cooperation in the health care system, physicians should be extremely reluctant to compromise this obligation by allowing third-party concerns to override it. Again, this is not to say that the public interest can never override confidentiality. But it should only be allowed to do so in cases where the danger posed by the patient's condition is demonstrable and immediate. And even here, physicians who judge that they must share information are presumably bound to (1) reveal as little as necessary, protecting the identity of the patient where possible; and (2) obtain the patient's consent where this is at all possible. However, the physician's most compelling obligation—and, perhaps, the hardest to meet—is his obligation to be as certain as possible that the negative consequences he is attempting to avert are sufficiently serious and likely to outweigh the damage to the ideal of strict confidentiality that inevitably follows any compromise regarding that ideal.

Notes

1. American Medical Association, Office of General Counsel, Division of Health Law, "Patient Confidentiality," 1998, http://www.ama-assn.org/ama/pub/category/4610.html (23 June 2003).
2. American Medical Association, Council on Ethical and Judicial Affairs (CEJA), *Fundamental Elements of the Patient-Physician Relationship*, 1994, http://www.ama-assn.org/ama/pub/category/2510.html (23 June 2003).
3. Michael H. Kottow, "Medical Confidentiality: An Intransigent and Absolute Obligation," *Journal of Medical Ethics* 12 (1986): 117–22; D. K. Milholland, "Privacy and Confidentiality of Patient Information: Challenges for Nursing," *Journal of Nursing Administration* 24, no. 2 (1994): 19–24; but compare to Mark Siegler, "Confidentiality in Medicine: A Decrepit Concept," *New England Journal of Medicine* 307 (1982): 1518–21.
4. See note 1, above; see Milholland and Siegler, note 3, above.
5. See note 1, above; and Milholland, note 3, above.
6. See note 1, above.
7. See note 2, above.
8. D. S. Hargrove, "Ethical Issues in Rural Mental Health Practice," *Professional Psychology Research & Practice* 17, no. 1 (1986): 20–23.
9. Paul D. Ullom-Minnich and Ken J. Kallail, "Physicians' Strategies for Safeguarding Confidentiality: The Influence of Community and Practice Characteristics," *The Journal of Family Practice* 37 (1993): 445.

An Emergency Physician's Analysis

Elizabeth Ann Lindberg, MD,
and Kenneth V. Iserson, MD, MBA

What is Dr. W morally obligated to tell Mr. F's employer? In answering this question, we will consider both the breach of privacy during his visit to the emergency department (ED) and questions of confidentiality that ensued.

Privacy

EDs are obligated to balance safety and privacy. Privacy includes (1) a physical sphere in which others may not intrude, (2) freedom of choice for important decisions, and (3) control over personal information.[1] Providing patient privacy is generally an institutional responsibility, since the ED's architecture often determines the amount of privacy patients have at any point during their stay. However, nursing decisions to put patients in hallways or other open areas also contribute to a lack of privacy. For patient and staff safety, suicidal, violent, or aggressive patients are often placed in very public areas so they can be closely observed. In these cases, privacy is sacrificed for safety. The moral justification for this trade-off is, for suicidal patients, that patient safety takes precedence over privacy, just as mandatory treatment trumps liberty. For dangerous patients, health care workers' (HCWs') safety takes precedence over patient rights; although in a "rescue" profession, no emergency

HCW should ever unwillingly sacrifice personal well-being on the altar of patient civil liberties.[2] Some EDs that have only drapes between beds may, in fact, be safer for some patients since nurses may have better visual access to them. This affords physical privacy, but auditory privacy is obviously lacking.

The Joint Commission on the Accreditation of Healthcare Organizations[3] lists among patients' rights the right to be interviewed and examined in an area that provides reasonable visual and auditory privacy. Yet, it may not always be clear to clinicians (or admitting clerks) what information is sensitive and needs such "reasonable" privacy. Certainly, in Mr. F's case, no one could have expected that the information would be sensitive.

In small towns, while privacy of space and choice can be maintained, informational privacy may be especially problematic. Where most people know each other (yes, those places still exist), it is more likely—despite new Health Insurance Portability and Accountability Act (HIPAA) regulations, developed to further protect patient privacy and confidentiality—that sensitive information may become public.[4] This, though, should be the exception, and not be due to HCWs' breaching patient confidentiality.

Lack of space is common in EDs as patient volumes grow. Parallel with the demise of the U.S. health care system—including EDs replacing primary care providers for many people (insured and uninsured), a nursing shortage leading to holding more admitted patients in EDs, and a greater sense of entitlement to health care—privacy suffers. Increasing patient volume means the lack of patient privacy in EDs is getting steadily worse, with routine use of "hallway beds," rows of chairs or benches, and open bays for initial patient interactions. Physicians, nurses, and medics now must routinely ask patients about their medical histories, perform invasive and painful procedures, and examine them in nonprivate settings. These nonideal conditions make protecting patients' privacy difficult, if not impossible.

This hospital clearly failed to protect confidentiality, since others were able to overhear conversation pertaining to Mr. F's medical care. We cannot pretend this situation is unusual, except that Mr. F was unfortunate enough to have prying ears in close proximity. The question Dr. W faced was whether, after the lapse, to compound it by revealing information discovered within the context of the physician-patient relationship—that is, further breach his confidentiality.

Confidentiality

Confidentiality has long been the hallmark of the physician-patient relationship.[5] Since ancient times, as exemplified in the Hippocratic Oath, confidentiality has precluded health care professionals (HCPs) from divulging information without the patient's consent. Emergency physicians' primary obligation is to meet their patients' medical needs. Close behind is preserving the secrecy of information they gain about patients through the medical history, physical examination, or laboratory tests.

Physician-patient confidentiality can be breached only if the patient or surrogate gives permission; a specific law requires doing so (in the case of infectious disease reporting, child or elder abuse, or specific injuries such as gunshot wounds); or an *identifiable* third party is at risk of harm if the information is not released. None of these exceptions applies in this case.

Of course, we need also to ask if Dr. W had just cause to test Mr. F for alcohol and drugs. Without evidence of altered mental status, why did he need that information to treat his patient? (Incompetent medical practice comes to mind, but that is beyond the scope of this discussion.) Seen in its best light, perhaps Dr. W smelled alcohol on Mr. F's breath and was concerned about using sedation for wound exploration and closure—although this would be unlikely, as adults rarely need any sedation for simple wound closures; they only require local anesthesia.[6]

Conditions of Employment

Regardless of Dr. W's obligation to keep his patient's information confidential, a number of situations may lead to Mr. F's medical records being available to his employer. Most common among these would be a clause in Mr. F's work contract requiring that he supply blood or urine samples for drug/alcohol testing (or the results of such tests) for cause or, in some cases, simply at the employer's request. In addition, if Mr. F makes an industrial claim seeking compensation for the hospital bill or time off work, he might be required to waive his right to confidentiality. His medical records might then become available to his employer.[7] Industrial Commission rules and regulations vary from state to state, and current state laws regarding release of patient information may change due to new rules established by HIPAA.[8]

In addition, occupational medicine clinics where employees may be sent after relatively minor injuries may actually work for the employer, rather than the patient. This significantly reduces—and may, in fact, obliterate—the usual obligations of providers to protect privacy or confidentiality, regardless of any expectations the employee-patient may have.

In any event, Dr. W is morally obligated not to give Mr. F's results to his employer. Rather, he should refer the employer to the hospital's medical records department. The employer may have a right to view the records there (depending on the legal situation) or may view them with Mr. F's written permission, but those issues lie outside Dr. W's purview.

Notes

1. Kenneth V. Iserson, Arthur B. Sanders, and Deborah Mathieu, *Ethics in Emergency Medicine,* 2nd ed. (Tucson: Galen Press Ltd., 1995).
2. Kenneth V. Iserson, "Ethics of Wilderness Medicine," in *Wilderness Medicine,* 3rd ed., ed. Paul Auerbach (St. Louis: Mosby, 1995), 1440.
3. See note 1, above, 154.
4. U. S. Department of Health and Human Services, Office for Civil Rights–HIPAA, "Medical Privacy—National Standards to Protect the Privacy of Personal Health Information," 15

May 2003, http://www.hhs.gov/ocr/hipaa (30 July 2003); Leslie G. Aronovitz, "Health Privacy: Regulation Enhances Protection of Patient Records but Raises Practical Concerns" (Testimony before the U.S. Senate, 8 Feb. 2001), http://www.gao.gov/new.items/d01387t.pdf (25 June 2003).

5. "Hippocratic Oath." The exact date of Oath is not known. It is believed to date from the sixth or fifth century BCE to the first century CE.
6. Bonnie Goodman, MD, Staff Physician, Concentra Occupational Medical Clinic, interview by author, Tucson, Arizona, Feb. 2003.
7. Linda Smith, Clinical Risk Consultant and Jim Richardson, In-House Counsel, Risk Management Department, University Medical Center, discussion with author, Tucson, Arizona, Feb. 2003.
8. See Aronovitz, note 4, above.

A Physician's Organization Analysis

Edward M. Spencer, MD

This case illustrates a number of important and pervasive problems associated with the issue of confidentiality in today's health care delivery system. It clearly demonstrates the frequent conflict between the best interests (and rights) of the individual and the needs of society to have adequate information to protect its citizens. There are almost daily examples of just this dilemma in today's media.

From an organization ethics perspective, however, this case is thin gruel. Most involved in the development of an organization ethics structure in a health care organization would agree that the purpose of developing and supporting such a structure and the activities it sponsors (policy development, education, consultation, coordination concerning ethics activities in the organization) is to help the organization define the values it espouses as well as the mission and goals these values support. In addition the organization ethics structure is expected to develop and support mechanisms to inform appropriate stakeholders of observed deviations from espoused values and to analyze and advise on specific cases involving real or potential deviation from stated values and/or mission. I see no evidence of this case corresponding to any of these mandates.

Of course a health care institution may have policies concerning confidentiality which are based on its fundamental values, and these policies may or may not be adequate to address the issue presented in this case. But even if such policies exist and are pertinent to the problem at hand, this case should present little or no threat to the institution's fundamental values or how they are articulated and applied within the institution.

If the institution espouses values which may conflict in this situation, this case may call attention to this conflict and, in this circumstance, the case may need to be considered by the organization ethics process as it attempts to correct the potential for conflict among the institution's values. For instance, if the institution espoused absolute confidentiality for its patients (an unlikely circumstance in today's health care system) and at the same time had a contract with the company which required sharing of confidential information concerning the company's employees, then a values-based conflict exists and the organization ethics group could be involved. This case, however, represents no real conflict among fundamental values or a systemic threat to any particular value, only a question of how these values are to be applied in this particular situation. This type of question, in my opinion, needs to be addressed by the stakeholders directly involved in the problem and should not become an issue for consideration by the organization ethics program.

I believe the most acceptable answer to the problem posed is for Dr. W to honor Mr. F's confidentiality since he was not legally intoxicated at the time and since he had not been informed that a blood alcohol level had been ordered. However the physician's obligations do not end there. He should inform Mr. F that it was obvious that he had been drinking prior to the accident, that this information would be placed in his medical record, and that the record would likely be legally discoverable if he was involved in a second accident which led to injuries to others. Dr. W should urge Mr. F to refrain from drinking on the job and offer to refer him to an alcohol rehabilitation program if Mr. F desires. Dr. W should continue to refuse to divulge confidential information to Mr. G.

Mr. G may also have a less-well-defined obligation to talk with Mr. F when he returns to work to explain that the company can not tolerate any drinking on the job and, although not accusing him of drinking on the job, the accident acted as a trigger to reiterate this policy for Mr. F and all other employees. (A memo to this effect could be circulated.)

Although this case presents a common and difficult dilemma, the traditional ethical mandate for a physician to honor his patient's confidentiality should be given priority since no laws were broken and no imminent threat to another person is present. This case has little relationship to the health care organization's mission or values or to the application of the mission or values and therefore is not a case to be considered by the institution's organization ethics program.

Further Reflections

General

1. This case takes place in a small hospital with limited privacy and limited resources. What role should this fact play in determining if the physician and the hospital have a moral duty to protect patient confidentiality? Would the morally appropriate response be different in an urban center where patients are less likely to encounter other patients or personnel who know them?

Consequences

2. What important goods/benefits are sacrificed if the physician breaks patient confidentiality?

3. Lindberg and Iserson claim that privacy and confidentiality can be outweighed by the need to protect HCPs and the obligation to benefit patients. Why might these consequences morally restrict the obligation to protect patients' confidential information?

Autonomy

4. Do persons in jobs that put others at risk or that require specific levels of mental and visual acuity consent (if only implicitly) to relinquish at least some claim to confidentiality in much the same way as drivers give "implied consent" for breathalyzer tests?

Rights

5. Do persons have a moral right to confidentiality? If so, what is the basis of that right? What is it a right to? Who has the responsibility to protect that right? In what circumstances (if any) does a person forfeit or lose that right?

Virtues

6. What is the relationship between professional fidelity to the patient (to promote his best interests) and confidentiality? (Jollimore)
7. What is the relationship between institutional fidelity to the patient (to promote his best interests) and confidentiality? (Spencer)

Equality/Fairness (Justice)

8. If, as Jollimore suggests, "physician-patient confidentiality can be especially difficult to maintain in small-town and rural settings," what measures would be required to protect confidentiality in small communities? Do the typically limited resources of health care institutions in small communities limit the measures that must be undertaken to respect confidentiality? What role should nonspecific risks to others (e.g., coworkers) play in a justice-based analysis?

Chapter 16

Daddy Dearest

Mr. J is a 78-year-old Puerto Rican American* male with long-standing hypertension and recurring congestive heart failure. Twelve months ago he was hospitalized for acute pulmonary edema (fluid in his lungs). At that time he was admitted to the intensive care unit (ICU) and spent two days on a ventilator before his symptoms were controlled. After his hospitalization, Mr. J completed a Power of Attorney for Health Care (PAHC).**

Mr. J's PAHC is odd in two respects. First, he did not name a surrogate decision maker; he only specified that he wanted all care necessary to sustain his life. He specifically indicated he wanted CPR, intubation, a ventilator, and medical nutrition and hydration, should these modalities be needed. Second, Mr. J gave his rationale for aggressive care: his concern that his wife and three adult daughters would be unable to manage their affairs without his guidance. He stated in a narrative that these women depended on him and thus he felt obligated to make every possible

---

* Whenever possible, refer to Latinos with the term they prefer, in this case, "Puerto Rican." The general term "Latino" is usually preferred over "Hispanic" (which originated as a U.S. census term) and refers to persons from Mexico, Puerto Rico, Honduras, Cuba, and other countries in Central and South America.

**A PAHC is a legal document whereby one person can name another person as a surrogate decision maker if—and only if—he or she is unable to make his or her own health care decisions. In most states, a surrogate can consent to any and all treatment—and refuse any and all treatment, even if the refusal will cause the death of the person. Health care professionals (HCPs) who respect the decisions of surrogates are protected by law, just as they are if they respect a patient's choices, however much they may disagree with those decisions. If, however, the patient has left instructions in the PAHC form requesting or refusing specific treatments, the surrogate and, by extension, the HCPs, must respect these instructions.

effort to resume his position as head of his family. Mr. J did not discuss his PAHC or its contents with his wife or daughters; he merely gave copies to his physician and the local hospital.

Three weeks ago Mr. J suffered a massive hemorrhagic stroke. He has been comatose since he was admitted to the ICU. As his PAHC specified, he was intubated and placed on a ventilator; medical nutrition and hydration were begun. A CT scan of his head shows widespread brain destruction; he has made no attempt to breathe on his own since his admission to the hospital. His neurologist and intensivist believe his death is inevitable, though both agree that, barring medical catastrophes, his life can be sustained indefinitely—perhaps for several months.

Mrs. J died several months ago. Mr. J's three daughters, all of whom live out of state, have been present at his bedside. Each has been informed of Mr. J's request for continued life support; each objected to the physicians' plan to provide all life-sustaining therapies in accordance with Mr. J's specified wishes. The daughters point out that the claim that Mr. J used to justify his request—that his wife and daughters would be unable to manage their affairs without his assistance—is false. Their mother is dead and the daughters all have careers and families that are thriving without Mr. J's input. Indeed, the daughters all indicate that they left the state in part to avoid Mr. J's interference in their affairs. They find the life-sustaining interventions particularly ironic, given the virtual impossibility that Mr. J would ever recover sufficiently to give them advice or guidance (should they desire it, which they do not). So, if the goal of the life-saving interventions is their welfare, the interventions are useless. The daughters request that the life-saving interventions be stopped.

What would be an appropriate moral response to the daughters' request?

Introduction

This case raises two intricately integrated moral concerns:

1. The relation between personal identity (with special attention to values developed outside mainstream middle-class white American culture) and moral obligation (with special attention to decision making).
2. The competing moral claims of autonomy (doing what a patient requests) and utility (maximizing good outcomes).

The AJ Method

Step 1: Information Gathering   What facts are relevant to this dilemma? What is the purpose of a Power of Attorney for Health Care (PAHC)? What restrictions may a PAHC contain? What motivated Mr. J's PAHC? (Silva) What motivates his daughters? his caregivers? Were the particulars of his PAHC autonomously chosen?

PAHCs were developed to protect (and give evidence of our society's powerful commitment to) patient choice, patient autonomy, and the right to make decisions about one's life. Recognized by all 50 states, PAHCs enable persons to specify in advance their wishes regarding health care, thus providing direction to their families and health care professionals (HCPs).[1] But, equally important, a PAHC can identify *who* should speak (as surrogate decision maker) for a patient who can't speak for himself.

In Mr. J's culture, *men* (and parents) make decisions—facts that may in part explain his failure to name a surrogate.[2] Interestingly, Latinos often hesitate to name surrogates. One study found that 32 percent of Latinos preferred to name *no* surrogate,[3] a common reason being a belief that PAHCs were unnecessary in the presence of a loving, involved family.[4] Other studies have found a reluctance among Latinos to name family members as surrogates, feeling that surrogacy (1) places an unacceptable burden on the person named, (2) poses an inappropriate (role-related) burden on a child, or (3) singles out one family member inappropriately, suggesting that the surrogate is favored over others.[5]

More broadly, a 1992 study found that a majority of patients preferred that their surrogates override specific instructions in their PAHCs if doing so would better promote their (the patients') best interests.[6] A 1999 study discovered that 54 percent of patients would prefer to have their surrogates make their own choices to being bound by their (the patients') stated requests.[7] But a 1993 study found that 72 percent of patients ". . . wanted their preferences honored regardless of what their family wanted. . . ."[8] Asked to specify treatment desires if they were comatose with "only a small chance of full recovery," Latinos were most likely to request ICU care, CPR, artificial nutrition and hydration, and ventilators.[9]

Step 2: Creative Problem Solving   Any creative solution would have to respect the decisions—which are incompatible—of the father and his children.

Step 3: Pros and Cons   Survey CARVE principles to identify important moral reasons that support conflicting options for resolving this case.

Consequences   Will Mr. J be harmed or benefitted if HCPs comply with his requests? if they do not? How will his daughters be affected? Who else will be affected? Will these effects be negative or positive? How likely are they to occur? (Flescher; Schneiderman; Tarzian)

If Mr. J is beyond benefit and harm, maximizing good or minimizing bad consequences to all considered would appear to support terminating treatment. After all, the daughters' dismay will be relieved earlier than if their father lingers for months. Of course, we can wonder if Mr. J *is* harmed by the failure to follow his PAHC (much as we think people who make wills are harmed if those wills are not followed). Further, if HCPs override the expressed wishes embodied in Mr. J's PAHC, will they erode the professional commitment to the care of all patients who make odd requests? Will patients—present and future—whose PAHCs conflict with the desires or intuitions of HCPs, family, or health care institutions fear their directives will be ignored (whether they will or not) and lose trust in the system? Will Latinos and other minority racial or cultural groups—whose conceptions of benefits and harms often differ from the conceptions held by their caregivers—become even more wary of a system that too frequently fails to appreciate their values and culturally preferred methods for achieving them? Finally, will HCPs themselves come to view PAHCs as "mere suggestions" rather than binding indications of considered preferences? In short, what are the extended consequences of overriding Mr. J's explicit request?

Autonomy   Recall that autonomy, most broadly understood, applies to choosing the values in terms of which to live one's life, as well as the means to achieve those values. Whose autonomy will be respected if the HCPs comply with Mr. J's requests? if they do not? Whose autonomy is morally compelling? (All commentators)

One's identity and values are shaped by one's upbringing. Role-related responsibilities—including familial obligations—are both culturally conditioned and culturally diverse; so shared values can give rise to different behavior, even as different values can prompt similar behavior. Failure to assume one's duties or protect important values can expose one to social and moral condemnation.

When patients have not appointed a surrogate, HCPs usually turn to the family. This approach seems especially apt for Latino patients, who typically embrace a family-centered approach to health care decision making.[10] But Mr. J's directive seems to preclude this approach. After all, his rationale for his request—based on his culturally constructed conception of *who* has decisional authority—is that his family members are *unable* to make difficult decisions. Even if his daughters (or his HCPs) dispute his evaluation of their decisional ability, we have reason to believe Mr. J would simply ignore their assessments.

Patients in health care settings where few practitioners share their cultural assumptions may find that justifications for—or even the nature of—their requests are misunderstood, unappreciated, or deemed misguided or silly. Even so, Mr. J's case is a new version of an old moral conundrum: how strong is the duty to respect patients' choices and their right to self-determination in the face of personal or professional intuitions to the contrary? If the rationale for a PAHC is respect for patient autonomy, is respect still owed when the patient's goals or values can no longer be achieved? if others would be harmed by respecting a patient's wishes? if the patient himself would be harmed?

If *factual* answers to these questions are difficult to determine (see Step 1), *moral* answers are even more difficult to discern. First, are some choices—even when autonomous—morally improper (thus generating no duty of others to follow them)? Cultural variance might provide one occasion to challenge a PAHC, but other issues might prompt the same challenge.[11] For example, HCPs typically believe they are not morally obligated to honor requests for futile care, whether requested in a PAHC or through another medium. Indeed, most believe they are morally obligated *not* to provide care that will yield no health benefit.[12]

Rights   Mr. J's right to self-determination is central. (Schneiderman) Rights to not be harmed and to be aided also apply. Are the rights to privacy and confidentiality still in force, given Mr. J's unconsciousness?

Virtues   Does professional fidelity indicate which option is better? (Flescher; Schneiderman) Does tolerance? compassion? Does fidelity to family-centered role-related responsibilities give any direction? (Tarzian)

Justice   If HCPs comply with Mr. J's request, do they unfairly deny scarce medical resources to others (for example, an ICU bed)? Are such considerations compatible with professional integrity? Is denying patients a requested intervention ever unfair?

The Law   In conclusion, the following legal considerations are relevant to this case: (1) Who, legally, holds authority for decisions concerning Mr. J's health care? (2) Do the HCPs breach Mr. J's confidentiality and privacy rights by discussing his case with his daughters? (3) Under what conditions (if any) and by whom can a PAHC be overridden? (4) Would the removal of life support constitute a violation of the physicians' legal obligations to Mr. J?[13]

The following commentaries examine the application of various moral principles to this dilemma, thereby assisting the reader to undertake *Step 4: Analysis* and *Step 5: Justification*.

Notes

1. Multiple advance directive forms can be found at California Coalition for Compassionate Care, "Advance Health Care Directive Forms," 21 May 2003, http://finalchoices.calhealth. org/advance_directive.htm (8 Aug. 2003).
2. R. Sean Morrison et al., "Barriers to Completion of Healthcare Proxy Forms: A Qualitative Analysis of Ethnic Differences," *The Journal of Clinical Ethics* 9, no. 2 (1998): 118–26.
3. Panagiota V. Caralis et al., "The Influence of Ethnicity and Race on Attitudes toward PAHCs, Life-prolonging Treatments, and Euthanasia," *The Journal of Clinical Ethics* 4, no. 2 (1993): 155–65.
4. See note 2, above, 121.
5. Ibid.

6. Ashwini Sehgal et al., "How Strictly Do Dialysis Patients Want Their PAHCs Followed?" *JAMA: Journal of the American Medical Association* 267, no. 1 (1992): 59–63.

7. Peter B. Terry et al., "End-of-Life Decision Making: When Patients and Surrogates Disagree," *The Journal of Clinical Ethics* 10, no. 4 (1999): 286–93.

8. See note 3, above, 158.

9. Ibid.

10. Maryann S. Bates, Lesley Rankin-Hill, and Melba Sanchez-Ayendez, "The Effects of the Cultural Context of Health Care on Treatment of and Response to Chronic Pain and Illness," *Social Science Medicine* 45, no. 9 (1997): 1433–47; Leslie J. Blackhall et al., "Ethnicity and Attitudes Toward Patient Autonomy," *JAMA: Journal of the American Medical Association* 274, no. 10 (1995): 820–25.

11. See, for example, "To Feed or Not to Feed," this volume, p. 326.

12. Tom Tomlinson and Howard Brody, "Futility and the Ethics of Resuscitation," *JAMA: Journal of the American Medical Association* 264, no. 10 (1990): 1276–80.

13. Jessica Berg, Paul S. Appelbaum, Charles W. Lidz, and Lisa S. Parker, *Informed Consent: Legal Theory and Clinical Practice,* 2nd ed. (New York: Oxford University Press, 2001), esp. Part II: "The Legal Theory of Informed Consent," 41–164; and "The Role of Informed Consent in Medical Decision-making," 167–87. Also helpful are George P. Smith, II, *Legal and Healthcare Ethics for the Elderly* (Washington, DC: Taylor and Francis, 1996), 107–20, re: legal issues related to end of life treatment, including withholding and withdrawing life sustaining treatment, legal distinctions, and criminal liability; and Jerry Menikoff, *Law and Bioethics* (Washington, DC: Georgetown University Press, 2001), especially chap. 10, "The Right to Refuse Care," 241–303, and chap. 12, "Futile Medical Care," 356–73. Relevant discussions of legal decisions can be found in American Medical Association, Council on Ethical and Judicial Affairs, *Code of Medical Ethics: Current Opinions with Annotations,* 2000–2001 ed. (Chicago: American Medical Association, 2000), § 2.035, "Futile Care," 10–11; § 2.037, "Medical Futility in End-of-Life Care," 11–12; and § 5.05, "Confidentiality," 105–17.

A Daughter's Analysis

Cecilia Silva, PhD

As the demographics of American society change, health care providers (HCPs) in the United States—even those working in small, rural communities—will be more likely to encounter families such as Mr. J's. In attempting to understand Mr. J's case we begin by looking at the changing Latino family culture and the problems—of which patient care is a subset—that arise when individuals incorporate different belief systems and customs into the fabric of a culturally diverse society.

While Mr. J's advance directive is "odd" and voluntarily limited in one sense (he did not name an agent to make decisions for him if incapacitated), he did unequivocally specify that he wanted all care necessary to sustain his life and, as a rationale for his request, he stated that his wife and daughters were unable to manage their affairs without him. His rationale for such a request is not "odd" if we consider his role as a father in a traditional patriarchy. Mr. J, a 78-year-old Latino male, viewed himself as the family's authority figure. In traditional Latino families, women are expected to respect the authority of husbands and fathers and accept this authority without question. Mr. J's unwillingness to recognize the women in his family as capable decision makers was not at odds with traditional Latino cultural values. His values were reflected in his decision and in his goals for requesting such an aggressive type of life-sustaining treatment.

In this particular case, the "oddness" of Mr. J's request contrasts with the "common sense" response of the daughters. First, they are aware of Mr. J's condition and, given the deterioration of his mental capacities and inevitable death, are likely to view the life-saving procedures as an exercise in futility. Second, they find their father's rationale for treatment in conflict with their more contemporary perception of the role of women in the family. Precipitated by changes in social, cultural, and economic relations, Latinas are more willing to question traditional family roles. Growing up in today's society, Latina daughters learn to negotiate contradictory roles. While being taught to become the *mujer del hogar* (woman of the home), Latina women also become skilled at negotiating oppressive gender roles as they learn to *valerse por si misma* (to be self-reliant).[1] Mr. J's daughters are self-sufficient and view themselves as capable of acting independently of their father.

They find the physician's plans and rationale for aggressive intervention especially ironic, given the unlikelihood that Mr. J will ever be able to resume his role as head of his family. Though the daughters' response could be attributed to the process of acculturation experienced by their coming in contact with a different set of role expectations for women in the United States, it is more likely to reflect the gender role changes that have occurred across most Western societies over the last decades. Contemporary women throughout Latin America would quite likely express similar points of view given this situation.

So: what would be the appropriate moral response to the daughters' request? Mr. J's advance directive appears to be a cultural anomaly. His directive does not fulfill the purpose that this type of document is generally intended to achieve; it does not name an agent to make decisions for him now that he is incapacitated. In spite of the cultural conflicts revealed in this situation, Mr. J's document is clear regarding his wishes about the care he wants in order to sustain his life. Though the daughters and HCPs may have personal values and views that do not agree with Mr. J's wishes, he has clearly spelled out his expectations and his directive must be honored.

Notes

1. Sofia Villenas and Michelle Moreno, "To *valerse por si misma*: Between Race, Capitalism, and Patriarchy: Latina Mother-daughter Pedagogies in North Carolina," *Qualitative Studies in Education* 14 (2001): 671–87.

A Nurse Ethicist's Analysis

Anita J. Tarzian, PhD, RN

When trying to figure out the right thing to do, health care professionals (HCPs) often reflect on various professional codes and theories to help elucidate morally right and wrong actions. The most commonly cited ethical principles are non-maleficence (do no harm), beneficence (promote good), respect for persons (i.e., respect the autonomy of self-determined persons and protect persons who are unable to make decisions for themselves), and justice (treat people fairly).[1] Yet, what constitutes "harm," "good," "autonomy," and "justice" is context-dependent and varies with one's political, religious, and cultural beliefs and values. In the dominant U.S. culture, respect for the autonomy of the competent individual typically takes priority over other principles. Likewise, the American Nurses Association's code of ethics[2] emphasizes the nurse's overriding obligation to respect the patient's right of self-determination. However, growing acknowledgment exists among bioethicists that the process of "self-determination," despite what the term implies, is situated within the context of family, culture, and human relationships. Even in the individualist U.S. culture, individuals whose needs and desires are unaffected by relationships with family members or intimate friends are rare. Thus, HCPs must be careful in particular patient care situations to apply principles like respect for a person's self-determination without oversimplifying and decontextualizing an individual patient's situation.

Mr. J's nurse is obligated to be sensitive to and aware of how Latino (specifically, Puerto Rican) values, beliefs, and practices may be playing out in this case. Relevant concepts may include those of *familismo* and *machismo*. *Familismo* refers to the importance of family, which often includes extended and "nonblood" kin. Family members are often involved in decision making and care of the ill individual. *Machismo* is defined as "a strong or exaggerated sense of masculinity stressing attributes such as physical courage, virility, domination of women, and aggressiveness."[3] Many Latinos point out that machismo is misunderstood by non-Latinos. For example, the male is often the dominating figure in public, but at home he is often open to the opinions of the woman. Furthermore, this value is slowly changing, particularly among Latinos acculturating to U.S. values.

Mr. J appears to espouse the traditional machismo value of men making important decisions for women—he thought of himself as the head of his family and sole protector and decision maker for his wife and daughters. In some cultures that ascribe decision making to males, this role may be passed on to an adult son (not an option for Mr. J). While this approach to decision making works for families in many cultures (the nuances and harmony of the ascribed gender roles may be difficult for those from more egalitarian cultures to see), it does not appear to be embraced by

Mr. J's daughters. This highlights the complexity of considering cultural contributors in a situation like Mr. J's: one has to consider cultural values of the family while recognizing that individuals within that family are at differing points in the continuum of acceptance-rejection of those values. To add further complexity, in times of crisis individuals may revert to values or behaviors they espoused in the past but have since abandoned. Thus, information about an individual culture may serve as a general guideline for how to understand the behavior of an individual patient or family member and what questions to ask for further insight or direction, but final validation should always reside with the individual.

With these points in mind, the HCPs can determine the morally preferable course of action. Mr. J's request to be maintained on life support was contingent on the likelihood that he would recover to the point of contributing to family decision making. Regardless of the fact that his daughters neither want nor need his guidance in their life affairs, HCPs are obligated to honor his wishes to the extent possible. However in this case there is no reasonable hope that Mr. J will regain consciousness or decisional ability through the use of life-sustaining medical technology, which is merely delaying his death (assuming he is not yet brain dead). As it is not medically possible to achieve his goal, his daughters who, as his nearest relatives, know *him* best and are most likely to promote his best interests, are justified in requesting that the life-sustaining interventions be stopped. One could argue that maintaining life support for someone in Mr. J's condition is morally unjustifiable, as the burdens to his daughters (emotional strain, time away from their families and work, etc.) and resource use (the allocated intensive care bed and the amount of money spent) are not worth the "gain" of delaying an inevitable death in someone who cannot interact with others. This is the basis for policies of "medical ineffectiveness" (i.e., policies that define and determine the moral justification of appropriate care based on medical futility) in some hospitals. Here, opposing cultural and religious values and beliefs may present more complex conflicts. For example, what care would be considered "ineffective" for respecting patients' values?

The next step would be to provide support and guidance to Mr. J's daughters to minimize their regrets about his death, keeping in mind that the loss of both parents in such a short period of time exerts a heavy toll. This loss may be intensified because of the value placed on *familismo,* but the latter could also be a resource for the daughters as they gain strength from each other and from extended family. The ethic of care requires nurses to view patients and family members as individuals within the context of the culture(s) in which they live and were raised, and to provide holistic care with sensitivity to the complexities that competing cultural beliefs and values can exert, particularly at the end of life.[4] To this end, nurses should be open to learning how values, beliefs, and practices of patients and family members differ among cultures, and how these differences may influence moral decision making in the health care setting.

RECOMMENDED READINGS

Department of Health Sciences, Cleveland State University. "Puerto Rican Health Information: Puerto Rican Population in the United States." n.d., http://health.csuohio.edu/healthculture/culture/puertorican/prhealth.htm (8 Aug. 2003).

Fernandez, Reuben D. and George J. Hebert. "Rituals, Culture, and Tradition: The Puerto Rican Experience." In Mary L. Kelley and Virginia M. Fitzsimons, *Understanding Cultural Diversity: Culture, Curriculum, and Community in Nursing.* Sudbury, MA: Jones and Bartlett Publishers, NLN Press, 2000.

Galanti, Geri-Ann. *Caring for Patients from Different Cultures: Case Studies from American Hospitals*, 2nd ed. Philadelphia: University of Pennsylvania Press, 1997.

Guarnaccia, Peter J., Melissa Rivera, et al. "The Experiences of *Ataques De Nervios:* Towards an Anthropology of Emotions in Puerto Rico" *Culture, Medicine and Psychiatry* 20, no. 3 (1996): 343–67.

Huff, Robert M. and Michael V. Kline. "Hispanic/Latino Populations." In *Promoting Health in Multicultural Populations: A Handbook for Practitioners* Thousand Oaks, CA: Sage Publications, 1999, 115–97.

"Latino Cultural Values." In eds. Deborah Bender and Andrew Cameron. *Proceedings: Providing Quality Health Care Services to Immigrant Latino Populations in North Carolina: A Working Conference*, May 1999, http://www.hhcc.arealahec.dst.nc.us/culturalvalues.html (8 Aug. 2003).

Lipson, Julienne G., Suzanne L. Dibble, et al. *Culture & Nursing Care: A Pocket Guide*, San Francisco: UCSF Nursing Press, 1996.

Torres, Jose B., "Masculinity and Gender Roles Among Puerto Rican Men: Machismo on the U.S. Mainland," *American Journal of Orthopsychiatry* 68, no. 1 (1998): 16–26.

Welcome to Puerto Rico! 2003, http://welcome.topuertorico.org/culture/folklore.shtml (8 Aug. 2003).

Notes

1. Tom L. Beauchamp and James F. Childress, *Principles of Biomedical Ethics*, 5th ed. (New York: Oxford University Press, 2001).

2. American Nurses Association, *Code of Ethics for Nurses with Interpretive Statements* (Washington, DC: ANA, 2001), 2003, http://nursingworld.org/ethics/ecode.htm (8 Aug. 2003).

3. *The American Heritage Dictionary of the English Language,* 4th ed. (Boston: Houghton Mifflin Company, 2000).

4. A. Botes, "A Comparison Between the Ethics of Justice and the Ethics of Care," *Journal of Advanced Nursing* 32 (2000): 1071–75; Rosemary Tong, "The Ethics of Care: A Feminist Virtue Ethics of Care for Healthcare Practitioners," *Journal of Medicine and Philosophy* 23, no. 2 (1998): 131–52.

A Physician's Analysis

Lawrence Schneiderman, MD

Does a patient—who has the right to reject any treatment—have the right to demand any treatment? For example, does Mr. J have the right to require physicians to attempt cardiopulmonary resuscitation or provide life-sustaining mechanical ventilation after his massive stroke? Must physicians obey his request to "do everything" though Mr. J has no realistic chance of surviving outside the intensive care unit or regaining consciousness? "How can you be absolutely certain the patient won't miraculously recover?" someone might say.

These questions become all the more critical given the powerful array of technology available today. They force us to address the fundamental question: What are the goals of medicine?[1]

A patient is neither a collection of organs and body parts, nor a customer seeking to satisfy idiosyncratic desires. Rather, a *patient* (from the Latin root "to suffer") is a person who seeks the healing (from the root "to make whole") powers of the physician. The physician's goal is to provide not merely an *effect* on some organ, body part, or physiologic function, but to produce an effect that the patient has the capacity to appreciate as a *benefit*. Because Mr. J is permanently unconscious, he is incapable of experiencing any benefit from life-prolonging treatments.

Although Mr. J's daughters are not seeking a miraculous cure, many times grieving family members will impose this demand. Physicians can listen, seek to understand, empathize with their desires, and encourage their prayers. But physicians cannot do more than nature allows. Indeed, the very meaning of *miracle* depends on the premise that "the things which are impossible with men are possible with God" (Luke 18:27, NAS).

Today, approximately 80 percent of Americans die in a health care setting (60 percent in a hospital). Thus, it falls on many caregivers to determine not only how long a person will be kept alive but also the manner of dying. For example, if physicians attempt CPR or continue tube feeding on a moribund, terminally ill patient, all they are likely to do is increase the patient's suffering (adding the pain of rib fractures and increasing respiratory secretions, incontinence, and the risk of death by aspiration) without changing the prognosis.

The above considerations—serving the goals of medicine and avoiding futile treatments—form the moral basis for engaging the daughters in discussions about Mr. J's treatments. But what about patient autonomy and the wishes of his daughters? I am dubious about the motives of the daughters. They do not strike me as rich with filial devotion. They give a resentful slant on their father's self-described sense of responsibility to his family. Indeed, if Mr. J had a realistic chance of recovering, I would feel obligated to resist his daughters' advice on the grounds that they do not seem to be acting either consistent with substituted judgment (conveying what Mr. J would want for himself) or in Mr. J's best interest (placing their father's benefits ahead of their own interests).

Though my choice to withdraw life-sustaining treatments would concur with their wishes, my presentation to the daughters would make clear my dedication and determination to *care for the patient.* By presenting a plan of positive action, I would try to assure them that forgoing certain futile treatments does not mean abandoning the patient; rather that a course of treatment will be designed and carefully followed to assure a peaceful, pain-free, dignified death.[2] In other words—and in the words of an increasing number of hospital futility policies—although a treatment may be futile, care is never futile.

Futility policies, like all institutional policies, attempt to bridge the gap between the cultures of medicine and the law—doctors trying to say legal things, lawyers trying to say medical things. At a California conference in which health care professionals (HCPs), laypersons, lawyers, and judges reviewed a large number of futility policies, it became apparent to me that the HCPs, hoping to avoid doing things to patients that they considered to be futile, inappropriate, or burdensome, tended to seek specific *definitions* of circumstances and treatments. By contrast, the lawyers and judges were more concerned about putting in place a detailed *process* that will protect vulnerable patients.[3]

These two perspectives have persuaded me that *both* process and definition are required to achieve a workable futility policy. Definitions alone, although providing necessary grounding for actions, raise fears that important and compassionate communication between the involved parties will be neglected. On the other hand, a process-based approach without underlying principles and definitions, runs the risk of ending up with ethically problematic decision making, guided not by medical circumstances and standards, but more capriciously, by the demands of the most powerful, uncompromising, and threatening parties.

Some have argued that society has not reached a consensus on medical futility.[4] Medicine, however, like any profession, cannot expect society to define its goals and standards. The profession itself must propose these goals and standards of practice, which society may then accept, modify, or reject by court decisions and legislative statutes. Indeed, a strong case can be made that patient protection and optimal decision making would be better achieved by procedures carried out within health care institutions themselves. Judges are largely unfamiliar with the complexities of medical treatment and are neither expected nor even able to follow up medical outcomes once they have entered judgment. By contrast, physicians struggling to decide whether to discontinue a life-sustaining treatment have to live with the decision. For example, a judge who orders that a severely disabled child be kept alive rarely sees firsthand the long-term consequences of that decision, which remain a continuing vivid experience for the HCPs who must provide care for the child.

In any case, physicians should not expect the courts to give them prior permission to forgo futile treatment since the courts will want the opportunity to examine all the facts *after* the action is completed in order to judge its rightness or wrongness. Was the decision based on the best available clinical evidence? Was it taken after scrupulous attention to principles and professional standards, along with a respectful application of procedures that provide an opportunity for all values and wishes to be expressed? If so, the courts have shown themselves ready to accept decisions after the fact rather than give advance permission to withhold life-sustaining treatment.[5]

Notes

1. Lawrence J. Schneiderman and Nancy S. Jecker, *Wrong Medicine: Doctors, Patients, and Futile Treatment* (Baltimore: Johns Hopkins University Press, 1995).
2. Lawrence J. Schneiderman, Kathy Faber-Langendoen, and Nancy S. Jecker, "Beyond Futility to an Ethic of Care," *American Journal of Medicine* 96 (1994): 110–14.
3. Lawrence J. Schneiderman and Alexander M. Capron, "How Can Hospital Futility Policies Contribute to Establishing Standards of Practice?" *Cambridge Quarterly of Healthcare Ethics* 9, no. 4 (2000): 524–31.
4. Daniel Callahan, "Medical Futility, Medical Necessity: The Problem-without-a-name," *Hastings Center Report* 21, no. 4 (1991): 30–35.
5. Sandra H. Johnson et al., "Legal and Institutional Policy Responses to Medical Futility," *Journal of Health and Hospital Law* 30, no. 1 (1997): 21–47.

An Ethicist's Analysis

Andrew Flescher, PhD

Are a patient's expressed wishes more or less significant than the rationale upon which these wishes depend? In the case of Mr. J, the seemingly humane and commonsensical course of action—discontinuing his care—is precluded by an order plainly articulated in Mr. J's advance directive. This problem is complicated by two further competing considerations:

1. Mr. J's daughters, whom Mr. J loved dearly and for whose sake he apparently instructed his health care professionals (HCPs) to give him all treatments necessary to sustain his life, are the very ones poised to endure the brunt of the expense and the emotional hardship that will result from following their father's expressed wishes—an outcome Mr. J likely neither intended nor would support (were he fully aware of the situation).
2. Had Mr. J never drawn up an advance directive, nor elsewhere indicated what he would have liked done in the event of his incapacitation, he would nonetheless have been intubated and placed on a ventilator following a hemorrhagic stroke. That is, Mr. J's expressed wishes overlap with what the doctors would have done by default, arguably making the course of action that has been followed more, rather than less, justified.

The problem can be redescribed as follows: While the daughters' request that life-saving interventions be stopped is clearly reasonable (insofar as "reasonable" pertains to common sense), honoring it potentially erodes whatever "power" is thought to inhere in an advance directive.[1] Additionally, ignoring accepted medical protocol, when doing so is the most expedient course of action, sets a troubling precedent. Can we avoid the evil of "medical vitalism" (the blind policy of prolonging life whenever possible) without compromising *both* the value of autonomy that an advance directive allegedly ensures *and* the value that many place on a medical system that, unless otherwise indicated, engages in lifesaving and life-sustaining treatment?[2]

To justify ending the interventions which the daughters oppose, it will be helpful to address both issues just mentioned. First, consider the binding nature of a advance directive. Are HCPs ever justified in disobeying its contents? Here, we must reflect on the consequences of making such an exception. The concern is that if in even one case the answer to this question is "yes"—if an advance directive has a "vote" but not a "veto," then all future advance directives will lose their overriding authority. As a result, the autonomy of future patients who depend on advance directives to express their wishes will be compromised. On the other hand, instructions which make sense at one time may make no sense at another. In this case the patient explicitly announced his desire to release his wife and daughters from undue burden. As things have turned out, undue burden seems to take the form of Mr. J's being kept alive rather than being allowed to die.

Unfortunately for the daughters, however, a problem arises in trying to argue that the rationale for Mr. J's instructions supersedes the instructions themselves. While we may grant that Mr. J (were he aware of his own situation, his wife's death, and his daughters' success and independence) would likely no longer desire to be kept alive, we may not unconditionally presume that this represents his thinking. It is at least possible that Mr. J's stated rationale was only partial, and that he secretly wished—for additional reasons unstated in the advance directive—to be kept alive, should he fall ill and become unconscious. In filling out his advance directive perhaps he felt embarrassed, for example, about the perceived selfish nature of a sheer desire not to die (and consequently about a desire to prolong life as long as possible). In this case, it would be plausible to consider that, for privacy's sake, Mr. J wished to convey only the "acceptable" rationale for his chosen course of action: that he had his family's best interests in mind. Now, we may grant that this explanation is improbable. The point, however, is that when we start assessing Mr. J's rationale (or that of anyone else) we are inevitably engaging in interpretation—which is not an exact science—and thus potentially contravening the autonomy of an advance directive author. What *is* unambiguous in this scenario is the specific directive Mr. J gave to be kept alive. For this reason, on the grounds of autonomy, the daughters' request to cease their father's life-saving intervention should be denied.

There is an additional reason that lifesaving interventions should not be stopped: the potentially poor precedent of stopping treatment when recovery is still possible, even if unlikely. Will removing Mr. J—and other equally critical patients—from life support erode the default principle of providing care and medical assistance to those still ailing (i.e., not dead), regardless of what that ailment happens to be? This is a "slippery slope" concern: once common sense is introduced to dictate when ending care is reasonable, the serious commitment implied by the Hippocratic Oath—nonmaleficence and patient-centered beneficence—starts to erode.[3] Common sense is a fluid notion and, if offered as an overriding criterion, will be unpredictably appropriated in future cases to justify terminating care. The Hippocratic Oath does not permit convenience to override the presumption that doctors will act in the best interests of their patients. "Widespread brain destruction" is not the same as brain death, and so, failing explicit instructions to the contrary, every good faith effort ought to be made on behalf of Mr. J.

Notes

1. Note that problems of translation are present with some advance directives. The Spanish phrase for "health care proxy"—*apoderado para casos de assistencia medica*—indicates a person who has power in circumstances of medical need. Many Latinos indicate a reluctance to name a surrogate who is understood to then have power over them. See R. Sean Morrison et al., "Barriers to Completion of Healthcare Proxy Forms: A Qualitative Analysis of Ethnic Differences," *The Journal of Clinical Ethics* 9, no. 2 (1998): 121.
2. For an excellent discussion of advance directives, including the many nuanced distinctions they compel the astute moral theorist to make when rendering judgments about the value of autonomy, see Tom L. Beauchamp and James F. Childress, *Principles of Biomedical Ethics*, 4th ed. (New York: Oxford University Press, 1994), 173–78.
3. Consider the following, taken from the Oath of Hippocrates: "I will follow that system of regimen which, according to my ability and judgment, I consider for the benefit of my patients, and abstain from whatever is deleterious and mischievous." Clearly the subject of the sentence is the health care provider; it is his or her judgment, *not that of the patient*, which is crucially to be consulted in the evaluation process. The idea that the reasoned judgment of the physician takes precedence over that of the patient is so firmly established in the Hippocratic Oath that physicians are given leeway with respect to how much they are beholden to divulge to the patients they are treating. The tension between the values promoted in the Hippocratic Oath and the virtue of veracity is discussed by Beauchamp and Childress; see note 2, above, 395 *ff*. For full text of the Hippocratic Oath, see Hippocrates, "The Oath," trans. Francis Adams, n.d., http://classics.mit.edu/Hippocrates/hippooath.html (16 Aug. 2003).

Further Reflections

General

1. Discuss the ways in which Silva, Schneiderman, and Flescher relate *factual assumptions* about Mr. J's prognosis to their *moral assessments* of physician obligations and of the degree of decisional authority they give (or do not give) to the daughters.
2. How should Mr. J's Puerto Rican identity determine the health care professionals' (HCPs') response to the daughters' request? In other words, does this family's Puerto Rican heritage change in any significant way what is morally required in this case? If so, what and why?

3. Although the case focuses on the physician and the family, other HCPs are involved in Mr. J's care. What are the implications of this dilemma for the nurses caring for Mr. J? (Tarzian) What role should nurses play in determining what to do and in carrying out the final decision? How might nurses be a resource in this case that is presently not appreciated?

Consequences

4. Consider the following four sets of consequences and determine what each includes and how each should be weighed. Would appealing to these consequences morally support overriding Mr. J's expressed wishes?
   a. Enacting or ignoring patients' desires about (non)treatment
   b. Doing what will be best for the patient
   c. Enacting or ignoring the family's desires about (non)treatment
   d. Doing what will be best for family members other than Mr. J

Autonomy

5. Until about 20 years ago, *formal* advance directives for health care were quite rare; health care decisions for incompetent patients were made *informally* by physicians and family members. What moral principles support the move to advance directives? Why, from a moral point of view, would patient advocacy groups initially—and now physicians and nurses groups—enthusiastically support their implementation (as they have done)? What moral principles might challenge such documents?

Rights

6. Medical care can have a variety of effects on a patient: cure, relief without cure, change in physiological functioning with neither relief nor cure, preservation of physiological functioning without relief or cure, and satisfaction of patients' desires. What is the relationship of these possible effects to the well-recognized right of patients (and their surrogates) to participate in decisions about the health care they receive?

Virtues

7. If medical intervention is able to maintain a comatose patient's life but without hope of improvement or cure, what are the obligations of his HCP to his care? As HCPs have promised (in their various codes of ethics) to promote their patients' welfare (beneficence) or at least not harm them (nonmaleficence), what do they owe (based on professional integrity) Mr. J in terms of ongoing care and treatment? Does satisfying Mr. J's wishes count as a benefit?

Justice

8. When a patient is in an irreversible state of physical decline and death is inevitable (*if not necessarily imminent*), is expending resources (un)just? Why (not)? Would your analysis change depending on who will pay for the care, for example, the patient, private insurance, Medicare? If so, why? If not, why not? What are the implications of your decision for the rest of society?

Chapter 17

But You Need
a Real Doctor

Ms. R is a 36-year-old attorney and the founding partner of a successful law firm that specializes in commercial law. She is married and has a son, age 4, and is hoping to have another child. The family is very busy, but the couple prides itself on its involvement with their son's school, their church, and the larger community (Ms. R is also the treasurer of the local bar association).

Over the past three years Ms. R has increasingly suffered from severe headaches. They began as sporadic events. At first, Ms. R simply managed them with some exercise and over-the-counter medications (ibuprofen). Later, she found resting in a quiet, dark room provided temporary relief. At times the headaches seemed less severe (though never disappeared completely) for a few days or a couple of weeks, only to return with even greater force. Over the past 18 months the headaches have increased in severity and frequency, and in the last 4 months the situation has deteriorated to the point where her physician, Dr. N (an experienced general practitioner who has worked in town for about 20 years) felt some serious interventions were needed.

Based on a CT scan, X-rays, and lab tests (sedimentation rate and white blood cell count to check for inflammation/infection) her physician was unable to determine the cause of Ms. R's headaches. Her physician prescribed Fiorinal (a combination of nonsteroidal anti-inflammatory and sedative drugs), assuming she might be suffering from tension headaches. This gave some relief initially, but not permanently. Biofeedback also failed to offer sustained relief. Over four months Dr. N has prescribed various medications designed to relieve what might be migraine head-aches, including Amerge, Sumatriptan (Imitrex), and Zomig ("designer drugs" made specifically to treat the underlying pain mechanism occur-ring in migraine headache)—none of which has kept her pain-free. At her most recent visit, Dr. N referred her to a neurologist at the medical center an hour's drive away: "I think a neurologist will probably be able to help you. There are lots of things he can try, including physical therapy, elec-trical nerve stimulation, and even some antidepressants. If those are not effective, perhaps even acupuncture or botox injections in trigger point ar-eas might help. But I believe that one or more of these therapies will pro-vide you with some relief."

Ms. R considers her options. As her suffering increases, any option be-gins to look good. But the idea of injections into her nerves scares her and her faith in conventional therapies has already begun to weaken. She re-calls that a friend who had suffered from a similar problem attained sig-nificant relief from a chiropractor. In fact, several of her friends swear by a local chiropractor as providing the best therapy for relief of a variety of complaints. Ms. R checked with her medical plan to find out whether they would cover chiropractic care. The agent she spoke with at the health maintenance organization confirmed that the medical plan covers chiro-practic treatment, but only if the patient is referred to the chiropractor by a primary care physician.

Ms. R, finding now that her concentration at work, her interactions with her family, and even her performance at simple tasks are all suffer-ing, meets with Dr. N to discuss this alternative and get a referral. But Dr. N is quite critical of the chiropractic referral: "You've got a serious prob-lem here. You need to be careful with chiropractors and those interven-tions. Some evidence shows they can help some folks with lower back pain for awhile, but they aren't really headache people, and I'm not sure I'd trust my patients with this problem to them. There's no scientific proof that head and neck manipulations would offer much relief in your case. You'd be much better off to stick with physicians who have extensive expe-rience treating these problems and with the therapies we have already discussed."

All Ms. R wants is relief and a normal life. Should Dr. N refer Ms. R. to the chiropractor?

Introduction

Resolution of this dilemma requires decisions about:

1. The extent to which the virtue of professional integrity and the moral principle of beneficence obligate physicians to maintain currency about nontraditional treatment modalities.
2. The extent to which the virtues of honesty, integrity, and fidelity and the principle of autonomy support much fuller and franker discussions with patients about alternative therapies.
3. The appropriate hierarchy of commitments by physicians to individual patients vs. to patient populations.

The AJ Method

Step 1: Information Gathering   What facts are necessary for resolving this case? How likely is chiropractic to relieve Ms. R's headaches? (Parry; Rothfeld) How likely is a neurologist to relieve Ms. R's headaches? Is Ms. R (capable of) making an autonomous choice about a chiropractic vs. neurological consult? Is Dr. N a reliable resource regarding probable outcomes of chiropractic? of neurology? What motivates Dr. N's reluctance to refer? What explains the health maintenance organization's (HMO's) policy regarding chiropractic referral? What is Dr. N's obligation to the HMO?

The vast majority of Americans suffer from headaches at some point in their lives; 4 percent report daily or near-daily headaches. Among patients who see physicians, tension and migraine headaches are most prevalent. Migraines, which disproportionately affect women, are misdiagnosed or undertreated half the time.[1]

A recent survey revealed that 42 percent of U.S. residents use CAM (complementary and alternative medicine, including chiropractic, osteopathy, traditional Chinese medicine, acupuncture, herbal medicine, therapeutic massage, homeopathy, and naturopathy).[2] Chiropractic patients report very high levels of satisfaction with this modality.[3]

Step 2: Creative Problem Solving   Any creative solution would have to relieve Ms. R's headaches without violating Dr. N's professional integrity.

Step 3: Pros and Cons   Survey CARVE principles to identify important moral reasons that support conflicting options for resolving this case.

Consequences   What risks does Ms. R face if she undergoes a neurological assessment? (Clum; Zimbelman) if she undergoes chiropractic? (Clum; Rothfeld) What risks does Dr. N face if he refers against his better judgment? (Zimbelman) Are others likely to be affected by Dr. N's decision? If so, who and how?

Action consistent with patient-centered nonmaleficence and beneficence depends heavily on if Dr. N knows, for example, whether chiropractic is efficacious, dangerous, has had even limited success in relieving headaches, or is unlikely to benefit *or* harm the patient. (He should also consider whether the referral might benefit Ms. R via a placebo effect.) At this point the virtue of integrity, which incorporates a broad commitment to critical honesty, avoiding self-delusion, overcoming bias, and committing oneself to the patient's welfare is critical. Dr. N must ask himself whether he has sufficient data to make a recommendation. Is his evaluation of chiropractic based on recent and valid data of this modality, or merely a long-held bias in favor of his own approach?

Autonomy Patient choices—e.g., of care providers—are often limited when patients are insured by HMOs. Are such restrictions a limitation of autonomy? Since referral is an option, should Dr. N or Ms. R have decisional authority? (Clum; Rothfeld; Zimbelman)

The principle of autonomy, operationalized in the practice of informed consent, obligates physicians to provide patients with the information they need to determine, for themselves, the best course of treatment.[4] Information is critical for respecting the moral principle of autonomy, which requires HCPs to fully and accurately inform their patients about the burdens and benefits of all reasonable treatment options. Respect for patient autonomy and the right to self-determination imply a freedom to choose one's health care professionals and the treatments one wishes to undergo. A more robust understanding of these values suggests that physicians must strive to understand their patients' ultimate goals.[5] Patients are presumed to seek healing, but they also often desire information about coping with a chronic or debilitating problem, and taking a more decisive and active role in decision making or their treatment.[6] They may have ambivalent attitudes about medications, invasive therapies or diagnostic procedures, or referrals to other providers. For example, the medications typically prescribed for migraines must be taken on a limited basis to avoid serious complications, and may not provide complete relief. At the very least, respect for autonomy requires Dr. N to explain the burdens and benefits of referral to a neurologist as contrasted with referral to a chiropractor. If Dr. N has limited knowledge of chiropractic, he should explain that too.

Rights Within the patient-professional relationship, Ms. R has a right to be aided and a right to self-determination. She also has a right to not be harmed.

Virtues The virtue of integrity requires physicians to promote the patient's welfare, a requirement that mandates reasonable familiarity with treatment options. (Clum; Parry; Rothfeld) The virtue of compassion requires Dr. N to attempt to relieve Ms. R's suffering; while the virtue of tolerance requires him not to dismiss out of hand less common therapeutic approaches. Honesty requires him to admit any educational deficits he may have. (Clum; Parry; Rothfeld)

Insufficient clinical training or continuing education, as well as entrenched diagnostic and referral patterns among physicians, may partly explain the frequent misdiagnosis of headaches. (Note that the extent of Dr. N's appreciation of CAM—including chiropractic—is not specified in the case.) Physicians and patients may not see a physician's lack of educational currency as a moral dilemma so much as a mere fact of life (if they recognize it at all). But failure to appreciate the nature of available treatment for patients' problems; to recognize the limitations of one's own knowledge or diagnostic abilities; to refer patients to specialists earlier rather than later; and to establish a comprehensive and intimate knowledge of one's patients can be (if sufficiently significant) a moral failing, specifically, of fidelity to one's patients and of professional integrity. The American Medical Association (AMA) code of ethics explicitly requires that "A physician shall continue to study, apply, and advance scientific knowledge, maintain a commitment to medical education, make relevant information available to patients, colleagues, and the public, obtain consultation, and use the talents of other health professionals when indicated."[7]

Because no one can know everything about everything, we must consider under what circumstances and to what extent physicians might be excused from these professional and moral obligations without charges of infidelity. Perhaps practitioners need not familiarize themselves with nonefficacious treatments. But this raises the *problem of defining "efficacious,"* as well as the related *problem of evaluating efficacy*.[8] Patients, who often report relief with CAM, may be less inclined than physicians to grant the alleged superiority of "accepted," "evidence-based," "orthodox" therapies and "real" doctors over "complementary," "unproven," or "unorthodox" therapies and "alternative" practitioners.

A pluralistic, postmodern society that affirms pragmatism, scientific progress, and freedom of choice should at least tolerate patients who want to try something new or unproved. What, we might wonder, would make such unorthodoxy illegitimate? After all, currently accepted therapies were once experimental; moreover, many have never been subjected to rigorous scientific experiments themselves. Even long-accepted medical dogma is routinely debated and sometimes rejected (e.g., hormone replacement therapy, treatment of prostate cancer and ulcers). Today's alternative therapies may become tomorrow's accepted interventions. Our cultural commitment to scientific and evidence-based medicine and empirical observations of the failures of both conventional and alternative therapies suggests a moral obligation, founded on professional integrity and beneficence, to further test the efficacy of both.[9]

To complicate this issue, insistence on traditional Western-prescribed scientific investigation may be inappropriate for many CAM systems. Either patients need to be actively involved for a therapy to work *at all* (e.g., behavioral therapy) or knowledge may only be available in ways typically eschewed by randomized clinical trials (e.g., subjective perceptions rather than quantifiable outcomes, such as blood levels of physiologically active substances).[10] Further, such knowledge, even when achieved, may be of greater value to clinicians, who typically focus on the management of *disease* (i.e., discrete pathology) than to patients, who typically focus on *illness* (i.e., functional limitations).[11]

A further complication for both fidelity- and autonomy-based decision making is Dr. N's relationship to Ms. R's HMO. If Dr. N is simply Ms. R's doctor, whose *only obligation* is to *her health*, then the referral to the chiropractor may be merely a question of Dr. N's considered medical judgment and Ms. R's autonomous choice. But if Dr. N has an additional obligation to the HMO to benefit not only Ms. R but other insured patients by serving as a gatekeeper to specialists, he must engage in some rationing that fosters cost-containment in order to preserve resources for the entire population and ensure that the HMO remains solvent (a moral dilemma familiar to all physicians who work with third-party payers).[12] In some (but not all) HMOs, Ms. R would be required to personally assume financial responsibility for chiropractic care unless (or even if) Dr. N refers her. If Dr. N thinks chiropractic is nonefficacious, thus a waste of the HMO's limited monies, he has some reason to not refer Ms. R (though he should still discuss his concerns with her). But does his fiduciary relationship to Ms. R override his obligation to other covered patients or to the HMO if referral has at least some potential for relieving her symptoms? If so, how effective must the treatment be? Does the American Medical Association's stricture—"[a] physician shall, while caring for a patient, regard responsibility to the patient as paramount"—resolve this conflict?[13]

Equality/Fairness (Justice) Is restricting referrals an unfair burden on patients? Is rejecting CAM unfair to its practitioners? (Zimbelman)

The Law In conclusion, the following legal considerations are relevant to this case: (1) Given the general obligation to advance the best interests of patients, does Dr. N's action constitute negligence? (2) To whom do HMO HCPs have primary legal obligation—their patients, or the HMO with whom they have contracted? (3) Who has ultimate decisional authority in HMOs regarding treatment decisions and medical referrals? And under what conditions can patients demand decision-making authority or self-referral rights?[14]

The following commentaries examine the application of various moral principles to this dilemma, thereby assisting the reader to undertake *Step 4: Analysis* and *Step 5: Justification*.

RECOMMENDED READINGS

Callahan, Daniel, ed. *The Role of Complementary & Alternative Medicine: Accommodating Pluralism.* Washington, DC: Georgetown University Press, 2002.

Jonas, Wayne B. and Jeffrey S. Levin, eds., *Essentials of Complementary and Alternative Medicine.* Philadelphia: Lippincott, Williams & Wilkins, 1999.

Notes

1. Robert Kaniecki, "Headache Assessment and Management," *JAMA: Journal of the American Medical Association* 289, no. 11 (2003): 1430–33.

2. David M. Eisenberg et al., "Trends in Alternative Medicine Use in the United States, 1990–1997: Results of a Follow-up National Survey," *JAMA: Journal of the American Medical Association* 280, no. 18 (1998): 1569–75.

3. Richard A. Cooper and Heather J. McKee, "Chiropractic in the United States: Trends and Issues," *The Milbank Quarterly* 81, no. 1 (2003): 107.

4. Michael Weir, "Obligation to Advise of Options for Treatment—Medical Doctors and Complementary and Alternative Medicine Practitioners," *Journal of Law and Medicine* 10 (2003): 296–307; Jeremy Sugarman, "Informed Consent, Shared Decision-Making and Complementary and Alternative Medicine," *Journal of Law, Medicine & Ethics* 31 (2003): 247–50.

5. Eric Cassell, *The Nature of Suffering and the Goals of Medicine* (New York: Oxford University Press, 1991).

6. Franziska Trede and Joy Higgs, "The Clinician's Role in Collaborative Clinical Decision Making: Re-thinking Practice Knowledge and the Notion of Clinician-patient Relationships," *Learning in Health and Social Care* 2, no. 2 (2003): 66.

7. American Medical Association,"E-Principles of Medical Ethics: Preamble" (Principle V), 15 July 2002, http://www.ama-assn.org/ama/pub/category/8292.html (2 Apr. 2004).

8. Bonnie B. O'Connor, "Personal Experience, Popular Epistemology, and Complementary and Alternative Medicine Research," in *The Role of Complementary & Alternative Medicine: Accommodating Pluralism*, ed. Daniel Callahan (Washington, DC: Georgetown University Press, 2002), 54–73; Loretta M. Kopelman, "The Role of Science in Assessing Conventional, Complementary, and Alternative Medicines," in *The Role of Complementary & Alternative Medicine: Accommodating Pluralism*, ed. Daniel Callahan (Washington, DC: Georgetown University Press, 2002), 36–53; and Tom Whitmarsh, "The Nature of Evidence in Complementary and Alternative Medicine: Ideas from Trials of Homeopathy in Chronic Headache," in *The Role of Complementary & Alternative Medicine: Accommodating Pluralism*, ed. Daniel Callahan (Washington, DC: Georgetown University Press, 2002), 148–62.

9. See Weir, note 4, above, 298.

10. Kenneth F. Schaffner, "Assessments of Efficacy in Biomedicine: The Turn toward Methodological Pluralism," in *The Role of Complementary & Alternative Medicine: Accommodating Pluralism*, ed. Daniel Callahan (Washington, DC: Georgetown University Press, 2002), 1–14.

11. Arthur Kleinman, Leon Eisenberg, and Byron Good, "Culture, Illness, and Care: Clinical Lessons from Anthropologic and Cross-Cultural Research," *Annals of Internal Medicine* 88 (1978): 251–58.

12. Baruch Brody, "Costs and Clinicians as Agents of Patients," in *Bioethics: Readings and Cases,* eds. Baruch Brody and H. Tristram Engelhardt, Jr. (Engelwood Cliffs, NJ: Prentice Hall, 1987), 226–28.

13. See note 7, above, Principle IX.

14. The legal issues surrounding relationships with and referrals to CAM practitioners, as well as issues governing physicians' relationships with HMOs, are discussed in American Medical Association, Council on Ethical and Judicial Affairs, *Code of Medical Ethics: Current Opinions with Annotations*, 2000–2001 ed. (Chicago: American Medical Association, 2000), § 3.01, "Nonscientific Practitioners," 87–89; § 3.04, "Referral of Patients," 91–92; § 8.05, "Contractual Relationships," 154–55; § 8.051, "Conflicts of Interest under Capitation," 155–56; and § 8.13, "Managed Care," 175–81; most relevant to this case is § 8.132, "Referral of Patients: Disclosure of Limitations," 181–83. See also Michael H. Cohen, *Beyond Complementary Medicine: Legal and Ethical Perspectives on Health Care and Human Evolution* (Ann Arbor: The University of Michigan Press, 2000), chap. 3, "The Informed Consent Obligation," 37–45, and chap. 4, "Referrals to Complementary and Alternative Medicine Providers," 47–58; and Jerry Menikoff, *Law and Bioethics* (Washington, DC: Georgetown University Press, 2001), chap. 7, "The Doctor-Patient Relationship," 151–84. For legal compliance issues for CAM practitioners by state see Alternative Link Systems, Inc., ed., *The State Legal Guide to Complementary and Alternative Medicine* (Albany, NY: Delmar Learning, 2001).

A Neurologist's Analysis

Joel Rothfeld, MD, PhD

The case history of Ms. R supports a diagnosis of mixed musculoskeletal and migraine headaches. As often occurs with untreated headache sufferers, the patient starts with intermittent headaches and progresses to a chronic daily headache type. Headaches exist on a spectrum, ranging from intermittent migraines to chronic daily headaches. Migraine is defined as an episodic, incapacitating headache disrupting daily activity. A chronic daily headache is one which does not incapacitate (prevent performance of daily activities) but causes continual daily pain. Often an individual will cycle between these types of headaches, and an untreated migraine can transform into an intermittent migraine with an overlay of chronic daily headaches.

Appropriate medication depends on the type of headache being treated. Often an individual with a mixed headache disorder (as depicted in this case) will require intermittent use of tryptan medications (e.g., Imitrex, Zomig, Maxalt) specifically designed to treat the underlying pain of migraine headache. However, when such patients are in the phase of chronic daily headache these medicines won't prove as effective.

The workup initiated by Dr. N (CT scan of brain, X-rays, and lab tests) is typical for patients evaluated by practitioners with little experience in headache diagnosis and management. A detailed history with careful neurological exam and use of appropriate laboratory studies can lead to the correct diagnosis, which is necessary before therapeutic intervention is initiated. Incomplete or missed diagnosis of headache types occurs with inadequate history or exam findings.

Given Ms. R's detailed history, most internists would refer first to a neurologist rather than to a chiropractor. Referral to a chiropractor is not unusual in the scenario described and would be acceptable, provided the chiropractor in question has experience in dealing with this type of patient and can establish the correct diagnosis. Referral patterns are frequently dictated by patient requests and are based on information from friends, popular press, Internet bulletin boards, etc. Such sources, while sometimes helpful, often rely on anecdotal success stories that omit pertinent medical details. Some chiropractors will correctly diagnose a musculoskeletal component to the headache and treat appropriately with light stretching and massage. However, even if the correct diagnosis is made, chiropractic intervention alone may not adequately address the chronic headache symptoms. Given that chiropractors are not headache or pain specialists, a second missed diagnosis is possible.

Ms. R is frustrated, doubts the abilities of her physician, and is experiencing significant disruptions to her life. She wants a cure, hasn't found it, and now wants to seek relief from anyone she thinks can help her (even when there may be little evidence of likely efficacious treatment). Failure of traditional mainstream medicine to "cure" an illness can lead people to try nontraditional unproven therapies (as in seizure treatment and multiple sclerosis) that have no established efficacy. However, in this case treatment failed in part because the medications were improperly utilized. While alternative therapies have clearly gone more mainstream and in some cases have proven effective, inappropriate self-referral is more prevalent among patients who have been misguided in their preliminary contact with the medical community.

What are the moral issues here?

First, Dr. N has failed in his professional responsibility. With the growing complexity of medical therapies and advances in our understanding of disease processes, it is the responsibility of the physician to guide the patient toward a resolution of this problem. To be effective, this guidance must be based on the correct diagnosis and proven treatment options (both traditional and holistic).

Second, patient autonomy plays an important role. In the current medical environment the physician-patient relationship is evolving rapidly. With an increasing abundance of information readily available to the lay public, the traditional relationship in which the physician acted as informed advisor to uninformed or poorly informed patients has been replaced by a collaboration in which both parties bring information to the encounter. There exists an even greater pressure on physicians to get the diagnosis and treatment right, perhaps because patients see the process as easier ("just look it up on the Web") than it really is. An incomplete therapeutic course by a physician inexperienced in the treatment of headache has raised doubt in the patient, leading her to utilize her own resources to solve the problem. This doubt has led to lack of confidence in Dr. N. The shaman, the medicine man, and the mystic all lacked the armamentarium of potions we have currently. Despite this, they had the unwavering loyalty and confidence of their followers. Why? The answer: creation of a therapeutic trust through an alliance with the patient.

Dr. N is still in a position to guide Ms. R, providing he can regain her trust. Acknowledging that her headache pattern is beyond his level of expertise, he should clearly explain why his referral pattern is the most appropriate intervention for solving her problem. Dr. N should choose the route he supports and carefully explain why, while at the same time admitting his inability to solve the problem. At that point it ultimately becomes the patient's choice as to how to proceed. In a setting of mutual respect between patient and physician, knowledgeable, humanistic guidance on the part of Dr. N hopefully will provide Ms. R with the trust needed to follow the recommendations of her doctor.

RECOMMENDED READINGS

Goadsby, Peter J., Richard B. Lipton, and Michael D. Ferari. "Migraine—Current Understanding and Treatment." *New England Journal of Medicine* 346 (2002): 257.

Macklin, Ruth. "Treatment Refusals: Autonomy, Paternalism and the 'Best Interest' of the Patient." In *Ethical Questions in Brain and Behavior,*" ed. Donald W. Pfaff. New York: Springer-Verlag, 1983.

Sacks, Oliver. *Migraine* (with special attention to chap. 14, "General Measures in the Management of Migraine"). New York: Vintage Books, 1992.

A Philosopher's Analysis

Susan Parry, MA, PhD(c)

Dr. N is reluctant to refer Ms. R to a chiropractor because "there's no scientific proof" that such treatment will relieve her headaches. The American Medical Association (AMA) code of ethics states that "A physician may refer a patient for diagnostic or therapeutic services to a chiropractor . . . whenever the physician believes that this may benefit his or her patient."[1] So it seems that Dr. N is clearly following the AMA's ethical guidelines. He argues that there is no scientific evidence that chiropractic care will benefit Ms. R. But is his judgment based on sound medical judgment? He might be misinformed or influenced by his profession's historical prejudice against chiropractors.

Physicians have a long history of hostility toward chiropractic and other alternative and complementary medicines (CAM). From 1963 to 1974 the AMA had a special committee to focus on eliminating chiropractic, and until 1980 the AMA code prohibited members from consulting with chiropractors.[2] Dr. N might be biased in his assessment of chiropractors, thinking they are not "real" doctors because they do not follow the same scientific standards as MDs, or that they are only helpful in treating back pain; but this professional bias might be obscuring the facts. Even if not biased, Dr. N might be misinformed about current research in chiropractic care.

Recent clinical studies suggest some evidence for chiropractic's effectiveness for headaches. For example, a literature review by researchers at Duke University found some evidence for spinal manipulation's efficacy in treating headaches originating in the neck and tension-type headaches.[3] Even the AMA's Council on Scientific Affairs on alternative medicine acknowledges that "manipulation has been shown to have a reasonably good degree of efficacy in ameliorating back pain, headache, and similar musculoskeletal complaints."[4] The National Institutes of Health National Center for Complementary and Alternative Medicine (NCCAM) sponsors clinical research on the efficacy of a wide range of alternative therapies.[5] Like traditional clinical research, some therapies are proved and others disproved. Chiropractic has only recently been studied using randomized, placebo-controlled research methods, so there is not yet enough evidence to defend the general conclusion that chiropractic is always an ineffective treatment for headaches. As a gatekeeper to some of these therapies, Dr. N has a professional obligation to familiarize himself with current research literature so he can make fully informed recommendations to his patients.

If Dr. N is familiar with this literature, he has chosen to accept some evidence and dismiss other evidence. His reluctance to refer Ms. R to a chiropractor reflects a double standard. Every treatment he offered her failed. Would Dr. N conclude that these therapies are ineffective? No, he would only conclude that they were ineffective for Ms. R. Dr. N would not dismiss the scientific or clinical validity of treating some headaches with biofeedback or Imitrex. As an experienced practitioner he understands that clinical medicine is an imperfect science requiring adaptation and persistence. Dr. N does not conclude that, because he has failed to relieve Ms. R's headaches, the treatments used are scientifically invalid. The burden of proof he requires of chiropractic treatment is inconsistent with the proof required of mainstream treatments. In fact, only about one-third of standard clinical treatments have been subjected to rigorous scientific investigation (e.g., double-blind studies). This does not lead Dr. N to conclude that most standard clinical treatments are invalid. He should use empirical evidence as well as clinical experience to guide all treatment decisions, rather than assuming that chiropractic or any therapy that has not been tested by traditional scientific methods is invalid by default. If he fails to do this, he is guilty of ignoring evidence and holding chiropractic to a standard unmet by traditional medicine.

The AMA code is ambiguous; it simply states that a physician *may* refer a patient to a chiropractor. If Dr. N thinks that this referral could harm Ms. R, and this position is based on strong evidence, then he clearly has an ethical obligation to *not* make the referral and to warn Ms. R not to seek treatment at her own expense. But if there is some chance of benefit to Ms. R, Dr. N has an obligation to refer. Ms. R has been experiencing debilitating pain for three years with no improvement, despite aggressive medical treatment. While some might argue that her frustration makes her desperate and vulnerable, it does not necessarily make her request unreasonable.

Dr. N's reluctance might be fueled by concern that Ms. R is choosing chiropractic treatment over specialized treatment by a neurologist. He is concerned that she has not exhausted the domain of traditional medical therapies and that he also has an ethical obligation to protect Ms. R from "the hazards that might result from postponing or stopping conventional treatment."[6] Dr. N seems to have more confidence in the scientific standards of someone within his own profession. This is understandable since it is what he is most familiar with, but this should not entail having *no* confidence in alternative therapies. If his chief concern is Ms. R's well-being, he should agree to the referral but also encourage her to see a neurologist.

The claim that "there's no scientific proof" that chiropractic will relieve Ms. R's headaches is unjustified. The evidence for its efficacy may seem small, but it is not nonexistent. Dr. N may be professionally biased or misinformed about chiropractic treatment for headaches. While Dr. N has an obligation to encourage Ms. R to see a neurologist, this should not preclude a chiropractic referral.

RECOMMENDED READINGS

American Chiropractic Association, n.d., http://amerchiro.org (12 Aug. 2003).

Kaptchuk, Ted J. and David M. Eisenberg. "Chiropractic: Origins, Controversies and Contributions." *Archives of Internal Medicine* 158 (1998): 2215–224.

Notes

1. American Medical Association, "Current Opinions of the Council on Ethical and Judicial Affairs," (§ 3.041), 1995–98, http://www.ama-assn.org/ama/pub/category/2503.html (12 Aug. 2003).
2. Norman Gevitz, "The Chiropractors and the AMA: Reflections on the History of the Consultation Clause," *Perspectives in Biology and Medicine* 32 (1989): 281–99.
3. Douglas C. McCrory et al., *Evidence Report: Behavioral and Physical Treatments for Tension-type and Cervicogenic Headache* (Des Moines, IA: Foundation for Chiropractic Education and Research, 2001).
4. American Medical Association, "Report 12 of the Council on Scientific Affairs (A-97): Alternative Medicine," http://www.ama-assn.org/ama/pub/article/2036-2432.html (12 Aug. 2003).
5. National Center for Complementary and Alternative Medicine, 12 Aug 2003, http://nccam.nih.gov/ (12 Aug. 2003).
6. See note 4, above.

A Chiropractor's Analysis

Gerard W. Clum, DC

This case raises a series of clinical and ethical questions.

Clinically speaking, Ms. R has failed to receive relief of her pain or resolution of her underlying problem from Dr. N, who is quite unsure about the true nature of her problem, and who appears to have reached the limit of his ability to help Ms. R. Nonetheless, he balks at referring her to a chiropractor. His reluctance raises several ethical issues.

First, one might question whether Dr. N truly has Ms. R's welfare foremost in his mind. The types of interventions he suggests the neurologist might pursue are all well within the ability of an experienced general practitioner. Dr. N's failure to provide or secure these services himself raises a question in and of itself: the referral to the neurologist begins to look like a ploy of "moving the patient along" rather than a sincere referral for a higher level of evaluation and care.

Further, he potentially places his patient at risk and undercuts his ability to provide her with beneficial treatment options when he dismisses the chiropractic referral out of hand. Dr. N does not know why Ms. R is experiencing headaches. Rather than be candid with Ms. R about her circumstances and the limits of his knowledge, he asserts that a neurologist "will probably be able to help"—a conclusion which simply does not follow from what Dr. N knows about this patient. He would be better advised to research the benefits of chiropractic, rather than condemning it without further investigation.

Second, one might question Dr. N's intellectual honesty. He is clearly uncomfortable with the suggestion that chiropractic care might be appropriate for Ms. R. His response is to assert the need for "scientific proof" of its efficacy before he will make a referral. In contrast, the suggested antidepressant therapy or botulism toxin injections have scant evidence—let alone "proof"—of their effectiveness for the problems demonstrated by Ms. R. The interventions he proposes are themselves highly speculative. In fact, for each and every intervention attempted or proposed by Dr. N, no definitive scientific "proof" exists to support the effort. There is a measure of scientific evidence for each of the interventions, but no clear "proof." The evidence for chiropractic care in this environment is every bit as compelling—or more so—than the evidence associated with many of Dr. N's recommended interventions. To pretend otherwise reflects a deepening confusion on the part of the physician about which he is not being honest. In fact, if Dr. N has concerns about unproven therapies, he should abandon his own recommendations.

Third, Dr. N fails to demonstrate respect for Ms. R as a person. Her response to the neurological referral can be characterized as tepid and Dr. N's response to chiropractic referral could be considered harsh to hostile. When Ms. R expressed the desire for a chiropractic referral, Dr. N responded that Ms. R was misguided and that her desire to be referred to a chiropractor was foolish and unjustified. But Ms. R is a learned person. She is accomplished personally and professionally. She is used to being involved in situations that require complex levels of decision making. She has sought counsel from her physician and received a patronizing and patriarchal response. Her input and inquiry have not been given due consideration, even when she has shown a remarkable level of consideration of the input and feedback of Dr. N.

Fourth, Dr. N's commitment to professional currency (professional integrity) seems unduly weak. Dr. N, like most physicians, in fact knows very little about chiropractic care. He is likely to be uninformed about its indications and contraindications, of which none of the latter is present in this case. Further he is not likely to be aware of the education and training of a doctor of chiropractic and he has likely drawn his conclusions from rumor more than fact.

The ethical issues in this situation, which arise in large part from Dr. N's unwillingness to admit the limits of his own knowledge, include a high level of condemnation for a given clinical intervention without adequate investigation; a willingness to explore highly speculative interventions because of the party providing them as opposed to the information behind them; a general dismissal of the input of a well-informed and actively involved patient; and finally, a failure to respect the rights of a patient to be an active player and party in her recovery and well-being.

In summary, every health care provider has a responsibility to seek the most effective and least intrusive solution/response to a patient's health care problem. This responsibility should not be limited by the worldview of the provider, cultural bias, or an assumption of clinical totality. This responsibility should include the perspectives and experiences of provider and patient alike. This consideration did not occur between Dr. N and Ms. R.

Ms. R should be referred to the chiropractor. The chiropractor and general practitioner should have a dialogue about Ms. R, and the providers in question should set aside their respective biases and act in the patient's best interest.

An Ethicist's Analysis

Joel A. Zimbelman, PhD

How is sense to be made of the fact that a large and prestigious group of clinicians and biomedical researchers seems so utterly hostile to [complementary and alternative medicine] while a large portion of the public (and the educated public at that) seems so attracted to it?

—DANIEL CALLAHAN[1]

The Rise of Modern Medicine

Medicine, as it is practiced in the United States, is indebted to ancient Greek culture for two of its most enduring characteristics. First, medicine is humanistic; it exhibits a desire to respond to the tangible needs of patients who suffer. Second, it is inquisitive and exhibits a desire to determine what it is that ails patients who suffer. In the modern period, beginning with the Enlightenment in the eighteenth century, medicine melded these earlier commitments to the tools of the new scientific method. The scientific method makes important theoretical assumptions about the nature of the world; the nature of health, disease, and illness; how we come to know the forces that undercut human flourishing; and the actions one must embrace if one is committed to healing.[2] In its attempt to treat disease and illness, the scientific method embraced a commitment to reason and rationalism—and to empirical, evidence-based, and experimentally defined methods of assessing medical efficacy.[3]

The society's tendency toward professionalization and specialization further established medicine's place and importance in society. Modern medicine, with the support of society and governments, established mechanisms for research into basic science and applied medicine, regulatory oversight of the training of practitioners and the provision of health care, mechanisms for the distribution of health care re-sources, and a framework for the division of labor among nonmedical health care professionals (HCPs). As a result of these commitments, it is convenient to speak with some accuracy of Western Biomedicine (WB) as the dominant paradigm of mainstream health care in the United States.

Postmodernism and the Rise of Complementary and Alternative Medicine (CAM)

In spite of the importance of and respect for WB in our society, a growing interest in and a commitment to CAM has appeared in recent years. Both WB and CAM claim proficiency in restoring or maintaining health and relieving suffering, albeit via different approaches.

CAM is a catch-all phrase that is often used by its proponents as shorthand for practitioners, medicines, therapies, and practices that are often grounded in philosophies of health and healing at odds with or outside the accepted methods and tools of WB. These include non-Western philosophies of healing (from In-dian, Chinese, and aboriginal cultures), vitamin therapies, therapeutic touch, herbal remedies, and body massage and manipulation therapies, to name a few. CAM advocates claim that even though their approaches may be difficult to as-sess, patient responses are consistently positive. Critics of CAM, alternately, assert that such approaches are not genuine therapeutic alternatives; that they are grounded in pseudoscience or—even worse—not grounded in science at all, and that their use is opportunistic quackery of the worst sort.

In spite of these criticisms, the popularity and growing use of CAM are signifi-cant.[4] Alternative therapies are used most frequently by Americans for chronic con-ditions. 629 million visits to CAM practitioners were made in 1997, exceeding the total visits to all U.S. primary care physicians. Expenditures to CAM *practitioners* in 1997 were estimated at over $21 billion (half paid out-of-pocket). Expenditures for all CAM *therapies* were over $27 billion (exceeding all out-of-pocket expendi-tures for all U.S. hospitalizations in the same year).[5]

CAM challenges WB on many levels, most significantly by introducing alterna-tive metaphysical systems and advancing different epistemic foundations for under-standing and appreciating health and disease.[6] CAM also employs empirical and ev-identiary foundations of modern science in ways which often conflict with the orthodoxy of WB,[7] asserts divergent perspectives on the status of patients and heal-ers,[8] and introduces alternative practices and therapies which cannot be explained in the evidentiary framework of WB.[9]

Where the legitimacy of WB is established in the framework of the Enlighten-ment and modernism, the use of CAM is justified from the perspective of a *postmodern* mentality—a changed view of the world in which we live. David B. Morris indicates three important traits of postmodernism relevant to our discussion:

First, the postmodern era coincides with the rise of late consumer capital-
ism. . . . Health care too is aggressively marketed as a product. . . . Second,
postmodern thinkers regard all knowledge as historically situated and cul-
turally inflected, so that we stand deprived of an outside, wholly objective,
God's-eye view of Truth. Even the most accurate science does not supply
pure facts, knowledge in a vacuum, but reflects time-bound distinctive po-
litical and social desires. . . . Third, experience for postmodern thinkers is
always mediated by organized discourses that amount to systems of repre-
sentation. Along with individual genes and biological processes, it is collec-
tive social discourses and codes (including the ultrapowerful discourses of
medicine) that help shape human health and illness.[10]

In the postmodern world, medicine is often seen by its critics as an extension
of capitalism and as a tool—appropriated by the rich and powerful—to advance
their own interests. Supporters of CAM often argue that proponents of WB assert
their personal and professional interests at the expense of good patient care as a
way to hold on to the social status and the economic benefits WB confers on its
practitioners. The presuppositions of objectivity and of rationalism in medicine as
tools that help human beings better their situations are also challenged by CAM.
The monolithic nature and control of the "medical industrial complex" is seen by
some as choking off alternative perspectives and resources for thinking about human health, happiness, and well-being.[11] Charges of quackery leveled at some
CAM professionals by WB sometimes define a contentious relationship between
traditional physicians and the practitioners of CAM. These attacks marginalize ancillary health professionals (e.g., nurse practitioners and midwives among more
"mainstream" practitioners and individuals—herbalists, shamans, acupuncturists,
therapeutic touch specialists—with identities in traditional, folk, or new age
communities).

WB's Response to Postmodernism

Supporters of WB argue that postmodern critiques are always aimed at whatever or
whoever embraces any established, significant, and successful method of healing. In
short, it's easy to take potshots at modern medicine because of its undeniable success,
support by many social institutions, and broad appeal among the general public. But
the proof of WB's legitimacy, its supporters argue, is in the pudding: WB provides a
legitimate and scientifically testable explanatory framework for understanding disease, cure, and patient-based beneficence. Modern medicine—by its very presence,
durability over centuries, and documented outcomes—is able to respond to the
needs of contemporary patients in ways that are helpful, life-changing, and desired
by most patients who are given the option of modern medical treatment. Who could

oppose the significant inroads in public health; the miracles of blood transfusions and organ transplants; the use of antibiotics against infection; the research into treatments for AIDS, SARS, malaria; the lifesaving interventions of trauma medicine and surgery? In the end, the response to the question "Are human beings helped by these interventions?" is the ultimate test of medicine's validity—whether CAM or WB. And if they believe that various alternative therapies prey on the ignorance or desperation of terribly ill patients, then medical practitioners are morally obligated to root them out and to encourage the use of truly efficacious therapies.

The Counterchallenge to WB

Supporters of CAM recognize the legitimacy in many of these claims by WB, but respond with several counterclaims. First, CAM supporters assert that WB responds inappropriately to the needs of patients. CAM supporters note the widespread decline and frequent failures in the quality and efficacy of WB. Often attacked are the expense of conventional therapies and the highly invasive surgical, pharmacologically intense, and technical character of much modern medicine—all combining to as frequently harm as benefit patients. This is not to say that patients, when the chips are down and their options appear to have dwindled, won't take advantage of the promise—in spite of the perils—of WB. But the oversubscribing of and developing resistance to antibiotics; the failure to provide adequate and appropriate pain relief to suffering patients; the training of physicians in narrow specialties that fail to meet the most important health care needs of the population; and the failure to support national health care plans that would improve patient access and medical outcomes are simply the most visible examples of the failure of WB to be faithful to foundational commitments.

Second, supporters of CAM argue that many of the therapies and conventions of WB have failed both to undergo the rigors of testing, or, when they have undergone such testing, have failed to measure up to their own standards of efficacy.[12]

Third, CAM retains its popularity because its approach is viewed by many consumers as more "humane," "personalist," and "patient-centered" than the technocratic, impersonal delivery of WB. Modern medicine, so the argument goes, has lost its soul and its patient-centered approach by treating patients as bodies, by treating disease (pathology) rather than illness (patients' functional limitations), and by refusing to allow patients to take ownership both of their illnesses and their management. The moral failings of WB are hubris, self-indulgence, and erroneous attitudes about patients and disease.

WB, CAM and Ms. R

The debate surrounding the "mainstreaming" of CAM raises a host of issues that go to the heart of the tension that exists between Ms. R and Dr. N. What reasons explain Ms. R's attraction to and Dr. N's reticence regarding chiropractic? Is Ms. R's primary concern with illness—functional limitations—while Dr. N is primarily concerned with disease (etiology of Ms. R's symptoms)? Is Dr. N worried that a chiropractor will help Ms. R, thereby revealing his limited diagnostic or treatment skills? Does Dr. N view Ms. R's request as rejection of him? of the discipline to which he has devoted his life? something else equally noxious? Is Ms. R's request an autonomous one, based on an evaluation of an approach that, in her estimation, cannot leave her worse off than she currently is? Has she grown weary of the *science* of medicine to the extent that she wishes to embrace the *humanism* of CAM?

The answers to these questions cannot be answered unless Ms. R and Dr. N have an honest conversation about her motives and his capabilities. But the more important point is that each needs to take the other's perspective seriously. Both chiropractic and more mainstream medicine have helped many patients—and both have failed others. Neither has a lock on the truth.

In the end both WB and CAM can claim moral legitimacy only if they do well by patients. That means understanding patient problems; avoiding harms to patients; providing the best care possible; seeking the best resolution possible for *this* patient; appreciating—as a practitioner—the limits of one's knowledge and ability; and an openness to refer patients to other qualified practitioners who may be able to heal a person.

Notes

1. Daniel Callahan, Introduction, in *The Role of Complementary and Alternative Medicine: Accommodating Pluralism,* ed. Daniel Callahan (Washington, DC: Georgetown University Press, 2002), vii.
2. Paul Root Wolpe, "Medical Culture and CAM Culture: Science and Ritual in the Academic Medical Center," in *The Role of Complementary and Alternative Medicine: Accommodating Pluralism,* ed. Daniel Callahan (Washington, DC: Georgetown University Press, 2002), 163–71.
3. Paul Kurtz, "In Defense of Scientific Medicine," in *Science Meets Alternative Medicine: What the Evidence Says About Unconventional Treatments,* eds. Wallace Sampson and Lewis Vaughn (New York: Prometheus Books, 2000), 13–18; Kenneth F. Schaffner, "Assessments of Efficacy in Biomedicine: The Turn Toward Methodological Pluralism," in *The Role of Complementary and Alternative Medicine: Accommodating Pluralism,* ed. Daniel Callahan (Washington, DC: Georgetown University Press, 2002), 1–14. For examples of the contemporary tension between "evidence-based science" and "pseudo-science" and between Western biomedicine and CAM, see Arthur Wrobel, ed., *Pseudo-Science and Society in Nineteenth-Century America* (Lexington: University Press of Kentucky, 1987).
4. David M. Eisenberg et al., "Unconventional Medicine in the United States: Prevalence, Costs, and Patterns of Use," *New England Journal of Medicine* 328 (1993): 246–52.
5. David M. Eisenberg et al., "Trends in Alternative Medicine Use in the United States, 1990–1997," *JAMA: Journal of the American Medical Association* 280, no. 18 (1998): 1569–75.
6. See David J. Hufford, "CAM and Cultural Diversity: Ethics and Epistemology Converge," in *The Role of Complementary and Alternative Medicine: Accommodating Pluralism,* ed. Daniel Callahan (Washington, DC: Georgetown University Press, 2002), 15–35; and Bonnie B. O'Connor, "Personal Experience, Popular Epistemology, and Complementary and

Alternative Medical Research," in *The Role of Complementary and Alternative Medicine: Accommodating Pluralism,* ed. Daniel Callahan (Washington, DC: Georgetown University Press, 2002), 54–73.

7. Wayne B. Jonas, "Evidence, Ethics, and the Evaluation of Global Medicine," in *The Role of Complementary and Alternative Medicine: Accommodating Pluralism,* ed. Daniel Callahan (Washington, DC: Georgetown University Press, 2002), 122–47.

8. Douglas Tataryn, "Paradigms of Health and Disease: A Framework for Classifying and Understanding Complementary and Alternative Medicine," *The Journal of Alternative and Complementary Medicine* 8, no. 6 (2002): 877–92.

9. Micaela Sullivan-Fowler, Terry Austin, and Arthur W. Hafner, *Alternative Therapies, Unproven Methods, and Health Fraud: A Selected Annotated Bibliography* (Chicago: American Medical Association, 1988).

10. David B. Morris, "How to Speak Postmodern: Medicine, Illness, and Cultural Change," *Hastings Center Report* 30, no. 6 (2000): 7–8.

11. Ivan Illych, *Medical Nemesis: The Expropriation of Health* (New York: Knopf, 1982).

12. Loretta M. Kopelman, "The Role of Science in Assessing Conventional, Complementary, and Alternative Medicines," in *The Role of Complementary and Alternative Medicine: Accommodating Pluralism,* ed. Daniel Callahan (Washington, DC: Georgetown University Press, 2002), 36–53.

Further Reflections

General

1. Dr. N needs to balance the following four moral obligations: (1) respect Ms. R's wishes and her desire to participate in deciding about her health care; (2) do that which advances Ms. R's well-being; (3) make only efficacious and beneficial referrals to effective health care professionals; and (4) abide by the standards of care established by his profession. What moral principles support these commitments? Which commitments seem most important to Dr. N? to commentators Rothfeld, Clum, and Parry?

Consequences

2. Clum, Parry, and Zimbelman argue that many conventional treatments are scientifically unproven. What can be done in the future to determine what treatments are most effective for specific problems? To what extent should "proof" be required before treatments can be offered? What role should insurance companies have in testing and facilitating the availability of therapies?

Autonomy

3. Rothfeld suggests that referral to a neurologist is clinically indicated, in part because it is the course of action most likely to result in a correct diagnosis. How can Dr. N most effectively guide Ms. R (he cannot force her to follow his advice) to a course of action that will resolve her problem? What should be his response if she continues to insist on chiropractic?

Rights

4. Patients have a well-established right to participate in decisions about their health care. Does Ms. R's right to self-determination, which she exercised in choosing her health care plan and physician, entail a right to choose the practitioner to whom she is referred? What moral principles support Ms. R's claim to such authority? What argument against such patient decisional authority might be made by her physician or her health care carrier?

Virtues

5. Which virtues does Dr. N demonstrate? Which does he lack?

Equality/Fairness (Justice)

6. Is the insurance company's demand of a referral by a physician before it will pay for chiropractic just or unjust? Why?

Chapter 18

To Feed or
Not To Feed

Mrs. S is a 62-year-old with three daughters and two sons. She has been essentially healthy through her life, but has mild hypertension and was diagnosed three years ago with Parkinson's Disease (PD). The PD has affected her mobility and coordination. She has increasing muscle rigidity and difficulty initiating voluntary movements; occasionally she "freezes" in place, leaving her stranded until her muscles finally relax. She has also noted increasing problems with her balance and has fallen a few times. She lives at home with support from Meals-on-Wheels, a housekeeper who also does her laundry, and a high school student who runs errands for her twice a week. Her children all live within a two-hour drive and visit as frequently as they are able (typically once a month). During the visits the children make repairs or purchases as needed to ensure that Mrs. S's life is as trouble-free as possible. Still, maintaining her independence has become increasingly difficult.

Recently a neighbor suffered a stroke and was comatose for two months before dying. Mrs. S mentioned to her daughters, though not to

---

°A Power of Attorney for Healthcare (PAHC) is a legal document whereby one person (the PAHC author) can name another person as a surrogate decision maker to make health care decisions for the PAHC author if—and only if—the PAHC author is unable to make her own health care choices. In most states, a surrogate can consent to any and all treatment; he or she can also refuse *any and all* treatment, even if the refusal will cause the death of the PAHC author. Health care professionals (HCPs) who respect the decisions of a surrogate are protected by law, just as they are if they respect a patient's choices, however much they may disagree with those decisions. If, however, the PAHC author has left instructions in the document requesting or refusing specific treatments, the surrogate and, by extension, the HCPs, must respect these instructions.

her sons, that she would never want that to happen to her. She commented that she found being tube-fed particularly unappealing. None of her daughters pursued the conversation, so the reasons for Mrs. S's repugnance are unknown. One daughter suggested that Mrs. S should complete a Power of Attorney for Healthcare.* Mrs. S said she would "look into it," but she did not complete a document.

Two weeks ago Mrs. S fell and struck her head on the cement steps of her back porch. The fall caused an epidural hematoma (bleeding causing pressure on her brain). Following successful surgery to stop the bleeding and remove the collection of blood, she had a cardiac arrest. She was resuscitated, but failed to regain consciousness. She is now breathing on her own and shows no further cardiac irregularities, but she remains comatose (or possibly suffering from persistent vegetative state (PVS)) and her physicians do not expect her to awaken. Her only present treatment is intravenous (IV) therapy. The physicians agree that she could be maintained, perhaps for months or years, in this state as long as she receives adequate nutritional and other physical supports. They request permission to insert a gastrostomy tube (g-tube) into her stomach through which nutritional feedings can be administered.

The daughters relay to the treating team Mrs. S's comments about not wanting to be tube fed; consequently, they do not want the g-tube inserted. Her sons, however, not having been privy to these conversations, want the tube inserted. Both sons are horrified by the prospect of "starving mom to death." The discussion becomes heated and the treating team are, understandably, reluctant to proceed in the presence of deeply felt disagreement, especially in the absence of a designated surrogate decision maker. After three days the five children approach Mrs. S's primary physician and indicate that they all now want the g-tube inserted. A tube is placed and feedings are begun.

A week later Mrs. S's three daughters approach the primary physician and make the following unusual request: Please continue to feed our mother, but do not give her sufficient nourishment to meet her nutritional needs. The physician replies that this approach would result in Mrs. S's slow death from starvation. The daughters say that they appreciate this fact; indeed, it is their goal. The physician asks why the daughters agreed to the g-tube insertion if they were opposed to medical nutrition. The daughters reply that their brothers are so vehemently opposed to death by *starvation that they would never have forgiven their sisters for pursuing this approach. As a result, this very close family would suffer an irreparable rift. However the daughters believe they are betraying their mother who, even though she put nothing in writing, requested that she not be fed artificially—a request she made to three different people on three separate occasions. The daughters add that, as they understand their mother's condition, she will not be aware of her starvation and will not feel any discomfort. The daughters end by cautioning the doctor that, of course, their brothers must never know about this approach.*

The physician agrees to consider the daughters' request. Over the next several days, she discusses the request with Mrs. S's primary care nurse, the unit's nurse manager, and the head of the dietary department. The primary care nurse and the chief dietitian are vehemently opposed to starving Mrs. S to death, claiming that they would be required to lie to Mrs. S's sons. The nurse manager and physician note that Mrs. S's sons are unlikely to suspect that her nutrition is inadequate; and, in any case, Mrs. S's wishes should count for something, however understandable the sons' uneasiness.

Should the physician comply with the daughters' wishes?

Introduction

Three issues are important to a moral analysis of this case:

1. What criterion(a) should determine decisional authority?
2. What moral obligations do health care professionals (HCPs) have to patients' children?
3. What role does the distinction between "killing" (directly and immediately causing death) and "letting die" (failing to intervene to prevent death) play in defining professional integrity?

The AJ Method

Step 1: Information Gathering   What is Mrs. S's true condition? (Brakman; Ott) What are the actual treatment goals regarding Mrs. S? (Ott) What motivated Mrs. S's rejection of medical nutrition and hydration (MN&H)? Was her rejection autonomous? (Brakman; Ott) What were her actual preferences? Who has *legal* decisional authority about Mrs. S's care? What does fidelity to one's parents require? (Brakman) What motivates Mrs. S's children? (Brakman) What would be the effects on Mrs. S's HCPs if they participate in the suggested deception? What would be the effects on Mrs. S's children, considered as a family unit, if the deception were undertaken and discovered by her sons? (Brakman; Ott)

Readers can agree on a number of points. First, Mrs. S. repeatedly expressed a desire *not* to be tube fed and—evidently—not to be "kept alive" if she was ever in a situation similar to her neighbor's.

Second, if she is in a persistent vegetative state (PVS)—a diagnosis not yet unequivocally established—she has forever lost neocortical brain function and will never again experience pleasure, pain, suffering, or conscious thought.

Third, medical decision making for Mrs. S would be easier for HCPs—though probably no less contentious for her children—if she had completed an advance directive (AD). However even without such a document, the medical establishment and most citizens generally agree that withdrawing life-sustaining treatments from patients who are unlikely to regain consciousness or resume lives that they would value (particularly with evidence that the patient would not value the life predicted for her) is morally permissible. However, in March 2004, Pope John Paul II announced that artificial nutrition and hydration must be understood as basic care, rather than as optional medical treatment and, as such, are morally mandatory.[1] Whether and to what extent popular attitudes will change as a result of this pronouncement is as yet unknown.

However, two relevant facts are missing, complicating the decisional process: (1) No one knows *why* Mrs. S rejected the possibility of tube feeding or whether her rejection of tube feeding was based on an accurate understanding of its burdens and benefits. Without knowing whether her decision was autonomous or merely an expression of an unconsidered preference, HCPs cannot confidently determine her treatment goals. (2) If she could *now* choose, would her opposition to tube feeding be stronger, weaker, or unchanged—especially if she knew her family's reaction to her wishes?

Step 2: Creative Problem Solving   A creative solution would have to simultaneously respect the choices of Mrs. S, her daughters, and her sons (or get all of them to agree).

Step 3: Pros and Cons   Survey CARVE principles to identify important moral reasons that support conflicting options for resolving this case.

Consequences   What would be the effects on Mrs. S if her HCPs participate in the suggested deception? (Brakman; deLeon and Hodgkin) on the HCPs? on Mrs. S's children, considered as a family unit, if the deception were undertaken and discovered by her sons? (Brakman; Ott) Would these effects be positive or negative? How likely would they be to occur? Are long-term effects (including to future patients) possible? likely? (Brakman)

Autonomy   Recall that autonomy, most broadly understood, applies to choosing the values in terms of which to live one's life, as well as the means to achieve those values. Whose autonomy should be considered? (Brakman; deLeon and Hodgkin; Ott)

Since Mrs. S cannot speak, a host of moral questions arise: First, *who* should speak for her? When patients are unable to exercise their right to decisional authority and no surrogate has been *formally* named, decisional authority passes to someone who knows the patient's values and preferences; typically, though not always, this is the family. This approach is morally justified by the assumption that persons who know the patient best can best represent—and choose in concert with—her values and desires. But Mrs. S's daughters and sons represent these values and construe these desires differently.

Second, what standard should guide the surrogate? Three standards of surrogate decision making are possible:[2]

1. *Substituted judgment:* The patient has made no *unambiguous* statement about the option under consideration, but the surrogate knows the patient's values and postulates what the patient would choose (were she able) based on those values.
2. *Pure autonomy:* A surrogate knows and accurately reports the patient's considered and explicitly expressed decision about a particular option.
3. *Best interests:* The surrogate compares the burdens and benefits of each treatment option, then chooses the option with the best ratio—based on a dispassionate calculation—of benefits to burdens.

Tradition and convention suggest that Mrs. S's caring, conscientious children should act as her surrogate, but they cannot achieve consensus. Based on Mrs. S's explicit rejection of tube feeding, her daughters appear to embrace an autonomy standard. However, because her motivation and actual treatment goals are unknown, complying with her choice may not promote her best interests—the standard to which her sons appear committed.[3]

Rights   Which option(s) protect Mrs. S's right to self-determination? (deLeon and Hodgkin; Ott) to not be harmed? to be aided? (deLeon and Hodgkin) of privacy? of confidentiality? Do Mrs. S's children have rights of which the HCPs must take moral account? (Brakman)

Virtues   What does professional fidelity require regarding cessation of MN&H? (Brakman; deLeon and Hodgkin; Ott) Are compassion, honesty, (Brakman; deLeon and Hodgkin; Ott) or courage (Brakman) relevant? What does fidelity to family require? (Brakman; Ott)

To whom do the HCPs have a greater moral duty: Mrs. S or her children? Although HCPs explicitly promise to promote *the patient's* welfare, they might wonder whether—in her present state—promoting Mrs. S's welfare is possible in any meaningful sense. Granting the moral obligations to avoid harm, remove or reduce burdens, and provide the best chance of recovery and a meaningful life, one might still wonder how, exactly, to do these things for a patient who is unlikely to regain consciousness, experience pain or pleasure, or participate in meaningful relationships with others. HCPs undoubtedly have some moral obligations to Mrs. S, but what, exactly, are they?

Beyond their commitment to Mrs. S's welfare, do HCPs have moral obligations to her family? In the first place, the physician must decide whether lying to her sons is morally justifiable (see "Must Health Care Professionals Always Tell the Truth?" in this volume). But the more basic moral concern is to what extent alleviating the family's suffering is the responsibility of the HCPs. Mrs. S's children are not patients, yet the pain of this family is both real and immediate. Further, their pain appears to be partially driving their decisions. If their pain can be ameliorated by lying, ought HCPs lie?

Independent of particular obligations to Mrs. S, MN&H raises three thorny moral issues: (1) Does failure to provide MN&H constitute killing a person, or "merely" letting the patient die? (2) Is letting a patient die of "natural causes" *morally* different from killing? and (3) In either case, ought HCPs be instrumental in a patient's death?

Killing and letting die are sometimes distinguished by the *intent* of the agent.[4] For example, a physician can administer very high doses of narcotics to a terminally ill patient to relieve pain, even if doing so may hasten the patient's death. The physician *intends* pain relief, and merely *foresees* the possibility of the patient's earlier death. This distinction has become a mainstay in considering treatment options for patients with grim prognoses.[5] In this case, the physician could intend to honor Mrs. S's request, while merely foreseeing her death.

Nonetheless both the logical possibility and the moral propriety of the killing/letting die distinction have been challenged. How, critics ask, can one *remove* a feeding tube, knowing the patient will die, and claim not to be intending the death?[6] Further, if the patient is better off dead, and if HCPs should be committed to doing what is best for their patients, why not kill her rather than letting her die, a process that may be painful, undignified, or both?[7] Others believe that even if someone's death would be beneficial, causing (whether by omission or commission) that death is morally wrong.[8]

Cessation of MN&H raises another moral conundrum: Is the symbolic importance of food and fluid morally relevant?[9] Even if one supports withholding some medical interventions (e.g., CPR), "starving a person to death" has a heinous connotation.[10] Food and water are the most basic human needs, and denying them to the helpless seems particularly callous.

These questions must be asked in the context of professional integrity.[11] Even if death is preferable, can killing or allowing the death of *a patient* ever fall within appropriate moral behavior for HCPs? In other words, even if *some* persons might be allowed to kill persons or let them die, does participating in death violate some important professional commitment? Is causing or allowing death a failure of compassion, courage, fidelity?[12] Thus, even if Mrs. S would herself neither benefit from MN&H nor be harmed by its withdrawal, might society in general and HCPs and families in particular be horribly harmed by anyone's—but especially HCPs'—failing to meet these most primary needs?

Equality/Fairness (Justice)   Is continued care of Mrs. S an unfair use of resources?

The Law   The following legal considerations are relevant to this case: (1) Who, legally, has decisional authority for Mrs. S? (2) How must Mrs. S's expressed wishes (both verbal and written) be legally accounted for in the treatment decisions made by her family and her physician? (3) Under what conditions may HCPs legally override decisional authority of a (presumably) competent patient or her surrogate(s)? (4) Are HCPs legally obligated to avoid deceiving (presumably) competent patients or legal surrogates? (5) If Mrs. S is not adequately nourished, could the hospital or its HCPs be held legally liable for her medical deterioration or her death (due to negligence or intentional homicide)?[13]

The following commentaries examine the application of various moral principles to this dilemma, thereby assisting the reader to undertake *Step 4: Analysis* and *Step 5: Justification.*

Notes

1. Cathy L. Grossman, "Pope declares feeding tubes a 'moral obligation,'" *USA Today*, 2 Apr. 2004, 1A.
2. Tom L. Beauchamp and James F. Childress, *Principles of Biomedical Ethics*, 5th ed. (New York: Oxford University Press, 2001), 98–103.
3. K. A. Bramstedt, "Ethics in Medicine: Questioning the Decision-making Capacity of Surrogates," *Internal Medicine Journal* 33, no. 5–6 (2003): 257–59.
4. President's Commission for the Study of Ethical Problems in Medicine and Biomedical and Behavioral Research, *Deciding to Forego Life-Sustaining Treatment: Ethical, Medical, and Legal Issues in Treatment Decisions* (Washington, DC: U.S. Government Printing Office 1983), 60–73; James Rachels, *The End of Life: Euthanasia and Morality* (Oxford: Oxford University Press, 1986), especially chap. 7.
5. See President's Commission, note 4, above, 77–89.
6. Paul Ramsey, "Should Physicians Hasten the Death Angel When She Pauses in her Flight?" in *Covenants of Life: Contemporary Medical Ethics in Light of the Thought of Paul Ramsey,* eds. Kenneth L. Vaux, Sara Vaux, and Mark Stenberg (Dordrecht, The Netherlands: Kluwer Academic Publishers, 2002), 237–46.
7. Ibid.; Margaret Pabst Battin, "The Least Worst Death," *Hastings Center Report* 13, no. 2 (1983): 13–16; and Peter Singer, *Rethinking Life and Death: The Collapse of our Traditional Ethics* (New York: St. Martin's Press, 1994), 75–80.
8. Leon Kass, "Death With Dignity and the Sanctity of Life," in *Last Rights: Assisted Suicide and Euthanasia Debated,* ed. Michael Uhlman (Washington, DC: Ethics and Public Policy

Center and Grand Rapids, MI: Eerdmans, 1998), 199–222; and Gilbert Meilander, "Euthanasia and Christian Vision," in *Last Rights: Assisted Suicide and Euthanasia Debated*, ed. Michael Uhlman (Washington, DC: Ethics and Public Policy Center and Grand Rapids, MI: Eerdmans, 1998), 237–48.

9. Joanne Lynn and James F. Childress, "Must Patients Always be Given Food and Water?" *Hastings Center Report* 13, no. 5 (1983): 17–21.

10. Daniel Callahan, "On Feeding the Dying," *Hastings Center Report* 13, no. 5 (1983): 22; and Daniel Callahan, "Feeding the Dying Elderly," *Generations* 10, no. 2 (1985): 15–17.

11. Loretta M. Kopelman and Kenneth A. De Ville, eds., *Physician-assisted Suicide: What Are the Issues?* (Dordrecht, The Netherlands: Kluwer Academic Press, 2001).

12. Franklin G. Miller and Howard Brody, "Professional Integrity and Physician-Assisted Death," *Hastings Center Report* 25, no. 3 (1995): 8–17; and Lynn and Childress, see note 8, above.

13. For a general overview of legal considerations, see George P. Smith, II, *Legal and Healthcare Ethics for the Elderly* (Washington, DC: Taylor and Francis, 1996), 107–20. Theoretical and some legal issues related to decisional authority are discussed in Jessica Berg, Paul S. Appelbaum, Charles W. Lidz, and Lisa S. Parker, *Informed Consent: Legal Theory and Clinical Practice*, 2nd ed. (New York: Oxford University Press, 2001), esp. part II: "The Legal Theory of Informed Consent," 41–164; "The Role of Informed Consent in Medical Decision-making," 167–87; and "Consent Forms: Documentation and Guidance," 188–207. Basic medical guidelines and recent judicial rulings in related cases are summarized in American Medical Association, Council on Ethical and Judicial Affairs, *Code of Medical Ethics: Current Opinions with Annotations*, 2000–2001 ed. (Chicago: American Medical Association, 2000), § 2.17, "Quality of Life," 50–52; § 2.035, "Futile Care," 10–11; § 2.037, "Medical Futility in End-of-Life Care," 11–12; and § 2.20, "Withholding or Withdrawing Life-sustaining Medical Treatment," 55–71. See also Robert A. Burt, *Death is That Man Taking Names* (Berkeley: The University of California Press and New York: The Milbank Memorial Fund, 2002), esp. chap. 6, "Choosing Death," 106–22, for a provocative discussion of conflicts among legal precedent, constitutional law, and cultural attitudes. To follow the evolving law relevant to skilled nursing facilities, see the monthly journal: *The Bulletin on Long-term Care Law*.

An Ethicist's Analysis

Sarah-Vaughan Brakman, PhD

At first blush, Mrs. S's daughters present a creative solution to this case. Mrs. S's wishes will be respected; she will feel no pain; the sons, unlikely to know about the plan, will not be upset; and sibling relationships will be preserved.

Regardless, the physician should not comply with the daughters' wishes for four reasons: (1) Two ambiguous facts cast doubt on the moral permissibility of discontinuing adequate nutrition; (2) The request violates trust between siblings; (3) Since all the children are moral as well as legal stakeholders in the decision-making process, this request unjustly violates the duties the physician has to the sons; (4) Most importantly, the long-term negative consequences for both the family and the practice of medicine from this act of deception are more compelling than the positive consequences the daughters envision. We will consider each of these concerns and propose an alternative.

One caveat: the *Cruzan* ruling upheld a state's right to set its own requirement for a "clear and convincing evidence standard in proceedings where a guardian seeks to discontinue nutrition and hydration of a person diagnosed to be in a persistent vegetative state."[1] In some states only written evidence meets this standard; others allow oral statements.

(1) Two facts are underdetermined here. First, the daughters could be mistaken about their mother's wishes and/or the strength of her preference. It is difficult to say from this slight case description that her statements constitute "clear and convincing evidence." *Unappealing* and *repugnant* might be solely an aesthetic judgment rather than a true moral preference.

Second, the nature of Mrs. S's condition is not clear. Persistent vegetative state (PVS) is "a vegetative state present one month after acute traumatic or nontraumatic brain injury or lasting for at least one month in patients with degenerative or metabolic disorders or developmental malformations."[2] Thus, the diagnosis of PVS is not definite.

(2) If these facts were addressed, three considerations might justify acceding to the daughters' request:

a. *The sons have not acted properly as surrogates.* The proper standards of surrogate decision makers are substituted judgment or best interests. The brothers may be disregarding both standards and deciding on their own values. If so, it might be morally acceptable to exclude them from this process, though that argument needs development. However, the sons might be invoking the best interest standard when claiming they will not starve their mother.

b. *It appears the brothers are not fulfilling their filial duties to their mother.* They may be violating respect and honor for their mother by making a decision based on their own interests. Filial relationships might even account for the striking gender difference present in the case: while both sons and daughters visited their mother, studies indicate that daughters tend to assist elderly parents with more intimate physical care, while sons tend to assist with household chores and less intimate types of care.[3] Intimate caregiving might lend itself to more intimate personal sharing—thus accounting for why Mrs. S disclosed her views to her daughters but not her sons.

However, the sons might claim refusing to allow "death by starvation" *is* fulfilling reverence and honor to their mother. It is worth inquiring about family members' religious backgrounds, as religious beliefs influence perceptions of filial obligations. For example, although PVS is not discussed specifically, the "dominant view in conservative Judaism is the obligation to continue treatment once it has been started."[4] Roman Catholicism holds that "There should be a presumption in favor of providing nutrition and hydration to all patients, including patients who require medically assisted nutrition and hydration, as long as this is of sufficient benefit to outweigh the burdens involved to the patient."[5]* This could, then, be a conflict between (a) the duties the sons believe they have to act on substituted judgment and (b) a perceived greater duty not to participate in causing their mother's death.

   c.   *The daughters claim open disagreement would fracture the family.* Even if the sons are acting wrongly, are the daughters justified in lying to them? It seems odd to define as "close" a family engaged in betrayal. If the daughters feel so strongly about their mother's wishes, they should be willing to put that concern before their brothers.

(3) Asking the physician to deceive the sons is asking the physician to violate her obligations to them by implicitly lying. The sons believe their mother is receiving adequate nutrition because they participated in making that decision and they see that their mother has a feeding tube when they visit. Since there is no formal advance directive, the team has a responsibility to the sons who have a right to be part of the decision-making process. This would not be a problem if violating obligations to truthfulness was the best way for the physician to fulfill her obligation to Mrs. S. However, if the team was "reluctant to proceed in the presence of deeply felt disagreement, especially in the absence of a designated surrogate decision maker," what makes this situation morally different? Again, we return to the fact that all of the children are, jointly, the surrogate decision makers.

(4) Providing inadequate nutrition is reminiscent of running "slow codes." The practice of responding slowly and incompletely to a code, thus providing the fiction of resuscitation, is roundly condemned. The daughters' request is morally similar—in effect, a "slow feed." These practices are cowardly because they are deceptions designed to achieve ends and avoid confrontation. The real damage, though, is that this would weaken trust in the profession.

Making and granting this request assumes the lie is necessary both to respect Mrs. S's wishes and to save the family unit. These assumptions are just not proven. Can any solution achieve the desired ends without significant violations of rights and obligations? The physician could propose an alternative: Mrs. S's situation will be reviewed at one month. If her neurological status is unchanged, she will be diagnosed with PVS and the decision to discontinue artificial nutrition will be revisited. Her children ought to be educated about what feeding can and cannot accomplish

---

*Editor's note: See endnote 1, "Introduction" to this case, p. 332, regarding Pope John Paul II's 2004 pronouncement on this topic.

and about the actual experience of patients for whom it is discontinued. The sons need to be made aware that (1) discontinuing artificial nutrition for a patient with no expectation of recovery may be a decision about the futility of treatment and not a decision to "starve to death"; and (2) that surrogate decisions must be based on one of the two standards discussed above. If applicable, a religious counselor ought to be involved to help the family. The team may be able to provide guidance to make the decision from a best interest standard. The brothers may come to see that they are not violating duties to their mother if they decide to discontinue artificial nutrition. They also may feel like they now have given their mother's recovery every chance. If the sons maintain their insistence on artificial nutrition and the daughters maintain their insistence against, then the physician could indicate that the team is willing to seek a court-appointed decision maker and/or a ruling on whether Mrs. S's statements meet the clear and convincing standard of *Cruzan*. At the very least, the "slow feed" is morally wrong.

RECOMMENDED READINGS

Council on Scientific Affairs and Council on Ethical and Judicial Affairs. "Persistent Vegetative State and the Decision to Withdraw or Withhold Life Support." *JAMA: Journal of the American Medical Association* 263 (1990): 426–30.

The Hastings Center. *Guidelines on the Termination of Life-sustaining Treatment and the Care of the Dying* (Briarcliff Manor, NY: Hastings Center, 1987).

Notes

1. Cruzan v. Missouri Department of Health, 497 U.S. 261, 25 June 1990, n.d., http://www.law.umkc.edu/faculty/projects/ftrials/conlaw/cruzan.html (16 Aug. 2003).
2. The Multi-Society Task Force on PVS, "Medical Aspects of the Persistent Vegetative State," *New England Journal of Medicine* 330 (1994): 1499–1506.
3. Elaine M. Brody, "Filial Care of the Elderly and Changing Roles of Women (and Men)," *Journal of Geriatric Psychiatry* 19, no. 2 (1986): 177–78; Older Women's League, "Failing American's Caregivers: A Status Report on Women Who Care," May 1989, www.owl-national.org (1 Apr. 2004).
4. American Dietetic Association, "Ethical and Legal Issues in Nutrition, Hydration, and Feeding," *Journal of American Dietetic Association* 102 (2002): 716–26.
5. United States Conference of Catholic Bishops, *Ethical and Religious Directives for Catholic Healthcare Services*, 4th ed. (Washington, DC: United States Catholic Conference, 2001), directive #58.

A Nurse's Analysis

Barbara B. Ott, PhD, RN

This dilemma cannot be resolved until the goals of care and treatment are established.[1] The current diagnostic uncertainty supports an initial goal of curing Mrs. S. Thus aggressive treatments—placing the feeding tube and monitoring Mrs. S for a change in her neurological condition—are appropriate. At the same time, her children feel the stress of their mother's uncertain future. Support and education about the probable trajectory of this injury is important for the family.

The physicians believe that Mrs. S will not awaken from this comatose state. If persistent vegetative state (PVS) is diagnosed, the goals of care would change. A diagnosis of PVS indicates neurological devastation, and cure or recovery from her injuries are impossible. However, Mrs. S could live for many years in a comatose state.

Is the goal to prolong Mrs. S's life for as long as possible? That depends on what Mrs. S wanted. Did she say she wanted all measures used to keep her alive as long as possible, despite her quality of life? No evidence suggests this. In fact, Mrs. S stated to her daughters that, unlike her neighbor, she would never want to be kept alive in a coma.

So for Mrs. S the goals of care after the diagnosis of PVS are to prevent harm and respect her human dignity. Harm from pain and discomfort are not of concern, since one characteristic of PVS is the lack of the ability to feel pain or discomfort. Respecting human dignity requires many things including cleanliness, safety, kind and compassionate care, truthfulness, and trustworthiness. Trust is a vital part of human and professional relationships. Trust allows us to rely on one another even when we are vulnerable.[2]

Understanding the goals of care still does not tell the nurse what to do about the feeding tube. At first blush, the health care professionals (HCPs) may wish to discontinue the tube feeding immediately. The Code of Ethics for Nurses reminds us that in order to respect human dignity, we must recognize the importance of patient self-determination.[3] The daughters relayed their mother's feeling that tube feeding was particularly unappealing, so the HCPs may want to honor the patient's autonomy by discontinuing it. This action could be ethically acceptable, but would cause great disagreement among family members—disagreement the daughters probably wanted to avoid by asking the physicians to decrease the nourishment and not tell the brothers.

Should the HCPs comply with the daughters' deceitful request? Truth-telling and integrity are important aspects of health care delivery. The nurse's integrity is threatened if he or she lies, deceives, or withholds important information from patients or families. Truthful communication is an essential part of professional nursing practice. Patients are susceptible to both help and harm. Through professional nursing practice help can come with truthful communication and harm can come from untruths. Only the nurse with integrity can be trusted by vulnerable patients. The nurse recognizes the patient's vulnerability and values her autonomy; he or she also values his or her own professional autonomy and judgments. The daughters' request is deceitful and a clear threat to the integrity of the HCPs. The request should not be honored.

So what should be done now? The gastrostomy tube is already inserted and feedings are proceeding. The daughters and sons are in stark disagreement about what is best for their mother now. People need help making life and death decisions. Although many HCPs see these decisions every day, they are strange and unusual for most people—and emotionally traumatic when a loved one is involved.

To complicate matters, both the daughters and the sons are suffering from grief. Grief can cause general problems with decision making, and treatment decisions that affect the dying process or lead to the death of the loved one can be devastating. Therefore, enabling the family to begin to process the grief may ultimately help with decision making. Professionals who specialize in counseling—palliative care professionals, chaplains, psychiatric liaison nurses, social workers, and psychologists—can help tremendously. Embracing the palliative care model would help the family adjust. On this model, professionals would focus on caring for (rather than attempting to cure) Mrs. S and providing care that she would want for herself now. Acknowledging the family's distress and grief and meeting them "where they are" will support and reassure them.

These siblings are close and care about their mother. Preserving their supportive relationship is important and probably something their mother would want very much. A counselor could help the children reevaluate their mother's situation frequently over the next days and weeks. The sons and daughters should visit their mother several times a week and stay for several hours to see how she is doing overall and how she is responding to the tube feedings.

Human life has great intrinsic value. Intending the death of Mrs. S is not ethically acceptable. But removing an impediment to an inevitable natural death is acceptable when that impediment is an ineffective or burdensome treatment.[4]

The proper criterion for whether to withdraw treatments is a comparative analysis of burdens and benefits of treatment in terms of the goals of care. Benefits include meeting the goals of therapy. Tube feeding would effectively prolong her life, but because Mrs. S previously stated she would never want to live in a coma being fed by a tube, she would not endorse the goal of saving her life. Thus, she would not find tube feeding beneficial. Instead, the tube feeding is the source of many burdens: prolonging a life she found unattractive; interfering with a natural death; probable aspiration pneumonia; and monetary and emotional costs to her family.[5] In this case, the burdens of life-supporting fluid and hydration outweigh the benefits.

When the burdens of any treatment outweigh its benefits, the treatment can be withdrawn. As the family visits Mrs. S several times a week, they may come to see that the burdens of tube feeding outweigh the benefits. The family should also be reminded that Mrs. S's right to accept or reject medical treatments does not end with her incapacity. Her right to decide is exercised through surrogate decision makers—here, the daughters—who are privileged to know her wishes.

Ideally, the family will come to a unanimous decision. The brothers' grief may make it difficult for them to discontinue their mother's life-sustaining treatments. But if professionals share the burden of the decision with the family, the family may begin to work through their grief and decide to discontinue the feeding tube out of respect for their mother's wishes.[6]

If disagreement continues, HCPs should seek help from an ethics committee or other professionals such as lawyers, hospice workers, grief counselors, chaplains, community services, or others skilled in conflict resolution.

Notes

1. Albert Jonsen, Mark Seigler, and William Winslade, *Clinical Ethics* (New York: McGraw-Hill, 1992).
2. Annette Baier, "Trust and Anti-trust," *Ethics* 96, no. 2 (1986): 231–60.
3. American Nurses Association, *Code of Ethics for Nurses with Interpretive Statements,* (Washington, DC: ANA, 2001), § 1.4.
4. Edmund Pellegrino, "Decisions to Withdraw Life-sustaining Treatment," *JAMA: Journal of the American Medical Association* 283, no. 8 (2000): 1065–67.
5. Thomas E. Finucane, Colleen Christmas, and Kathy Travis, "Tube Feeding in Patients with Advanced Dementia," *JAMA: Journal of the American Medical Association* 282, no. 14 (1999): 1365–69.
6. Thomas J. Prendergast and Kathleen A. Puntillo,"Withdrawal of Life Support: Intensive Caring at the End of Life," *JAMA: Journal of the American Medical Association* 288, no. 21 (2002): 2732–40.

A Dietitian's Analysis

Milenne L. deLeon, MPH, RD,
and Georgia E. Hodgkin, EdD, RD, FADA

The case of Mrs. S is truly tragic. Not only is this relatively young woman of 62 dealing with a terminal illness (Parkinson's Disease), but her life has been complicated by the recent fall, leading to a probably irreversible coma. Now at this moment of crisis, her children are having great difficulty making medical decisions on her behalf.

In this particular scenario we cannot ignore the fact that the patient expressly stated to her daughters, individually and separately, that she would never want to live in a comatose state. She witnessed the final months of suffering in her neighbor's life and based her decision on her perceptions of the discomfort endured by her neighbor. After observing her neighbor, she chose death over life in a coma. In addition, Mrs. S specifically mentioned tube feeding as a particularly unappealing medical treatment.

Although preserving and prolonging life (beneficence) is one goal of medical care and of dietetics, not all patients perceive prolonging life as beneficent.[1] Thus a second principle, autonomy (being in charge of one's own health care), forces us also to consider the patient's right to refuse treatment, regardless of how family or clinicians personally may feel about the patient's decision.[2] According to the Code of Ethics of the American Dietetic Association (ADA), "The dietetics practitioner provides sufficient information to enable clients and others to make their own informed decisions." The Code also calls for honesty (Principle 1), professional judgment (Principle 3), and providing "professional services with objectivity and with respect for the unique needs and values of individuals" (Principle 8).[3]

Once the medical considerations of treatment have been addressed, two questions surface: *can* the treatment be implemented, and *should* the treatment be implemented? Once we have established what can be done medically for the patient, we must consider the patient's wishes. In this case the patient did state a clear preference (against the use of a feeding tube). Subsequently, we follow the concept of *substituted judgment*: doing precisely what the patient wanted.° Following a patient's wishes is morally justified if we know them with certainty, even if that involves stopping a treatment that is already in place.[4] Individuals do have the right of self-determination, which may be expressed through another person. Patients have a more reliable opinion of their acceptable quality of life than caregivers, offspring, or any suitable proxy.[5] Thus, treatment plans need to be aligned with the wishes of the patient.

Unlike Mrs. S, many patients have no record of clearly stated opinions about gastrostomy tubes or life support prior to a severe illness. In such cases, the medical team must apply the concept of *best interests*: choosing the level of treatment that most people in similar medical circumstances would want to have. This, of course, is often a difficult and highly subjective task, since all of us prioritize values somewhat differently. At the same time many, though not all, would agree that a person in a persistently vegetative or permanently comatose condition, as Mrs. S is likely to be, would probably not see her best interests served by long-term life prolongation through medical nutrition therapy.

Dietitians play an interesting role in these cases. As part of the multidisciplinary health care team we are often placed in a delicate position of negotiation between patient and family and/or patient and the health care team. In this case the nurses and dietitian are understandably uncomfortable about lying to the patient's sons about their sisters' proposed plan of administering minimal nutrition in order to hasten their mother's death.

We are morally obligated to respect Mrs. S's wishes and discontinue her medical nutrition therapy as mandated by the principle of self-determination. This principle is appropriately applied in this situation, since the patient had previously verbalized a choice. However, upholding the moral principle of substituted judgment in a backhanded way by lying to some of her children is inappropriate. The ADA Code of Ethics places great importance not only on the idea of patient autonomy, but also on *fidelity*. However, the need to uphold one principle of moral conduct should not negate or diminish our responsibility to act in an *honest* manner with *integrity*. As stated in the first principle of the ADA Code of Ethics:

°Editor's note: Historically the "substituted judgment" standard was synonymous with the "pure autonomy" standard, as defined in the introduction to this case.

"The dietetics practitioner conducts himself/herself with honesty, integrity, and fairness."[6] Therefore, the medical team's duty, with assistance from the dietitian, is to help the sons understand that their mother's prior statements have great moral weight, and that following proper protocol for withdrawing medical nutrition and hydration is painless. Physiologically, even in conscious persons, feelings of hunger diminish and loss of appetite results from a state of ketosis that follows food restriction.[7]

In summary, Mrs. S presents the health care team with indisputable challenges. We must treat the patient with compassion and professionalism, and we must address the fears and the emotional needs of her sons and her daughters. In addition to these duties, our ethical code mandates first that we honor the patient's autonomy and decision-making privilege as expressed by her clear prior statement to her family. Our second duty as dietitians and members of the health care team is to be instrumental in helping the physician explain the palliative treatment plan (including the details of nutritional withdrawal), so Mrs. S's children may understand that quality of care will not be compromised in these tough final days.

Notes

1. M. Rosita Schiller, Julie O. Maillet, and Judith A. Gilbride, *Handbook for Clinical Nutrition Services Management* (Gaithersburg, MD: Aspen Publishers, 1991).
2. Ibid.
3. American Dietetic Association, "Code of Ethics for the Profession of Dietetics" [adopted 18 Oct. 1998], *Journal of the American Dietetic Association* 99, no. 1 (1999): 109–13, Principles 3 and 6, http://www.eatright.org/Public/index_8915.cfm (11 Aug. 2003).
4. Albert R. Jonsen, Mark Siegler, and William J. Winslade, *Clinical Ethics: A Practical Approach to Decisions in Clinical Medicine*, 5th ed. (New York: McGraw-Hill, 2002).
5. J. A. Myers et al., "Duration of the Condition Is Unrelated to the Health-state Valuation on the EuroQoL," *Clinical Rehabilitation* 17, no. 2 (2003): 209–15.
6. See note 3, above.
7. Eleanor N. Whitney, Corinne B. Cataldo, and Sharon R. Rolfes, *Understanding Normal and Clinical Nutrition*, 6th ed. (Belmont, CA: Wadsworth Thomson Learning, 2002).

Further Reflections

General

1. Both Brakman and Ott suggest that whether Mrs. S is simply in a coma or suffering from PVS is an important factual consideration. What is the moral relevance of Mrs. S's physical state?
2. What moral principles might serve to justify treatment? nontreatment?
3. When a surrogate speaks for a patient, to whom do HCPs have primary responsibility—the patient or the surrogate?

4. What *process* would you recommend to resolve this dilemma?

Consequences

5. Identify and comparatively evaluate the burdens and benefits that will be experienced by Mrs. S, the daughters, the sons, the physician, other HCPs, the hospital, and society if the physician accedes to the wishes of the daughters *and* if the physician decides not to go along with their wishes and instead continues to feed Mrs. S indefinitely.

Autonomy

6. An autonomous choice is made by a competent person who is informed and understands her therapeutic options, and who is not coerced to choose a particular course of action. Was Mrs. S's choice autonomous, as deLeon and Hodgkin claim? If you think it was not, is there moral justification for respecting it anyway?
7. Was the daughters' decision autonomous? Was the sons'?

Rights

8. Brakman claims the sons have a right to participate in decisions about their mother's care. Do the sons have such a right? Why (not)?

Virtues

9. Is starving Mrs. S "cowardly" as Brakman claims? Why (not)?
10. Ott believes that lying could undermine the integrity of the nursing profession. Why might this happen? How likely is it?
11. Why is lying to the brothers so problematic? Discuss this issue in terms of role-related responsibilities of HCPs *and* family members. What *virtues*, if any, morally support lying to the brothers?

Equality/Fairness (Justice)

12. Would continuing to feed Mrs. S be unfair? If so, to whom?

Chapter 19

Is My Obligation to My Client or My Neighbors?

Ms. T is the owner of and the pharmacist at a small independent pharmacy in a rural town in the Midwest. Her pharmacy is the only one in the area and serves several small communities with a population of about 30,000. The nearest significant competition for her business is about 40 minutes away.

Recently Mr. L, a 55-year-old male, came to her pharmacy with a prescription for Viagra (sildenafil) written by a new physician in town. Normally the dispensing of Viagra is not a problem for Ms. T: the pharmacy stocks a ready supply of the drug; patients have in general complied with the instructions for use; and no significant adverse side effects have occured among individuals in this community. However, Ms. T recognized Mr. L as an individual who had been convicted some years ago of two counts of sexual assault of a minor, and incarcerated.

Mr. L's request for Viagra has made Ms. T suspicious and worried. She knows nothing about his present circumstances, but she has many questions. For example, how long has Mr. L been out of prison? Is he married or living alone? Is he still a sex offender or has treatment solved this problem? Is he currently in a parole-type arrangement? If he is under parole supervision, is he under the care of a physician as part of that program, and are there stipulations and restrictions on his movement or what he can purchase, including Viagra?

Ms. T is fearful of having Mr. L back in the community; she worries (as, presumably, would most parents) about the safety of her own

9-year-old daughter. She contemplates calling the police and checking on some of these questions, but wonders whether such an action would violate any professional obligations to Mr. L or his civil rights. Furthermore, she realizes that even if she had access to this information, her concerns would not be assuaged. She would still worry that a known sex offender taking Viagra might lead to intolerable damage to the individuals—especially young girls—in her community. She considers not filling the prescription, but wonders what justification she could give to the patient and to herself.

What should Ms. T do?

Introduction

This case raises three important moral issues:

1. What are the fundamental moral obligations of pharmacists when the interests of patients conflict with the interests of the community, the profession, or one's personal moral commitments?
2. What is the appropriate relationship between pharmacists as health care professionals (HCPs) and local law enforcement agencies?
3. Would a decision not to fill the prescription be unjust treatment of Mr. L; specifically, could it count as further punishment for a crime for which he has already paid (with jail time)?

The AJ Method

Step 1: Information Gathering   What facts are necessary for resolving this case? Has Mr. L been treated successfully? Is he likely—and, if so, how likely—to reoffend? Why does Mr. L want to take Viagra? If he takes the drug, who (if anyone) is likely to be harmed? What would be the nature of the harms? What are the conditions of Mr. L's parole?

Over 100,000 cases of sexual abuse of children were documented in the United States in 2000.[1] Sex abuse of children is a matter of tremendous concern to Americans.[2] Witness the strident demands for nationalizing the Amber Alert response to kidnaping, at least in part as a means to preventing sexual abuse of children who are abducted. Witness, too, the horror with which most citizens have followed the media reports regarding abuse of children by Catholic priests. This heightened public awareness, concern, and vigilance may sometimes lead to the moral dilemma described in this case.

Sexual abusers of children are often considered to be mentally ill.[3] This form of psychopathology has posed an especially knotty therapeutic challenge. The causes of sexual abuse are incompletely understood; until causal mechanisms are better understood, constructing reliable therapy is difficult. Knowing this, Ms. T must wonder if Mr. L has received effective treatment or if he is still a risk to society.

The moral obligations that govern the practice of pharmacy are similar to those prescribed for other HCPs. These include obligations to avoid harm to and advance the well-being and interests of patients; to respect patient confidentiality, freedom, and self-determination; and to dispense goods and services justly.[4] In a pharmacist's context, these obligations refer to dispensing medications and information.[5] For a patient to autonomously choose to (not) take a drug, he or she needs to know the drug's intended actions and its potential benefits, burdens, and risks—including specifically its side effects. The pharmacist is professionally obliged to ensure that these facts are in the patient's hands.

Step 2: Creative Problem Solving   Any creative solution would have to provide Viagra to Mr. L without risking harm to others.

Step 3: Pros and Cons   Survey CARVE principles to identify important moral reasons that support conflicting options for resolving this case.

Consequences   Who would be harmed if Mr. L receives the Viagra? What would be the nature of those harms? (Buerki and Vottero) Who would benefit if Mr. L receives the Viagra? What would be the nature of those benefits? Who would be harmed (or benefited) if Ms. T contacts the police?

To determine how to maximize benefit and minimize harm, the pharmacist needs to know whether the drug is appropriate to the patient's condition. To adequately assess the prospective burdens and benefits, the pharmacist needs to know something of the patient's health history—at the least, his general health status, why the doctor prescribed the drug, and what other drugs the patient is taking. Without this information, the pharmacist is unable to advise the patient appropriately. Further, she would be helped by knowing whether Mr. L is a pedophile or a child sexual abuser, as the motivations and treatments for these two conditions differ.[6] Note, however, that the patient is under no obligation to divulge any information to the pharmacist—even if doing so is in his best interests. This observation is relevant because if Mr. L were a complete stranger to Ms. T, she would have no way of knowing his past history, nor any claim—or even concern—that he share it with her. Put differently, Ms. T would have no qualms about dispensing the drug, except that, as a member of a small community, she has "extra" information about Mr. L. If Ms. T confines her professional evaluation to Mr. L's prescription, she has no reason not to fill it.

Autonomy   Do Ms. T's professional practice standards allow her to ignore or overrule a patient's autonomous request for medication? (Buerki and Vottero)

Rights   Within the patient-professional relationship, Mr. L has a right to be aided and a right of self-determination. He also has a right to not be harmed. He also has rights of privacy and confidentiality that might limit Ms. T's consultation with or questioning of local law enforcement authorities. (Buerki and Vottero; Graybosch) Is the general right to not be harmed relevant here? (Graybosch)

Mr. L has a right of confidentiality that may be threatened if Ms. T consults with other persons likely to have relevant information about the risk Mr. L poses to the community.[7] She might enlist the aid of local law enforcement agencies. Mr. L is probably on parole and parole usually includes particular restrictions a parolee must meet. If the conditions of his parole restrict his activities and/or medications that he can—or is required—to take, Ms. T may be able to assess the risk he poses and further determine whether filling his prescription would have any effect on the risk. Or she might consult with the physician who wrote the prescription to ascertain if that doctor knows about Mr. L's past offenses, prosecution, incarceration, and parole status. If the physician was uninformed, he might, in the presence of new facts, revise his therapeutic approach, perhaps even revoke the prescription. In either case, however, her cooperation would violate Mr. L's right to medical confidentiality.

Virtues   Does Ms. T have an obligation of fidelity to her profession or of compassion to Mr. L to dispense the Viagra? (Buerki and Vottero; Graybosch) Would refusing to dispense the drug demonstrate courage?

Given that Ms. T possesses additional (albeit incomplete) information about Mr. L, she has a non-patient-centered professional duty because ". . . the obligations of a pharmacist may at times extend beyond the individual to the community and society."[8] How does this duty to serve the community apply in this dilemma? Does serving the community require Ms. T to refuse to fill the prescription? to fill it, but "get the word out" to her neighbors? Sharing information about Mr. L's access to Viagra would surely violate the pharmacist's duty to respect patient confidentiality. Precisely how should Ms. T balance the interests of the community and of Mr. L?

Equality/Fairness (Justice)   Would failing to dispense the drug be unfair—that is, punish Mr. L for an earlier crime for which he has paid? Would it be inappropriately unequal treatment?

Finally, Ms. T might consider whether failing to fulfill the prescription would be unjust. Questions of consequences to others aside, would denying Mr. L this drug count as an extra and unwarranted punishment? After all, he has served his time and has been released. The judicial system has determined and administered what it took to be appropriate punishment. Why would Ms. T be justified in further burdening Mr. L for what are literally past crimes?

The Law   The following legal considerations are relevant to this case: (1) Do pharmacists have a legal obligation to prevent *potential harms to others*? (2) What is the extent of a pharmacist's legal obligation to patient confidentiality?[9]

The following commentaries examine the application of various moral principles to this dilemma, thereby assisting the reader to undertake *Step 4: Analysis* and *Step 5: Justification*.

Notes

1. David Finkelhor and Lisa Jones, "Explanation for the Decline in Child Sexual Abuse Cases," *Juvenile Justice Bulletin* (Office of Juvenile Justice and Delinquency Prevention), Jan. 2001, http://www.ncjrs.org/ojjdp/html/199298/contents.html (2 Apr. 2004); National Child Abuse Statistics, Childhelp USA, n.d., http://www.childhelpusa.org/abuseinfo_stats.htm (2 Apr. 2004).
2. See, for example, Wendy Root and Jennifer Zabniski, "How Americans Define Child Abuse" (1999), http://www.childrensinstitute.org (2 Apr. 2004).
3. American Psychiatric Association, *Diagnostic and Statistical Manual, Fourth Edition, Text Revision* (Washington, DC: American Psychiatric Association, 2000).
4. American Pharmacists Association, "Code of Ethics for Pharmacists," 27 Oct. 1994, http://www.aphanet.org/pharmcare/ethics.html (22 Apr. 2003).
5. For an excellent justification of the moral obligations of pharmacists to clients, see Richard M. Schulz and David B. Brushwood, "The Pharmacist's Role in Patient Care," *Hastings Center Report* 21, no. 1 (1991): 12–17. Though dated, in that it argues for obligations that have subsequently been adopted, its presentation of the moral reasoning for pharmacists as patient advocates and educators is excellent.
6. John B. Murray, "Psychological Profile of Pedophiles and Child Molesters," *The Journal of Psychology* 134, no. 2 (2000): 211–24; Peter J. Fagan et al., "Pedophilia," *JAMA: Journal of the American Medical Association* 288, no. 19 (2002): 2458–65.
7. See Fagan, note 6, above, 2461, 2464.
8. See note 4, above.
9. See Richard R. Abood and David B. Brushwood, *Pharmacy Practice and the Law*, 3rd ed. (Gaithersburg, MD: Aspen Publishers, 2004), chap. 16, "Legal Issues with Ethical Implications"; and Patricia Younger, et al., *Pharmacy Law Answer Book* (Gaithersburg, MD: Aspen Publishers, 1996), chap. 6, "Liability." Tarasoff continues to exert its influence in such scenarios; see Tarasoff v. Regents of the University of California, Supreme Court of California 51 P.2d 334 (Cal. 1976). Discussions of physician's tort liability for "failure to warn" in situations where known HIV disease may put others at risk may provide some insight into the legal implications of such a case; see American Medical Association, Council on Ethical and Judicial Affairs, *Code of Medical Ethics: Current Opinions with Annotations*, 2000–2001 ed. (Chicago: American Medical Association, 2000), § 2.23, "HIV Testing," 84–85; and § 5.05, "Confidentiality," 105–17.

A Pharmacist's Analysis

Robert A. Buerki, PhD, RPh, and Louis D. Vottero, MS, RPh

Traditionally, pharmacists have recognized a moral, even legal, duty to fill valid prescriptions. For decades this duty focused on pharmacists as self-appointed guardians of public health, protecting their patients from dangerous poisons, fraudulent patent medicines, and irrational or potentially harmful prescribed remedies.

More recently, as pharmacy practitioners struggle to meet their obligations in providing pharmaceutical care, they encounter prescribed therapies linked to cases involving issues such as pharmaceutically assisted death or the "morning after" pill, situations that generate profound clinical concerns that test pharmacists' ability to accommodate their rights of conscience in the dispensing of drugs without sacrificing the quality of patient care. These rights of conscience are grounded in the pharmacist's respect for the patient's right of self-determination as well as pharmacy's professional ethic, which remind us that the patient's autonomy should not be purchased at the price of the pharmacist's parallel rights. The pharmacist's basic values and beliefs would be violated by carrying out rigid, unchallenged prescribing requests.

In this case, the patient confronts Ms. T with a particularly disturbing dilemma, giving her grave concern about the potential for harm to unsuspecting members of her community if she dispenses the legitimately prescribed medication to a convicted sex offender. The geographic isolation of her pharmacy precludes referring the patient to another source, and in seeking a resolution Ms. T faces a difficult balancing act—namely, to respect the patient's autonomy and his right to confidentiality (and, more broadly, liberty), and to respect the need-to-know rights of the community, which should not be subjected to significant unconsented-to harms. Finally, she needs to comfort her conscience should she decide not to fill the prescription.

The legal duty for a health practitioner to warn patients about potential untoward effects from prescribed medications is well documented. Pharmacists have a duty to seek assurance that all patients have sufficient information about their prescribed medications so that they may give informed consent to the prescribed therapy. In this case, for example, the patient needs to be aware of the possibility of neurologic, emotional, or psychological disturbances or aggressive behavior that may occur with the intended sildenafil (Viagra) therapy.

However, the pharmacist's legal duty to inform (or alert) others, either single persons or large communities, about possible harmful actions that may occur because of dispensed medications could be problematic. The question of whether pharmacists have a legal duty to inform others about potential dangers is not a settled issue in case law: "The duty to warn is an esoteric body of law that establishes responsibilities and sets limits by using concepts such as superior knowledge and reasonable foreseeability of harm."[1] Nevertheless, pharmacists are as accountable to their service communities as are mental health therapists and other health professionals.[2]

In light of these observations, the pharmacist's moral duty to inform the community of potential harms from dispensed medications may be stronger than the moral obligation to protect the patient's confidentiality. That is, situations may arise where moral obligations to protect confidentiality must be overridden in the face of stronger moral demands, such as protection of the rights and interests of third parties. Such concerns suggest that stringent public policy protecting the confidential character of patient-pharmacist communications is not absolute, and must bow to the extent to which disclosure is essential to avert danger to others.

The Code of Ethics for Pharmacists establishes the pharmacist-patient relationship as a covenant based on "moral obligations and virtues," especially trust. Further, the Code adds a pledge of respect for patient "autonomy and dignity," all of which must be done in a "caring, compassionate, and confidential manner." At the same time the Code certifies that "a pharmacist serves individual, community, and societal needs."[3] This broad ethical platform provides a basis for whatever action Ms. T may ultimately decide, whether to fill the prescription as requested by the physician or to deny her services because of personally held concerns. Thus, various choices are available for consideration, based on both personally held moral standards or through professional pharmacy practice standards broadly expressed in a recognized code. Clarifying all the unknown aspects of the patient's lifestyle, including legal monitoring, will be essential for ethical decision making by the pharmacist. The right action, to serve the patient and not to put the community at peril, will require a careful balancing of benefit to risk.

Filling the sildenafil prescription for this patient creates a number of difficulties for Ms. T. Should she decide to pursue this action, she will need to seek more information and attempt to answer her many concerns about the stability of the patient and the possible consequences of dispensing the prescribed drug. In doing so, she ought to preserve the confidentiality of the patient-physician-pharmacist triad and communicate only with the patient and the physician. Going beyond this triad for information, such as calling the police, would break any bond of trust, violate the confidence of the patient, and reduce the event to a mere mercantile transaction.

The peculiar elements of this case strongly suggest that Ms. T should initiate a frank discussion with Mr. L's physician, a tactic that might yield an unbiased response concerning the nature and extent of Mr. L's problem and the possibility of recidivism. As a newcomer, this practitioner is possibly unaware of Mr. L's problematic history; and although it is difficult to imagine any emergency need for sildenafil, some clinical nuance could prompt the physician to prescribe such therapy. Speaking directly to Mr. L about her concerns may not provide Ms. T all the answers she needs, since Mr. L may obfuscate or lie to obtain the medication. However, if Ms. T chooses this course of action, it will demonstrate her respect for Mr. L's autonomy. Simply stating. "I can't fill your prescription because I don't have the medication," could be a justification if Ms. T's supply of sildenafil is exhausted; however, this is unlikely as she has several patients on this therapy.

Nevertheless, if Ms. T concludes from her reasoning that the best alternative for her is to refuse to fill the prescription, she needs to discuss her reasoning with her patient in a truthful and private manner. Her refusal may be linked to personal reasons or her suspicion of sexual deviance, both of which are linked to her concern for public welfare. In her discussion with Mr. L, Ms. T ought to point out her resolve to respect patient autonomy and the correlative respect she anticipates from the patient—that is, her right of self-determination and her prerogative to decide the extent of her professional services. This firm belief in the fundamental respect of the autonomous person provides ample justification for the denial of professional service.

Notes

1. David W. Brushwood, "The Duty to Counsel: Reviewing a Decade of Legislation," *The Annals of Pharmacotherapy* 25, no. 2 (1991): 203.
2. Tarasoff v. Regents of the University of California, California Supreme Court, 17 California Reports, 3d series, 425, decided 1 July 1976; Tom L. Beauchamp and James F. Childress, *Principles of Biomedical Ethics*, 3rd ed. (New York: Oxford University Press, 1989), 400–403; and see note 1, above.
3. Louis D. Vottero, "The 1994 Code of Ethics for Pharmacists and Pharmaceutical Care," in *Ethical Dimensions of Pharmaceutical Care*, eds. Amy Marie Haddad and Robert A. Buerki (Binghamton, NY: Pharmaceutical Products Press, an imprint of The Haworth Press, 1996), 161.

A Philosopher's Analysis

Anthony Graybosch, PhD

Viagra (sildenafil) is effective for treating male erectile dysfunction. With optimal dosing, successful attempts at sexual intercourse are markedly increased. Ms. T is confronted with a client whom she must presume has a legitimate therapeutic need for Viagra, since Mr. L has a prescription. And, undoubtedly, successful intercourse is conducive to a happy life and the maintenance of an intimate relationship with a sexual partner. Ms. T also realizes that Mr. L is a convicted sex offender. Since sexual assault is plausibly motivated by the stimulation of power and domination, Viagra could be part of a therapeutic plan to recondition Mr. L's sexual response. It also suggests that sexual assault may continue to occur without Viagra, since Mr. L's primary motivation may be power and not successful sexual intercourse. Ms. T is not in a position to know the reason Viagra was prescribed, and cannot acquire this knowledge without risking violation of confidentiality.

The American Pharmaceutical Association's (APA's) Code of Ethics (COE) stresses that the pharmacist's primary moral obligation is to the patient:

> *Considering the patient-pharmacist relationship as a covenant means that a pharmacist has moral obligations in response to the gift of trust received from society. In return for this gift, a pharmacist promises to help individuals achieve optimum benefit from their medications, to be committed to their welfare, and to maintain their trust. A pharmacist promotes the good of every patient in a caring, compassionate, and confidential manner.*[1]

This quote stresses the moral obligation to maintain confidentiality. It might be tempting to think that the duty to promote the health of the patient would include helping Mr. L stay out of prison by contacting the physician or the police. But the COE clearly construes health in a narrower sense. The COE recognizes that a pharmacist's primary duty is to the patient. It does provide for consultation with other health care professionals (HCPs) when appropriate, but it is not clear that such consultation is appropriate in this case.[2] Mr. L may have a legitimate need for Viagra, and there is no known definite causal role between use of Viagra and recidivism as a sex offender.

Ms. T's refusal to sell the drug would place Mr. L at a serious disadvantage in pursuing a good life and so is prima facie immoral. The location (a privately owned pharmacy), however, does open up another moral option. Many pharmacists, unlike physicians, consult with patients in public spaces. For example, there is no special private consultation room at Costco. Yet Ms. T has the opportunity to speak in private with Mr. L without violating confidentiality. The APA COE apparently makes this uncomfortable option morally mandatory:

> The primary obligation of a pharmacist is to individual patients. However, the obligations of a pharmacist may at times extend beyond the individual to the community and society. In these situations, the pharmacist recognizes the responsibilities that accompany these obligations and acts accordingly.[3]

Ms. T should choose her words carefully, expressing concern for both Mr. L and other members of the community, as she inquires about Mr. L's current intimate relationships, rehabilitation, ongoing treatment, and probation status. Ms. T must also use her professional judgment and common sense to decide how sincere Mr. L is. This is important in considering an additional step.

It appears that Mr. L is entitled to Viagra as an important contribution to his autonomous pursuit of a happy life. And Mr. L is entitled to a confidential relationship with the pharmacist. Mr. L may have chosen the new physician in town as a subterfuge; but he may just as easily have chosen the new physician because it is uncomfortable talking to people who know he has been convicted as a sex offender. If Mr. L is indeed reformed then a call to the physician may unfairly deprive him of the trust of another health care professional. It is not an unheard of occurrence for paroled sexual offenders to have to constantly move due to rejection by the community.

Ms. T will probably already know if local law places her under any special legal obligation to contact the police. I can only consult the laws of my state (California) and say that pharmacists are not currently under any special obligation to report the purchase of Viagra by paroled sex offenders. Ms. T probably would feel guilty if Mr. L did commit additional offense and perhaps even feel she had aided and abetted Mr. L. Given the lack of known causal connection between Viagra or successful erections and recidivism, such feelings would not be well founded. But California has recognized that the sexual abuse of minors is such a horrendous crime, with a significant recidivism rate, that sex offenders are required to register and regularly report to local police agencies. And police are permitted to contact facilities, such as daycare centers, when they reasonably suspect that children may come in contact with registered sex offenders. Using the police as the avenue of tracking past offenders and as a means of informing the public is meant to balance the rights of past offenders, such as confidentiality, and the rights of children to be protected from potential abuse. It also relieves Ms. T of making the decision of whether a Viagra purchase is a significant warning sign.

Certainly if I were a police officer I would take Viagra purchase as warranting reasonable suspicion. And because police officers do not convict offenders, they are held to a lower level of proof than judges and juries. It will be a useful measure for Mr. L to know that the police are aware of his purchases and have notified various institutions and agencies where children are found. Ms. T should not only speak with Mr. L, but also contact the local police as a means of balancing her responsibility to the patient and to society.

One final word: California officials have recently admitted that the database that tracks sex offenders is ineffective. If this mythical Midwest state is like California in this respect, then citizens like Ms. T have special knowledge and are in a unique position to aid children. It may be unpleasant to have to talk to Mr. L. But her unique position and professional competence make Ms. T the person who can do the most good in this situation. It is morally mandatory for Ms. T to talk to Mr. L and contact the police. She also should sell him the Viagra.

Notes

1. American Pharmacists Association, "Code of Ethics for Pharmacists" (27 Oct. 1994), http://www.aphanet.org/pharmcare/ethics.html (22 Apr. 2003), § I.
2. Ibid., § VII.
3. Ibid., § VII.

Further Reflections

General

1. This case takes place in a small community with a single pharmacy. What role should this fact play in determining the pharmacist's duty to Mr. L? Would the morally appropriate response differ in an urban area with easier access to pharmacists?
2. Independent of what you think about the legitimacy of Ms. T's concerns, is it within the purview of her professional responsibilities to worry about the risk that Mr. L poses to the community? What are the strongest moral and professional arguments that can be advanced for Ms. T to pursue this issue? What are

the strongest moral arguments for urging Ms. T to *not* pursue her concerns in this case?

3. If we concede for the sake of argument that Ms. T can morally and legally seek answers to her concerns, what are the legitimate sources that she can consult? Buerke and Vottero suggest these would be limited to the patient and his physician. Graybosch suggests that these would be limited to the patient and the police. What different arguments does each make for limiting inquiries to these different parties? Are there other sources you think could be queried (e.g., the parole board; other community members; other pharmacists) in pursuit of the truth concerning Mr. L?

Consequences

4. Determine and evaluate the consequences for Mr. L, Ms. T, and the larger community if Ms. T chooses to fill the prescription and if she chooses not to do so. Assess the likelihood of their occurrence.

Autonomy

5. Based on the concerns about Mr. L and knowing what is morally required of Ms. T as a pharmacist, do you believe, as Buerke and Vottero suggest, that Ms. T has a "right to self-determination" (autonomous choice) that gives her the prerogative to decide whether or not to supply Viagra to this patient?

Rights

6. Does Mr. L have a right to pursue a private life in this community, in which the circumstances of his past and of his present medications are held in strict confidence? Does the community have a *moral* right to be notified of his history and presence? What notification is the community due—from its government and/or police force (who are sworn to "protect and to serve") or from physicians or pharmacists who possess information that they believe the public ought to know?

Virtues

7. Buerke and Vottero note that for pharmacists "situations may arise where moral obligations to protect confidentiality must be overridden in the face of stronger moral demands, such as protection of the rights and interests of third parties . . . and to avert danger to others." Is this case one such exceptional situation? Why or why not?

8. Do you agree with Graybosch that Ms. T. cannot acquire the knowledge about why Viagra was prescribed without risking violation of the professional responsibility to respect patient confidentiality?

Equality/Fairness (Justice)

9. Given that broad respect for privacy and confidentiality are extended to all persons in the society for most previous immoral or illegal activity, what are the possible moral and practical justifications to single out child molesters and sex abusers for distinct censure?

10. Does singling out sexual abusers constitute a *moral* version of "double jeopardy"?

When Bad Things Happen to Good Doctors

Dr. J shook his head with concern as he examined the patient's chart. This was the second time in as many months he had been called to Labor and Delivery (L&D) by the charge nurse to check on a patient of Dr. K's and he didn't like what he saw. Ms. L had been admitted in labor, four weeks prior to her due date. She was short of breath and appeared very pale. Her hemoglobin (which measures the oxygen-carrying capacity of the blood) was 7.7 mg/dl—dangerously low. In reviewing her medical record, Dr. J could find no record of any previous test of her hemoglobin. This omission was deeply disturbing, as pregnant women are prone to anemia (low hemoglobin) which often requires treatment (iron supplements or, if the anemia is especially serious, blood transfusions). Because Dr. J had no record of a previous hemoglobin level, he was unable to determine if Ms. L's anemia was long-standing or acute (if acute, the anemia might indicate that Ms. L was bleeding internally). Why hadn't Dr. K ordered a hemoglobin at any point in Ms. L's pregnancy? Troubling. . . .

Dr. K is an institution in Coventry, a Southern town of 20,000. The only board-certified obstetrician in the region, Dr. K has been caring for babies and their mothers for decades. He was instrumental in establishing the community's small hospital, as well as ensuring that its services were as current and high-quality as any in the state. He obstructed its takeover by a (now defunct) health maintenance organization (HMO) five years ago. He has served for the last two years as the chief of the hospital's medical staff. He and his wife endowed a trust to attract and support five family practitioners. He recently retired as president of the county medical society. At 70 years of age, Dr. K still sees patients full-time. His patients love and respect him—for good reason. In short, Dr. K has had an illustrious and community-minded career.

All that having been said, the last six months have seen increasing problems with Dr. K's patient management. Errors and omissions in diagnosis, treatment, and patient follow-up have begun to arise at a disturbing rate. Dr. J last encountered one of Dr. K's problems when the L&D nurse, evaluating a new admission, identified two fetal heart beats. The patient said Dr. K had not mentioned twins as a possibility (though the patient's grandmother was a twin). She reported refusing an early routine sonogram as needless and expensive, and Dr. K hadn't pressed the point. An emergency sonogram revealed twins and, fortunately, extra personnel were available to help with the delivery and care for the twins at birth. Dr. J discussed the case with Dr. K, indicating "we dodged the bullet on this one; we could have been in trouble if the twins had had problems or we hadn't had enough staff." Dr. K just smiled and said quietly, "God handles these things."

Other smaller incidents have been noted by the L&D staff: A patient reported she had been "deathly" allergic to penicillin since she was a child, though Dr. K's record indicated she had no known allergies. Two patients had been admitted without having had pap smears or tests for syphilis or gonorrhea (two sexually transmitted diseases that put infants at risk). One patient reported she was taking prenatal vitamins four times daily, though the standard dose is once a day. And who knew what other as-yet-unidentified problems were waiting in the wings? On more than one occasion L&D nurses have opined "Dr. K seems to be slipping," or worried aloud that eventually some mother or child will suffer grievous harm.

Dr. J and the L&D staff have so far been able to manage the patients, but they are uncertain how to manage Dr. K—or even whether he should be "managed" at all. Dr. K's daughter was killed six months ago in an auto accident, and his wife has not yet fully recovered from this shock. Certainly Dr. K's family stresses could affect him, dilute his concentration, sap his energies. But the health care professionals (HCPs) are not certain that stress is the source of Dr. K's problems. Could his forgetfulness, errors, and lack of attention to detail be due to "old age" or a dementing disease? If his inabilities are temporary, his colleagues would hate to criticize his competence if what he really needed was support and understanding.

Further, one might question whether Dr. K actually poses a significant risk to most of his patients. True, he has made mistakes—but who doesn't. Some of his lapses have been minor; other concerns have had reasonable explanations (e.g., the woman's refusal of the sonogram) or may represent reasonable judgment calls (e.g., the vitamins). The medical system ensures that several HCPs interact to provide patient care, and every HCP cannot help but review the actions of colleagues. The checking and cross-checking of patients' records and conditions helps to prevent or catch mistakes or omissions before they become serious. And anyway, half a dozen incidents in a year don't seem outrageously excessive, and most of Dr. K's patients were managed well.

Then, too, Dr. K has always been a valuable professional resource. As the only local obstetrician, he has been the only referral opportunity for his colleagues' patients who are at high risk for obstetrical complications. Local family practitioners would be lost without his willing and (historically, at least) able consultation on their patients with diabetes, multiple fetuses, excessively high blood pressure, and the like. Without Dr. K as backup, high-risk patients would have to travel 80 miles to the nearest out-of-town obstetrician.

Nonetheless, some of Dr. K's actions have put his patients at risk for serious harm. The L&D nurses, as well as some of Dr. K's physician colleagues, feel that their luck cannot hold, that sooner or later something will go dreadfully wrong. Still, Dr. K could suffer serious harm if his career were inappropriately cut short or his reputation sullied. After all his good deeds, maybe he deserves the benefit of a doubt.

What is the moral responsibility of Dr. K's colleagues at this point?

Introduction

Two important moral issues merit attention in this case:

1. What are the consequences of interceding (if facts demonstrate a problem)?
2. To whom or what do the health care professionals (HCPs) have obligations of fidelity? How should they adjudicate possible conflicts between these obligations?

The AJ Method

Step 1: Information Gathering   What is Dr. K's true condition? (Hippen; Peter) Is he capable of competent practice? Is he capable of autonomous participation in structuring his professional future? What motivates Dr. K's colleagues? How many mistakes are "too many"? (Smith) Were the "mistakes" truly mistakes, or just differences in professional practice? (Hippen)

Dr. K's incompetence is suspected but unproven. Significant data (for example, whether tests were done) are missing. As facts help to define the nature of any dilemma, unwarranted assumptions or interpretations based on incomplete evidence need to be acknowledged. Without relevant facts, any suggested resolution is likely to miss the mark. Indeed, a careful collection of the facts may reveal that no dilemma exists.

Step 2: Creative Problem Solving   A creative solution would have to simultaneously respect Dr. K and protect patients from incompetent practice. (Hippen; Peter)

Step 3: Pros and Cons   Survey CARVE principles to identify important moral reasons that support conflicting options for resolving this case.

Consequences   What would be the effects on Dr. K if his colleagues take steps to restrict his practice? (Kraman and Hamm) if they do not? on Dr. J? (Smith) on Dr. K's colleagues? on Dr. K's patients? (Hippen; Peter; Kraman and Hamm) on the hospital? Are long-term effects (including to future patients) possible? (Smith) likely?

What is the central moral issue here? The most prominent concern is to avoid harm. HCPs, institutions, and various oversight committees are committed both to preventing harms to and advancing the well-being of patients. Yet in this case preventing harm to patients could harm a respected colleague, while avoiding harm to one's colleague risks harms to patients and the hospital.

While professional codes of ethics specify patient welfare as having priority, providing health care is a collegial enterprise. HCPs can only be effective if they have the support of and can rely on each other in the diagnosis and treatment of patients. Nurturing relationships among practitioners are essential for keeping practitioners in the profession and in a given community. This issue is especially critical in small towns, where attracting and retaining qualified specialists are typically difficult. Lacking urban amenities that many HCPs desire (easy access to the arts, a community of one's discipline-specific peers), small towns might understandably view a few (more?) errors as an unavoidable consequence of their restricted diagnostic or therapeutic environment, or as an acceptable trade-off for retaining a practitioner with specialized skills. Thus protecting a provider's reputation and, derivatively, his livelihood may be in the best interests of small communities—assuming, of course, that threats to patients are neither frequent nor severe. None of these remarks is meant to suggest that small towns should "settle" for mediocre health care; rather, they remind us that different circumstances can change a consequential calculus.

Then too, HCPs—like all persons—have self-interested concerns. If Dr. J or the Labor and Delivery (L&D) nurses are perceived as whistleblowers, their reputations might suffer and their positions—psychological and economic—may be threatened. At the least, collegial relationships will be tainted, perhaps irreparably.

The loss of friendships, mutual trust, and respect may be perceived as too high a cost to pay in an attempt to rectify what is arguably a minor problem against which the system's safeguards are usually adequate. Again, maintaining a congenial workplace is especially critical in small communities, where disharmony cannot be shed by moving one's practice to a different hospital or one's collegial affiliations to a new group. And the option of outrunning one's past is virtually nonexistent unless one is willing to leave town altogether. Since to err is human, perhaps collegiality requires tolerating not-too-frequent or not-too-serious mistakes.

In sum, future patients may be harmed by Dr. K's continued practice. The community—including Dr. K's colleagues—may be harmed by the loss of its only specialist in obstetrics and gynecology (ob-gyn). Particular patients whom Dr. K would have helped may suffer more complications. The loss of trust in Dr. K (should his reputation be sullied) may—or may not—be balanced by increased trust in the general health care community. If forced from practice, Dr. K may lose his financial stability; if he is allowed to continue in practice, more patients may suffer preventable harm. This dilemma quickly becomes one of balancing Dr. K's interests with those of his patients and colleagues.

Autonomy   Recall that autonomy, most broadly understood, applies to choosing values in terms of which to live one's life, as well as the means to achieve those values. What role does autonomy play here? What might explain Dr. K's errors in judgment? (Hippen; Kraman and Hamm)

If Dr. K is likely to seriously compromise care to patients, what should patients be told? Any general warning may worry patients without providing sufficient information to evaluate their own risks. A more specific warning would violate the confidentiality owed to Dr. K, either as a patient himself or as a practitioner who is innocent until proven guilty.

Rights   Which option(s) protect Dr. K's right to self-determination? to not be harmed? of privacy? of confidentiality? (Smith) Do Dr. K's patients or colleagues have rights that the HCPs must take into account?

Virtues   What does fidelity to one's colleagues require? If fidelity to a colleague conflicts with fidelity to patients, which takes precedence? (Kraman and Hamm; Peter; Smith) How significant are the appeals to honesty and courage?

Who has the greater claim on the HCPs? Both the American Medical Association's (AMA's) Code of Ethics[1] and the American College of Physicians (ACP)[2] specify the patient's welfare as primary. The ACP notes: "Patient care must never be compromised because a physician's judgment or skill is impaired." Similarly, the American Nurses Association Code of Ethics mandates: "Nurses must be vigilant to protect the patient, the public, and the profession from potential harm when a colleague's practice . . . appears to be impaired."[3]

How extensive is professional fidelity in this regard? Surely one cannot be responsible for *every* patient, especially (perhaps) the patients of one's colleagues. Perhaps not, but HCPs have espoused obligations to maintain the public trust by exposing incompetent practitioners and limiting patient exposure to those who are likely to harm them. On the other hand, the community collectively owes Dr. K a debt of gratitude for his long-standing service to and promotion of a thriving medical community. Sabotaging his career seems like an odd way of repaying this debt.

Do HCPs have duties to institutions in which they practice? For example, should they act to minimize potential harms to the reputation or financial risk of their local hospital? Conversely, do institutions have obligations to protect the populations they serve? If a social contract exists between citizens (who are also taxpayers) and health care institutions, does the hospital itself have a duty to limit future foreseeable harms to as yet unidentified patients?

Morality is about doing the right thing, of course; but it is also about being a good person. A person is partly defined and shaped by the professional identity he or she assumes. The public in general, and patients in particular, have traditionally expected HCPs to demonstrate the virtues of fidelity (to include a general benevolence toward patients), courage (to confront colleagues whose practices fail to meet a recognized standard), and honesty (about identifiable risks to patients). Several commentators discuss character traits and virtues that we might expect from responsible professionals, usefully reminding us that HCPs should manifest certain characteristics.

Equality/Fairness (Justice)   Are Dr. K's patients or colleagues placed under an unfair burden if he continues to practice?

The Law   In conclusion, the following legal considerations are relevant to this case: (1) What legal obligations do HCPs have to prevent foreseeable harms to potential patients? Is a Tarasoff-like legal obligation (to inform potential and actual patients about potential harms by Dr. K) present? (2) What legal obligations do the physicians in Coventry have to Dr. K? (3) Under what conditions must or may HCPs legally override the decisional authority of a colleague? (4) Does Dr. J have a legal obligation of confidentiality concerning what he knows or suspects about Dr. K?[4]

The following commentaries examine the application of various moral principles to this dilemma, thereby assisting the reader to undertake *Step 4: Analysis* and *Step 5: Justification*.

Notes

1. American Medical Association, *Code of Ethics*, § 9.031, 18 July 2003, http://www.ama-assn.org/ama/pub/category/2416.htm (16 Aug. 2003).
2. American College of Physicians, "The Impaired Physician," *Ethics Manual*, n.d., http://imc.gsm.com/demos/dddemo/consult/imp_acp.htm (4 Apr. 2004).
3. American Nurses Association, *Code of Ethics for Nurses with Interpretive Statements* (Washington, DC: ANA, 2001), 15, 2001, http://nursingworld.org/ethics/code/ethicscode150.htm, § 3.6 (12 Aug. 2003).
4. Most helpful in sorting out the legal conundra of this case is American Medical Association, Council on Ethical and Judicial Affairs, *Code of Medical Ethics: Current Opinions with An-*

notations, 2000–2001 ed. (Chicago: American Medical Association, 2000), § 8.02, "Ethical Guidelines for Physicians in Management and Other Non-Clinical Roles," 141–42; and § 9.031, "Reporting Impaired, Incompetent, or Unethical Colleagues," 201–202. The obligation to warn third parties of foreseeable injuries under a Tarasoff-type scenario (Tarasoff v. Regents of the University of California; Supreme Court of California 551 P.2d 334 (Cal. 1976)), as well as related issues of tort liability for "failure to warn" are discussed in the context of HIV testing in § 2.23, "HIV Testing," 84–85.

A Clinical Ethicist's Analysis

Martin L. Smith, STD

A short list of suspected errors and omissions related to Dr. K's delivery of medical services is now known. The good news is that serious harms have not resulted. What is not known is how this list, compiled during the past six to twelve months, compares with previous, similar time periods of Dr. K's medical practice. A reasonable assumption is that Dr. K has a history of demonstrated competency and delivery of quality care; therefore the reported failures and lapses are not due to deficient knowledge, poor judgment, or substandard clinical skills, but possibly to other factors such as a disease, a disorder, or emotional distress.

Dr. J seems reluctant to intervene because of uncertainty that a sufficient pattern of error exists, or in deference to Dr. K's prestige and power, or due to feelings of loyalty to a fellow physician—or all three.[1] Despite his good intentions, should Dr. J choose to intervene, he risks possible retaliation or recrimination from Dr. K or from peers, counteraccusations, a lawsuit for defamation of character, or, at a minimum, Dr. K's anger.[2]

At stake in this case are the professional ethical duties of promoting patient well-being (beneficence) and not causing patient harm (nonmaleficence). At issue are the dual questions of whether standards of care are being violated and whether Dr. K is now an impaired professional.

In 1972 the American Medical Association's Council on Mental Health defined physician impairment as "The inability to practice medicine with reasonable skill and safety to patients by reason of physical or mental illness, including deterioration through the aging process, the loss of motor skills, or the excessive use or abuse of drugs, including alcohol."[3]

If Dr. K's errors and omissions result from impairment, they are likely to be repeated unless and until the impairment is corrected. If the staff is correct that "their luck cannot hold," it is simply a matter of time before serious harm comes to one of Dr. K's patients, with the accompanying consequence of serious damage to Dr. K's reputation and livelihood.

Dr. J and the Labor and Delivery (L&D) nurses need to determine first whether a sufficient pattern of violations of local or national standards for obstetrical care exists. Although Dr. J is not a board-certified obstetrician, he may have the expertise and resources (e.g., other physician colleagues whom he can consult confidentially) to evaluate the quality of care rendered by Dr. K and to make judgments about whether the standards have been followed. If Dr. K failed to adhere to standard procedures, protocols, and practices, there may be legitimate cause for concern. Dr. J and the L&D staff may have a unique opportunity to prevent future harm to patients, as well as to protect Dr. K.

In deciding whether to intervene with Dr. K, Dr. J should seriously consider the following directive from the *Ethics Manual* of the American College of Physicians: "Every physician is responsible for protecting patients from an impaired physician and for assisting an impaired colleague. Fear of being wrong, embarrassment, or possible litigation should not deter or delay identification of an impaired colleague."[4]

If Dr. K's patients are at serious risk, the L&D nurses have their own relevant and applicable directives from the second and third provisions of the 2001 Code of Ethics for Nurses:

"The nurse's primary commitment is to the patient, whether an individual, family, group, or community."

"The nurse promotes, advocates for, and strives to protect the health, safety, and rights of the patient."[5]

On a practical level Dr. J and the L&D staff should determine if there is a sufficient pattern of clear errors, omissions, and lapses to warrant a conclusion that Dr. K is functioning in an impaired condition. If not, they should continue to monitor his practice to see if such a pattern develops. If they conclude now or in the future that a pattern exists, someone (see below) should talk directly to Dr. K about the observed pattern, presenting him with specific instances and details. The aim of such a conversation need not be Dr. K's resignation from all clinical practice. Rather, a variety of assists or monitoring processes are available to protect patient safety, uphold standards of care, and continue to utilize Dr. K's expertise and skills. Further, depending on the causes of the impairment, resources may be available to Dr. K to compensate for, reverse, or slow the impairment process.

A direct conversation with Dr. K is more likely to have a good outcome if the information is presented to him in a supportive, caring manner by a colleague or friend whom Dr. K respects and trusts. Assistance from other internal mechanisms such as the hospital's quality assurance office or the ethics committee (if they exist) should be sought, if needed. Only as a last resort and only if Dr. K refuses to change practices in ways that protect his patients should Dr. J and the staff use the power or influence of external vehicles, such as the leadership of the county medical association or the state licensing board.

When a case such as this unfolds in smaller, community hospitals, some additional courage and cautions may be needed. Where professional staffs are smaller in number and may have a family-like closeness, there can be an even stronger reluctance and resistance to intervene with Dr. K, who may have a father-like status in the hospital both as an authority figure and as a well-known and beloved leader. Many of Dr. K's colleagues who have a close relationship with him may feel that they have a stake in the outcome of any intervention and therefore will want to monitor attempted resolutions closely. Further, because Dr. K is not shielded by the anonymity present in larger professional populations, information can spread rapidly among a significant percentage of the staff about Dr. K's pattern of suspected errors and omissions, as well as about evolving plans to intervene. The L&D staff and any other involved persons may need explicit reminders to protect Dr. K's reputation by adhering strictly to the confidential nature of the process.

Notes

1. Bernard Lo, "Impaired Colleagues," in *Resolving Ethical Dilemmas, A Guide for Clinicians* (Philadelphia: Lippincott Williams and Wilkins, 2000), 271–76.
2. Giles R. Scofield, "Impaired Professionals," in *The Encyclopedia of Bioethics,* rev. ed., ed. Warren T. Reich (New York: Simon and Schuster/Macmillan, 1995), 1191–94.
3. American Medical Association, Council on Mental Health, "The Sick Physician: Impairment by Psychiatric Disorders, Including Alcoholism and Drug Dependence," *JAMA: Journal of the American Medical Association* 223 (1973): 684–87.
4. American College of Physicians, *Ethics Manual,* 4th ed., *Annals of Internal Medicine* 128 (1998): 590.
5. Gladys White, "Code of Ethics for Nurses," *American Journal of Nursing* 101 (2001): 75.

A Physician's and a Lawyer's Analysis

Steve Kraman, MD, and Ginny Hamm, JD

To simplify: The only obstetrician in the area, formerly an excellent practitioner, is now apparently beginning to falter in his old age, due perhaps to a dementing illness, stress from a personal tragedy, or both. Most of the clinical needs in the county can be covered by other physicians, but not the high-risk obstetrics needs. Thus, depriving the community of Dr. K's services could endanger patients. His colleagues feel it is just a matter of time before a patient is terribly harmed by Dr. K's diminishing abilities. To complicate matters, they also want to avoid hurting an old friend and colleague who has given so much to the community.

Are there ethically acceptable alternatives that could ease the ethical tensions? What further information is needed to resolve these tensions? Can those involved even determine the appropriate action regarding Dr. K's behavior without clear information? Is compromise ever acceptable when there are competing ethical issues? What actions are within the ethical boundaries when problems arise?

One premise of ethics is to do no harm. Is Dr. K inflicting harm on his patients? We know he has a strong safety net with his practice. Shouldn't his staff "catch" these little oversights? What about potential harms to Dr. K himself? Is this a temporary problem that may resolve with the passing of the extreme grief Dr. K must be suffering? The confrontation with Dr. K could result in an exacerbation of the depression from his daughter's death. Is the risk of his suicide a factor to consider?

"Always resolve to do good" is a second ethical principle. Is Dr. K still doing good things? What about his potential benefits to future obstetrical patients with complicated problems?

The ethical principle of utility requires a comparative analysis of whether the harms outweigh the benefits of Dr. K's continued practice. The physicians in the family practice must weigh the impact of Dr. K's errors on the patients in their community against the good that he does. When is it ethically reasonable to withhold action and risk patient injury? Does his funding of five new family practice physicians outweigh the oversights in his patient care? What about the harm of depriving the local community of his services?

In analyzing the ethical tensions from a duty-based perspective we must determine who should assume responsibility for preventing or minimizing future harm. Does Dr. K have a right to make his own decisions about the conduct of his practice (and a correlative duty to insure his own competence)? Or does society have a duty to question (or strive to insure) his competence?

Further, what should patients be told? Do concerned professionals have a duty to inform the community about Dr. K's lapses? The truth is ethically the "gold standard" for informed consent, but the "therapeutic exception" is well recognized when the truth would likely generate more harm than good.

In fact, *all professionals* having knowledge about this dilemma have the duty to prevent foreseeable harms because they have promised, in their codes of ethics, to do so.

Clearly, the physician's primary responsibility is to the patient. The AMA, through their *Principles of Medical Ethics,* requires a physician to report "physicians deficient in . . . competence . . . to appropriate entities."[1] Such an entity might reasonably be the chief of the hospital's medical staff. However, Dr. K is that person. So, as we approach a plan of action, the dilemma is how to handle this in a way that protects patients, maintains necessary obstetric services, and spares Dr. K. This is not impossible, but if it can't all be worked out, we must decide what the priorities are. The responsibility to individual patients is paramount, but the other interrelated issues are important as well. This is how we would recommend handling this sensitive and complex problem:

First, determine if Dr. K's competence lapses are illness- or stress-related. Although Dr. J has tried to talk to him about one of these lapses, it did not lead to a productive conversation. A colleague of stature, whom Dr. K respects, should talk to him about the staff's concerns. Finding the right person for this job will best assure Dr. K's cooperation. He must see and accept that the rate of his errors is a real problem.

Second, if Dr. K's problems are stress-related (assuming that continuing to work is helping him deal with his grief), he can be offered assistance (e.g., written protocols for his office staff to use) to make sure that simple but important things are not overlooked, thereby helping him continue to practice safely. If organic mental illness is suspected, then he must be persuaded of the need to determine its cause, severity, and treatability. The goal is to support him emotionally, acknowledging the respect and affection of the staff while addressing a problem that is potentially serious and that could devastate Dr. K as well as a patient if he caused an adverse event. This is sincere concern for a colleague and the patients for whom all the staff are responsible.

Third, if after all efforts Dr. K refuses to see the problem, then the hospital staff have no real choice but to use their hospital policies to suspend his privileges and report their concerns to the State Medical Licensure Board. To do otherwise would expose Dr. K's patients, without their knowledge or consent, to risks of which the staff are aware. Preventing Dr. K from practicing would be unfortunate for him and most of his patients, but the patient's well-being is paramount and those needing high-risk obstetric services could choose to travel to other counties for their care.

A possible compromise solution might be to offer to aid Dr. K by relieving him of some of his stressors for a period of time to better determine his state of health without *permanently* sidelining him. Perhaps he could become the ob-gyn "emeritus" and engage strictly in consultation with the family practice group. This would give him time to recover or, with the group's guidance, accept his changing health.

Finally, succession planning: Dr. K is 70 years old. Regardless of how this goes, the community must plan to find a supplemental source of high-risk obstetrics services, perhaps to assist Dr. K at first and allow him to train his own successor. This will best assure a seamless provision of care whenever Dr. K is no longer able to practice.

Notes

1. Council on Ethical and Judicial Affairs, American Medical Association, *Code of Ethics: Current Opinions with Annotations* (Chicago: American Medical Association, 1997), xiv.

A Physician's Analysis

Benjamin Hippen, MD

Medical errors have become a hot topic for research in the medical literature. Several studies have examined ways in which errors can be identified, evaluated, and remedied, and recommendations for institutional reforms abound. Morbidity and mortality conferences, designed to review errors in diagnostic and therapeutic judgments in a didactic (and usually nonconfrontational) fashion, have been in existence for some time.

That being said, errors happen. The case of Dr. K describes a common scenario faced by contemporary practitioners. Implied, but never fully demonstrated, is that Dr. K is impaired. The reader is left with several tantalizing hints at impairment, such as Dr. K's age, his recent family trauma, apparently indifferent reaction when confronted with an oversight. However, the case for impairment is incomplete.

A striking feature of this case is the persistent voice of the author. While not written in first person, the internal monologue of Dr. J dominates the description of events. Dr. K's voice is entirely subordinated to Dr. J's concerns about Dr. K's clinical competence, made in striking contrast to the high regard for Dr. K's personal dedication to his patients and his professional contributions to a small community. This solipsistic[1] approach adequately presents the dilemma from Dr. J's perspective, but actually tells us little about Dr. K.

Did Dr. J ever *ask* Dr. K whether he had checked the hemoglobin of the patient in question? Is it possible that the patient did have her hemoglobin checked, but that it was part of the clinic record and not the hospital record? Small community hospitals may be less likely to have centralized computer records of laboratory studies, or they may exist in separate, incompatible databases. Perhaps the patient's laboratory studies were obtained by her primary care physician and passed on to Dr. K. All of these questions might have been answered with a phone call. As it stands, Dr. J's efforts to obtain this information are unclear. As a practitioner, I'm inclined to give Dr. J the benefit of the doubt on this point, but chagrined to find that Dr. J is not willing to give the same benefit to Dr. K, a clinician he otherwise holds in high regard.

Still, other oversights were noted by health care professionals (HCPs) other than Dr. J, who admits their observations to his narrative only toward the end of bolstering his own concerns. We are allowed that on one occasion, when Dr. K missed the presence of twins, that Dr. K "smiled" (benevolently?) and "said quietly, 'God handles these things.'" Is this supposed to be anecdotal evidence of Dr. K's indifference to error? A feature of his impairment? If so, this would seem to reflect the prejudices of Dr. J rather than the incompetence of Dr. K.

Obviously, Dr. J is a thoughtful, reflective physician. He has undertaken obligations to the patients under his care to ensure that they receive the high quality of care they deserve. His respect for Dr. K is evident. So too, unfortunately, is his solipsism, which leads him to a series of conclusions that, while plausible, are supported by limited evidence. The stakes for Dr. K (suspension of his medical license, loss of his practice and thereby his livelihood, personal and professional embarrassment) are quite high. Of course the stakes for Dr. K's patients, if Dr. J. is correct in his inferences, is much higher.

Dr. J has several professional and moral obligations that *require* him to discuss these issues with Dr. K directly. Prior to doing so, it is worth being certain that his facts are correct. Did Dr. K check the hemoglobin on the patient, or not? Did the patient taking several vitamins rather than one do so at the instruction of Dr. K, at the instruction of another health care provider, or of her own accord? Were the patients who were admitted without pap smears or tests for sexually transmitted diseases first seen at the beginning of their pregnancy, or just as they were approaching term? Dr. J allows that "most of Dr. K's patients were managed well." This observation *reinforces* the point that Dr. J must make every effort to ascertain the truth about the events troubling him, prior to making potentially actionable assumptions about Dr. K's impairment.

It is unlikely that medical errors will ever be completely eliminated, but institutional reforms to ensure checks and reviews would seem to be a good step toward eliminating many errors of omission. In initiating a discussion of his concerns with Dr. K, Dr. J has many approaches at his disposal. Let me suggest one:

"Dr. K, I noticed that on patients X and Y, there were no tests for syphilis and gonorrhea, and on patient Z, I was unable to locate a baseline hemoglobin. I've recently asked the hospital laboratory to put together an "OB panel" of laboratories, since I order the same tests on the majority of my preterm patients. That way, all the lab tests we need are sent to the same place, and are accessible through the same database. I think this would save a lot of time and effort in tracking down labs when patients are admitted to the hospital for delivery. Would you be willing to participate in such a protocol? I'm asking, because it has occasionally been difficult to find lab results on some of your patients when they are admitted to the hospital. I've found that this works very well for me. What do you think?"

This approach has the advantages of (1) initially offering Dr. K the benefit of the doubt, (2) solving the problem of omitted laboratory tests, (3) focusing on maintaining a high quality of patient care, and (4) avoiding dubious postulates about Dr. K's psychological and intellectual well-being. Discharging our obligations to patients and colleagues need not always, nor even often, be adversarial.

That being said, if Dr. J is proven right in his assumption that Dr. K is impaired, he has a moral and professional obligation to bring this to the attention of Dr. K, either himself or by way of respected colleagues. Should Dr. K prove to be completely unresponsive to these entreaties, Dr. J is obligated to refer the matter to his state medical board. I have argued that this ought to be the last, rather than the first, resort. Nevertheless, it is a logical extension of the premise that caring for patients is a physician's privilege, not a right. When impairment makes delivery of care impossible, the patients bear the cost of suffering, and the profession bears the cost of its credibility. That is something neither patients nor doctors can afford.

Notes

1. *Solipsism,* used here pejoratively, refers to positions that hold that the self is the primary source of insight in arriving at answers to philosophical questions. For a robust defense of methodological solipsism as a pillar of phenomenological reflection, see "Solipsism (Modali-

ties of the Strange)" in *Prism of the Self*, ed. Steven Galt Crowell (Dodrecht, The Netherlands: Kluwer Academic Publishers, 1995), 13–29. Coherent accounts of solipsism are defensible when they are a starting point, not an end point, of inquiry. Dr. J's attempts to explain and understand Dr. K's actions strictly through suppositions and interior monologue is, I argue, the indefensible kind of solipsism, since the facts of the case begin and end with Dr. J's many assumptions about Dr. K, untested by Dr. K's point of view.

A Nurse Ethicist's Analysis

Elizabeth Peter, PhD, RN

In this case, the Labor and Delivery (L&D) nurses have a fundamental moral responsibility to promote, advocate for, and strive to protect the health, safety, and rights of the patients.[1] Nurses "must strive to prevent and minimize adverse events in collaboration with colleagues on the healthcare team."[2] These adverse events can include physician and interdisciplinary team error. In working to minimize adverse events, nurses have a duty to address impaired practice in a compassionate and caring fashion.[3]

The case describes Dr. K as having had an exemplary career, but the details of the case also indicate that in the past six months "errors and omissions in diagnosis, treatment, and patient follow-up have begun to arise at a disturbing rate" in Dr. K's work. Specific errors have all had the potential to harm pregnant women. His colleagues wonder whether his family stresses have affected his concentration or whether his errors are the result of "old age" or a dementing disease, as Dr. K is now 70. Although his colleagues question whether his mistakes are minor or have a reasonable explanation, the facts of the case make it reasonable to conclude that Dr. K's practice is impaired to the extent that the health and safety of his patients are threatened.

Both the American Nurses Association (ANA) and the Canadian Nurses Association (CNA) codes of ethics provide clear direction for nurses in cases such as this one. First, the facts of the situation must be gathered and documented. Second, relevant legislation, policies, and guidelines for reporting incidents of incompetent care must be reviewed, and supervisory personnel normally should be consulted. Third, the impaired individual must be confronted in a supportive manner and be provided access to appropriate resources. The ANA code states that when "a nurse suspects another's practice may be impaired, the nurse's duty is to take action designed both to protect patients and to assure that the impaired individual receives assistance in regaining optimal function."[4] While the nurse's primary commitment is to patients, nurses have the broader obligation to advocate for respectful treatment of all people, including colleagues. Respectful and caring treatment is not only of moral importance in itself; it also leads to the development of health care environments that foster ethical practice and the well-being of all in those settings.[5]

With respect to this case, a colleague(s) who has a good rapport with Dr. K, someone Dr. K respects and trusts, would best be capable of approaching him. It is unknown whether Dr. K's impairment is temporary or progressive or even whether he has any awareness of his errors. Through this meeting, Dr. K could be supported while he is given the opportunity to learn about, and perhaps clarify, the observations of the team. He could also be given assistance in seeking help, getting rest, or retiring.

Although Dr. K is a prominent and powerful community member and he may deny his impairment and errors, it is essential that he be prevented from harming patients. It may be especially difficult to take action because Coventry is a small community. The withdrawal of Dr. K's services, even temporarily, could result in women needing to travel long distances to receive care, and could compromise the safety of emergency deliveries. Despite these inconveniences and potential harms, however, the likelihood of harm is greater if Dr. K continues to practice, given his recent history of errors. In addition, the integrity and trustworthiness of the L&D team will be compromised if they do not disclose and act upon their observations.

Because Dr. K cannot practice indefinitely, these incidents may also serve to hasten the inevitability of succession planning. The L&D nurses and Dr. J must also recognize that preventing Dr. K from practicing in an impaired state not only has the potential to prevent future harm to patients, but also could prevent harm to Dr. K himself. Dr. K has had an illustrious career. It would be tragic for him to end his working life in disgrace because of a grievous error. Such an error would likely be highly publicized, informally, if not officially, in a community like Coventry where reputations are easily built and lost through the words of others.

In conclusion, the L&D nurses and Dr. J must act on their observations of Dr. K's impairment and errors. In this way, they can prevent harm to both expectant mothers and Dr. K.

RECOMMENDED READING

Rubin, Susan B. and Laurie Zoloth. *Margin of Error: The Ethics of Mistakes in the Practice of Medicine.* Hagerstown, PA: University Publishing Group, 2000.

Notes

1. American Nurses Association, *Code of Ethics for Nurses with Interpretive Statements*, 2001, http://www.ana.org/ethics/ (14 Jan. 2003).
2. Canadian Nurses Association, *Code of Ethics for Registered Nurses*, 2002, http://www.cna.aiic.ca (14 Jan. 2003), 9.
3. See note 1, above.
4. Ibid., Provision 3.6.
5. See notes 1 and 2, above.

Further Reflections

General

1. This case takes place in a small community where physician specialists are in short supply. What role should this fact play in determining what should be done about Dr. K? Would the morally appropriate response differ in an urban center with easier access to more qualified physicians?

2. What factual issues need to be explored to determine what is really going on? On what basis should a conclusion of impairment be based? Compare the different assessments of Smith and Peter with that of Hippen.

3. Why is how Dr. K practices medicine Dr. J's business? Dr. J is *not* (a) Dr. K's employer, (b) in practice with Dr. K, (c) an administrator of the hospital in which Dr. K works, (d) a practitioner in Dr. K's specialty (and so might have trouble evaluating whether standards of care have been met), or (e) a patient of Dr. K.

4. Consider the strategies offered by Kraman and Hamm for determining if Dr. K is impaired and, if he is, for addressing his impairment. Who should be responsible for this undertaking?

Consequences

5. What are the likely effects and who is likely to be affected if Dr. K's problems are not investigated? if they are?

Autonomy

6. If Dr. K is impaired, can the appeal to autonomy require that his colleagues share this information with his own patients or with the general public?

Rights

7. Do patients *generally* have a right to know if their health care professionals are impaired? If not, why not? If so, who has the responsibility to provide this information?

8. If Dr. K is impaired, can he appeal to a right to confidentiality to preclude his colleagues from sharing this information with his own patients or with the general public?

Virtues

9. Which professional virtues offer guidance to Dr. J and the L&D nurses about how to proceed, both in determining Dr. K's level of ability and, if they discover deficits, responding to it?

10. Do virtues suggest that *any particular person* (e.g., Dr. J, an L&D nurse, the hospital administrator) has a responsibility to investigate or respond to the difficulties raised by Dr. K's recent practice? If so, who?

Equality/Fairness (Justice)

11. What weight should Dr. K's reputation and past performance have in this discussion?

Chapter 21

Do Health Care Professionals with HIV Disease Have a Duty to Warn Their Patients?

Ms. N is a registered nurse who works in the intensive care unit (ICU) of a small community hospital. She regularly inserts intravenous (IV) catheters, assists in the insertion of other tubes (e.g., chest, peritoneal, endotracheal), and gives wound care. She performs advanced cardiac life support (e.g., CPR, IV drug administration). Each of these procedures puts Ms. N and her patients at risk for exposure to each other's body fluids (saliva, sputum, blood).

Two years ago, while working in an urban emergency room, Ms. N was accidentally stuck with a needle while resuscitating a patient who was HIV-infected. An HIV test immediately after the puncture was negative. Occupational acquisition of HIV Disease (HIVD) is rare, but it has been documented. The probability of acquiring HIVD from a contaminated needle puncture is reportedly about 0.3 percent (~1 in 300 cases). Probability in particular cases varies with the level of virus in the blood of the source person and the extent of injury caused by the perforation.

In keeping with current therapeutic guidelines, Ms. N immediately began a prophylactic medical regimen that included a nucleoside analog (AZT) and a protease inhibitor (Indinovir) in an attempt to prevent her seroconversion. She has tolerated these drugs unusually well and has been able to continue working without any noticeable ill effects. Even with postexposure therapy, approximately 10 percent of persons exposed to HIV develop HIVD. Sadly, in spite of aggressive drug management, Ms. N's most recent ELISA, confirmed with a Western blot test, was positive. In short, Ms. N now has HIVD.

Ms. N immediately informed her supervisor, Ms. S, about her seroconversion. Ms. S worries that Ms. N's disease might put her ICU patients or coworkers at unacceptable risk of significant harm. She notes that while patients and health care professionals (HCPs) in urban medical centers might reasonably assume some of their caregivers, patients, or colleagues have HIVD, persons in this small, rural community have yet to see (so far as they know) anyone with HIVD. Consequently, when patients consent to admission and its generic risks, they are unlikely to assume they are consenting to HIVD exposure. Certainly any patient who acquired HIVD during hospitalization would be surprised and horrified.

Ms. S wonders if Ms. N should be transferred to a unit where she would not be required to perform invasive techniques. Perhaps Ms. N should be discharged. Ms. S is reluctant to embrace either of these options, as skilled critical care nurses are hard to come by in her small hospital. Ms. N is a very good ICU nurse, and her loss would be a hardship to the unit and, derivatively, its patients. Nonetheless, her presence does pose a risk to patients and colleagues. Ms. S, as a nurse, is morally obligated to protect patients from risk of harm. As a manager, Ms. S is obligated to protect her institution's welfare (e.g., its reputation), as well as ensure positive working conditions for her employees. But Ms. N is also one of her employees—and a patient, as well. Perhaps Ms. N's patients and coworkers should be told of her HIV status. If they consented to her continued presence in the unit, the dilemma would evaporate. Still, the likelihood that all would consent to this exposure is very small.

What should Ms. S do?

Introduction

This case raises five significant moral issues:

1. The moral relevance of risk.
2. Adjudicating harms and benefits (consequences).
3. The role of respect for autonomy and the right of self-determination.
4. Nurturing desirable professional virtues.
5. The role of justice.

The AJ Method

Step 1: Information Gathering   How likely is Ms. N to infect her patients? her coworkers? How likely is it that patients, if informed of Ms. N's HIV status, would refuse to be cared for by her? How likely is it that Ms. N's coworkers, if informed of Ms. N's HIV status, would refuse to work with her? Do patients legitimately assume a risk of HIV infection when they consent to hospitalization and treatment?

Between 800,000–900,000 persons in the United States are infected with the human immunodeficiency virus (HIV) and the number is increasing by 40,000 each year.[1] Health care professionals (HCPs) know that anyone—patient or HCP—may, perhaps unknowingly, be carrying the HIV or other potentially lethal pathogens. Most institutions require HCPs to use standard precautions (gloves, goggles, masks, and gowns) to protect patients and themselves whenever they anticipate exposure to a patient's blood or body fluids, though these precautions cannot absolutely prevent infection (e.g., accidental injury). Still, acquiring HIVD from a HCP has a very low probability (0.3% blood exposure; 0.09% mucous membrane exposure).[2]

Step 2: Creative Problem Solving   A creative solution would have to simultaneously respect Ms. N's right to confidentiality and protect her patients and coworkers from unacceptable risk. (White)

Step 3: Pros and Cons   Survey CARVE principles to identify important moral reasons that support conflicting options for resolving this case.

Consequences   What would be the effects on Ms. N if her supervisor restricts her practice? (Resnik) if she does not? on Ms. N's patients? (Drought; Resnik) on her colleagues? (Drought) on the hospital? Are long-term effects (including to future patients) possible? likely? (White)

Ms. N's HIVD poses a *risk* of infection to her patients and colleagues. Risk is not a guarantee of harm, but a probability that some outcome will occur. Risk is central to moral debate because when evaluating consequences one must consider *possible* as well as *actual* outcomes.

All health care is attended by risk. Patients are at risk for death or disability from failed treatment, for unwanted side effects from successful treatment, and iatrogenic (provider-caused) illness.[3] Risk has three dimensions: *probability* (likelihood), *magnitude* (severity and duration), and *materiality* (relevance) of harms (a risk is material if it causes one to choose differently than she would were the risk not present). Persons rarely worry about low-magnitude, high-probability risks (e.g., the common cold), but often worry about high-magnitude, low-probability risks. HIVD is a catastrophic disease (severe health effects of lifelong duration). Most people perceive exposure to HIVD as a risk to be avoided at all costs—that is, as a material risk. Most persons say the HIV status of their HCPs is a material risk.[4]

Other things being equal, a morally praiseworthy action minimizes both potential and actual negative consequences.[5] Negative consequences of HIVD are significant. Though death is no longer assured, drug regimens for health maintenance are intrusive, fraught with noxious side effects, and expensive—all significant burdens.[6] Nearly all patients still experience some social stigmatization and ostracism.[7]

The consequences of Ms. N's HIVD for her patients and colleagues are *potential*, but those for Ms. N are *actual*. In addition to those mentioned above, if Ms. N's HIVD becomes public knowledge, she may not be allowed to perform a job she enjoys and for which she is qualified. If she is forced to transfer to another department, especially one she does not enjoy or for which she is poorly qualified, the negative psychological effects will be great. If she is fired (or forced to resign), she loses her livelihood.[8]

Consequences for the hospital must also be considered. Whatever decision the hospital makes will have ramifications for its safety record, deployment of employees, liability under the Americans with Disability Act and The Patient's Bill of Rights, community reputation, and perhaps financial security/solvency. The magnitude and probability of these risks are difficult to predict, but are not zero.

Autonomy   Recall that autonomy, most broadly understood, applies to choosing the values in terms of which to live one's life, as well as the means to achieve those values. What role does autonomy play here? Whose autonomy should be considered? (White)

What about respect for autonomy and the right to self-determination? The obligation to inform persons before putting them at risk cannot be reduced to calculating harms and benefits, but requires that patients be apprised of and asked to consent to (at least) probable, severe, or material risks. Consequences of hospitalization are not uniformly benign; tens of thousands of patients suffer a complication during their hospital stays.[9] Because most patients are aware that some risk attaches to hospitalization, their consent to admission presumably includes consent to some risk of unspecified, prospectively unidentifiable harms—though patients' exact thoughts about this are unknown. However patients in rural hospitals are unlikely to assume they will be exposed to HIV.[10] Many patients and HCPs would choose to avoid all exposure to HIVD, no matter how remote the possibility of infection. If informed an HCP has HIVD, most patients would choose another provider.[11] If informed a patient has HIVD, many HCPs would avoid caring for the patient.[12] Thus, respect for autonomy and the right of self-determination may require that information about particular providers/colleagues with HIVD be divulged.[13]

Rights   Beyond patients' rights of self-determination, Ms. N also possesses rights—particularly the moral right to confidentiality and the legal right to not be discriminated against on the basis of a recognized disability (HIVD).[14] Which option(s) protect Ms. N's right to self-determination? to not be harmed? of privacy? (Drought) of confidentiality? (Drought; White) Do Ms. N's patients or colleagues have rights—for example, to self-determination—of which Ms. S must take moral account? (White)

Virtues   What does fidelity to one's colleagues require? If fidelity to a colleague conflicts with fidelity to patients, which takes precedence? To whom does Ms. S have a greater obligation: patients, employees, or the institution? (Drought; Resnik) How significant are the appeals to compassion, tolerance, honesty, and courage?

Right actions are morally important, but so are good persons and institutions. How might different responses to this dilemma affect important professional virtues? Ideally, actions encourage professional integrity and compassion in caregivers, supervisors, and institutions. Ms. N, already distressed by her disease, seems a likely candidate for compassionate treatment to which integrity commits all HCPs. Still, Ms. N might herself demonstrate compassion and integrity by voluntarily transferring to an environment (i.e., one with no invasive procedures) where she would pose less risk to patients. The professional virtues of integrity and honesty suggest keeping Ms. N's secret as a way of respecting professional promises to her as a patient, but these virtues might also counsel disclosure as a way to respect professional promises to other patients. Finally, the importance of strengthening trustworthiness in HCPs and hospitals may support a particular choice.

Equality/Fairness (Justice)   Are Ms. N's patients or colleagues placed under an unfair burden if she continues to practice in the ICU? Is Ms. N being treated unequally (as compared to other HCPs with infectious diseases)? (Resnik; White)

One would be hard pressed to claim Ms. N "deserved" her disease, so punishing her for it (by forcing another undeserved burden on her) would be unfair. Further, justice understood as equality requires considering whether Ms. N should be granted the same latitude as other HCPs carrying infectious diseases (or, conversely, placing other infected HCPs under greater restrictions). Is Ms. S justified in treating an employee with a disease of high magnitude, transmission of which is very improbable, differently from an employee whose disease is (usually) of lesser magnitude though more likely to be transmitted (e.g., hepatitis) to patients or colleagues?[15] Do these differences make Ms. S's discrimination morally permissible?[16]

The Law   In conclusion, the following legal considerations are relevant to this case: (1) What workplace modifications are required/precluded by the Americans with Disabilities Act? (2) Would revealing HIVD legally constitute a violation of confidentiality? privacy? workplace restriction? (3) If the supervisor does not transfer the nurse, is she legally liable for negligence, should a patient or coworker become infected? (4) To whom is the supervisor *primarily* obligated—patients, employees, her institution, other?[17]

The following commentaries examine the application of various moral principles to this dilemma, thereby assisting the reader to undertake *Step 4: Analysis* and *Step 5: Justification*.

Notes

1. Centers for Disease Control and Prevention, "HIV/AIDS Update: A Glance at the HIV Epidemic," n.d., http://www.cdc.gov/hiv/pubs/facts.htm#Surveillance (22 July 2003).
2. Centers for Disease Control, "Updated U.S. Public Health Service Guidelines for the Management of Occupational Exposures to HBV, HCV, and HIV and Recommendations for

Postexposure Prophylaxis," 29 June 2001, http://www.cdc.gov/mmwr/PDF/rr/rr5011.pdf (22 July 2003); Julie Louise Gerberding, "Occupational Exposure to HIV in Health Care Settings," *New England Journal of Medicine* 348 (2003): 826–33. For an illuminating comparison of HIVD to other risks, see Norman Daniels, "HIV-infected Professionals, Patient Rights, and the 'Switching Dilemma,'" *JAMA: Journal of the American Medical Association* 267, no. 10 (1992): 1368–81.

3. Institute of Medicine, Committee on Quality of Health Care in America, *To Err Is Human: Building a Safer Health System* (Washington, DC: Institute of Medicine, 2000), 1 Sept. 1999, http://www.iom.edu/ (22 July 2003).

4. Barbara Gerbert et al., "Physicians and Acquired Immunodeficiency Syndrome: What Patients Think about Human Immunodeficiency Virus in Medical Practice," *JAMA: Journal of the American Medical Association* 262, no. 14 (1989): 1962–72; see Daniels, note 2, above.

5. For an analysis of the social consequences of a duty to disclose, see Daniels, note 2, above.

6. See Gerbert, note 4, above.

7. See Daniels, note 2, above.

8. Ibid.

9. Ibid.

10. Rebecca Voelker, "Rural Communities Struggle with AIDS," *JAMA: Journal of the American Medical Association* 279, no. 1 (1998): 5–6.

11. See Gerbert, note 4, above.

12. Barbara G. Maguire et al., "Primary Care Physicians and AIDS: Attitudinal and Structural Barriers to Care," *JAMA: Journal of the American Medical Association* 266 (1991): 2837–42.

13. Lawrence O. Gostin, "A Proposed National Policy on Health Care Workers Living With HIV/AIDS and Other Blood-Borne Pathogens," *JAMA: Journal of the American Medical Association* 284 (2000): 1965–70. But compare to John R. Tuohey, "Moving from Autonomy to Responsibility in HIV-Related Healthcare," *Cambridge Quarterly of Healthcare Ethics* 4 (1995): 64–70.

14. Department of Justice, 28 CFR Part 35, "Nondiscrimination on the Basis of Disability in State and Local Government Services," 26 July 1991, http://search.usdoj.gov/compass (22 July 2003); see also Gerbert, note 4, above.

15. See Daniels, note 2, above.

16. Larry Gostin, "The HIV-Infected Healthcare Professional: Public Policy, Discrimination, and Patient Safety," *Law, Medicine & Healthcare* 18, no. 4 (1990): 303–10; see also note 13, above.

17. Though somewhat dated, the conceptual legal and ethical issues of testing proposals, rights to privacy and privacy law, testing health care workers, and warning patients are thoroughly discussed in eds. Martin Gunderson, David J. Mayo, and Frank S. Rhame, *AIDS: Testing and Privacy* (Salt Lake City: University of Utah Press, 1989). Joan C. Callahan and Jill Powell, "Nursing and AIDS: Some Special Challenges," 51–73, in eds. Elliot D. Cohen and Michael Davis, *AIDS: Crisis in Professional Ethics* (Philadelphia: Temple University Press, 1994) provides insightful nursing perspectives. Legal issues, particularly with respect to privacy concerns, are addressed by the Health Insurance Portability and Accountability Act of 1996 (HIPAA, Public Law 104-191). Accommodations in conformity with the Americans With Disabilities Act of 1990 (42 U.S.C.S. § 12101) are addressed by American Medical Association, Council on Ethical and Judicial Affairs, *Code of Medical Ethics: Current Opinions with Annotations,* 2000–2001 ed. (Chicago: American Medical Association, 2000), § 2.23, "HIV Testing," 84–85; and § 9.131, "HIV-Infected Patients and Physicians," 224–29. For some interesting international and comparative perspectives, see Alistair Orr, "The Legal Implications of AIDS and HIV Infection in Britain and the United States," 94–118, in

ed. Brenda Almond, *AIDS: A Moral Issue. The Ethical, Legal and Social Aspects*, 2nd. ed. (New York: St. Martin's Press, 1996); Paul Hampton Crockett, *HIV Law: A Survival Guide to the Legal System for People Living with HIV* (New York: Three Rivers Press/Crown Publishing, 1997), esp. chap. 16, "Discrimination: What are Your Rights?" and chap. 17, "A Survival Guide to HIV in the Workplace," which provide a pragmatic and realistic assessment of the challenges faced by HIV-positive individuals in the work environment, and the need for personal and proactive initiative.

A Nurse Ethicist's Analysis

Theresa S. Drought, PhD, RN

Ms. S is confronted with a dilemma of competing demands and obligations. She is obligated to treat her staff in a fair and compassionate manner, ensure that competent and skilled nursing care is provided by the staff, and provide an environment of care that is safe for patients and staff alike. Ms. N's occupational acquisition of human immunodeficiency virus (HIV) puts these obligations, which are usually closely aligned, into potential conflict.

Ms. S must first learn about the risks posed by HIV+ health care workers (HCWs). Transmission from an infected HCW to a patient is exceedingly rare; in a study of 22,000 patients cared for by 64 HIV+ workers (including surgeons and obstetricians), not a single incidence of transmission was documented.[1] Armed with factual knowledge about the real risks that Ms. N's HIV+ status poses, Ms. S can explore the moral issues she now confronts. *The Code of Ethics for Nurses with Interpretive Statements* (COE) can help her begin to sort through these issues.[2]

Fair and Compassionate Treatment of Staff

Ms. N informed Ms. S of her seroconversion voluntarily; there is no legal obligation to report one's HIV status. To both their credit, Ms. N felt the need to seek guidance from her supervisor and Ms. S has created an environment where her staff feel safe seeking her counsel. Provision 6 of the COE outlines this requirement for every nurse: "The nurse is responsible for contributing to a moral environment that encourages respectful interactions with colleagues, support of peers, and identification of issues that need to be addressed."[3]

Ms. S has an obligation to keep issues affecting a specific employee confidential, but she also has obligations to the other staff working on her unit. Compromising the rights of one individual can be justified only if failing to do so would result in serious, unavoidable harm to others.

Does Ms. N's HIV status pose sufficient risk to staff to justify divulging her HIV status? Although the community incidence of HIV might be lower in this rural area than in some urban areas, good nursing practice requires taking care in every case.[4] Universal precautions have been proposed as a method of protecting HCWs from exposure to infection from patients while protecting the patient from prejudicial treatment from HCWs who fear exposure.[5] Conceivably, the risk of exposure from a colleague would be much lower than from a patient with HIVD. The best way for Ms. S to protect her staff and maintain her obligation to Ms. N is to ensure that her staff are well-trained in and routinely use universal precautions.

Provision of Skilled, Competent Nursing Care

The nurse is advised to "be vigilant to protect the patient, the public, and the profession from potential harm when a colleague's practice, in any setting, appears to be impaired."[6] Ms. S acknowledges that Ms. N is a highly skilled critical care nurse and a valuable addition to her staff, and that her level of expertise is hard to come by in that geographic region. Ms. N has presumably given no indication that her practice is impaired; she would have a duty (see Provision 5 of the COE) to limit or quit her practice if her health created any challenge to her ability to provide skilled care. Likewise, Ms. S has an obligation to ensure that the nurses working on her unit possess the necessary skills to deliver competent nursing care, and she faces difficulty in finding skilled nurses to practice in the ICU in this rural setting. Ms. S should keep Ms. N unless there are compelling obligations to the contrary.

Maintaining a Safe Health Care Environment

We finally come to the crux of the issue: If Ms. N's HIV status poses any level of risk, aren't her patients and colleagues entitled to know of that risk?

While there is probably some statistical risk that Ms. N could expose her patients or colleagues to her blood or body fluids, that risk is exceedingly remote.[7] ICU nursing practice does not routinely create conditions that would expose patients or colleagues to an individual nurse's body fluids. Careful observance of infection control procedures, such as universal precautions, would further reduce the potential risk.

We might ask how we handle disclosure of other issues that might put patients or colleagues at risk. Many personal conditions risk the safety of patients and colleagues—the nurse with epilepsy or cardiac arrhythmias who could lose consciousness at a critical moment; the nurse preoccupied with an emotional crisis; the nurse whose prior, known, poor practice has placed her in a provisional status. Each of these situations risks the safety of patients as well as colleagues, yet we do not disclose these personal conditions nor gain consent from the patient for submission to that nurse's care. Does Ms. N's HIVD create a qualitatively different type of risk? I would say no.

While the patient has some interest in the personal conditions of the nurse, the nurse is also entitled to some level of privacy. The nursing license is a promise to the public that they can trust the nurse and the care he or she provides. Standards of practice set parameters of what constitutes care and safe practice. Policies guide the provision of that care, further delimiting the bounds and promise of safe practice. Finally, the COE provides guidance concerning the nurse's obligations within those standards and policies. Ms. N should be allowed to continue her professional practice, as long as it is squarely within these established standards. The standards for professional practice established through these regulatory and professional mechanisms provide justification for her continued practice. Ms. S has no obligation to disclose Ms. N's HIV status to her patients or colleagues.

RECOMMENDED READINGS

Friedson, Eliot. *Professional Powers: A Study of the Institutionalization of Formal Knowledge.* Chicago: University of Chicago Press, 1986.

Pellegrino, Edmund D., Robert M. Veatch, and John P. Langan. *Ethics, Trust, and the Professions: Philosophical and Cultural Aspects.* Washington, DC: Georgetown University Press, 1991.

Notes

1. Centers for Disease Control, "Surveillance of Healthcare Personnel with HIV/AIDS as of December 2001," 27 Jan. 2003, http://www.cdc.gov/ncidod/hip/BLOOD/hivpersonnel.htm (22 July 2003); and Laurie M. Robert et al., "Investigations of Patients of Health Care Workers Infected with HIV: The Centers for Disease Control and Prevention Database," *Annals of Internal Medicine* 122, no. 9 (1995): 653–57.
2. American Nurses Association, *Code of Ethics for Nurses with Interpretive Statements* (Washington, DC: American Nurses Association, 2001).
3. Ibid., 21.
4. Centers for Disease Control, "HIV/AIDS Surveillance in Urban and Nonurban Areas L206 slide series (through 2001)," updated 7 Mar. 2003, http://www.cdc.gov/hiv/graphics/rural-urban.htm (19 June 2003).
5. Centers for Disease Control, "Preventing Occupational HIV Transmission to Healthcare Personnel," updated 15 Feb. 2002, http://www.cdc.gov/hiv/pubs/facts/hcwprev.htm (18 June 2003); United States Department of Labor, Occupational Safety and Health Administration, "Safety and Health Topics: Bloodborne Pathogens and Needlestick Prevention," updated 9 July 2003, http://www.osha.gov/SLTC/bloodbornepathogens/index.html (22 July 2003).
6. See note 2, above, 15.
7. Centers for Disease Control, "Case-Control Study of HIV Seroconversion in Health-Care Workers After Percutaneous Exposure to HIV-Infected Blood—France, United Kingdom, and United States, January 1988–August 1994," *Morbidity and Mortality Weekly Report (MMWR)* 44 (50): 929–33 (22 Dec. 1995), 2 May 2001, http://www.cdc.gov/mmwr/preview/mmwrhtml/00039830.htm (18 June 2003); and CDC, "Surveillance of Healthcare Personnel" (see note 1, above).

An Ethicist's Analysis

Becky Cox White, PhD

In the minds of most persons, this case appears primarily to warrant a consequential analysis, comparing potential harms to a health care provider (HCP) (e.g., job loss, ostracism) against potential harms to patients and coworkers (e.g., inadequate staffing, contracting HIVD). However Ms. N poses only a minuscule threat to patients and colleagues.[1] This fact must be emphasized because the most common reason for restraining persons with infectious diseases is their threat to others. If threats to others are remote, a consequentialist appeal is less compelling.

I will argue that the primary moral dilemma is a conflict between the right of confidentiality (Ms. N) and the right of persons (patients and coworkers) to be informed of and consent to risks. In this case these rights directly conflict. The right to be informed and to consent can only be respected by violating the right to confidentiality, and vice versa. To resolve the dilemma we must determine which right is stronger.[2]

The *right to be informed* relies on a more basic right of persons to live their lives according to their own values and to make their own choices about how their lives will go. Call this the *right to self-determination*. Exercising this right requires good information because good lives depend on making good choices, and good choices depend on accurate data. This right justifies the practice of informed consent as the means by which patients acquire good information about treatment options (including their risks, benefits, burdens, and prognoses).[3] The right to be informed does not require access to every bit of relevant information—a practical and perhaps theoretical impossibility—but only information about probable, grave, or material risks.[4]

The *right to confidentiality* also enables persons to live their lives according to their own values. This right, also justified by the right to self-determination, allows persons to protect private information—especially salient to developing life plans and important relationships. Confidentiality contributes to a good life, at least in part, because persons might, upon learning our secrets, treat us differently—and not always better.

The right to confidentiality does not guarantee absolute freedom from interference. This right may be overridden if failure to share information has a high probability of seriously harming unconsenting others (e.g., failure to inform one's lifelong partner that one has HIVD). But we tolerate secrets if their protection does not *unreasonably* increase risks to others. So, for example, while unprotected sex with strangers carries the risk of sexually transmitted diseases, we assume competent adults know this risk and either have chosen to assume it or do not deem it material.

The conditions under which invasion of confidentiality is morally permissible—material risk of grave or probable harm, access to facts necessary for risk avoidance, or consent to the risk—suggest a resolution. If the right to confidentiality may be overridden in cases of probable risk to nonconsenting others who could avoid the risk if informed, Ms. N's confidentiality should be respected because she does not pose a *probable* risk to patients or colleagues. Moreover, knowing Ms. N has HIVD may not enable patients or colleagues to avoid the risk; if other HCPs with HIVD have not been forthcoming about their status, the risk remains. Concerns with consent can be *partially* respected if the general admission consent form includes an *explicit* statement that patients may face a risk of exposure to HIVD (similar to the statement on surgical consents that one faces a risk of anesthetic death). Presumably persons know that they can get sick(er) in hospitals, so this caveat will not come as a nasty surprise, but will serve to remind patients of this risk and, in so doing, partially meet the obligation to specify material risks.[5] As to the consent of Ms. N's coworkers, we may assume they are familiar with the risk of work-related infections and that their continued employment signifies consent to that risk.[6]

Note, though, that a general consent on admission only partially respects the right to be informed of and consent to risks. Ms. N poses a particular and identifiable (as opposed to a general or nonspecific) risk. The right of self-determination that underpins informed consent supports telling patients Ms. N is HIV+ and respecting their decisions about whether to have her care for them. Failure to share this fact counts as withholding information most patients would consider material. Yet HCPs often withhold material information. HCPs rarely tell patients they test positive for tuberculosis or carry the hepatitis virus, though these conditions also increase the risk to patients of both morbidity and mortality. HCPs withhold this information, not because it is immaterial to patients, but because the threat is acceptably low. This common practice suggests that Ms. N's right of confidentiality is buttressed by an appeal to equality. She should be treated no differently than are other HCPs with serious diseases that pose a small threat to patients.

Last, general consent on hospital admission makes possible partial respect of patients' right of self-determination. Conversely, respecting Ms. N's confidentiality is an all-or-nothing proposition. Thus, the breach of Ms. N's right with disclosure is more extensive than the breach of patients' rights with partial withholding of information about material risks.

In sum, Ms. N's right to confidentiality is more powerful than the right of patients and colleagues to be informed because the risk she poses to patients is extremely slight and because patients' general right to be informed of and consent to risk can be gained without breaching confidentiality. Ms. S may still offer Ms. N the opportunity to transfer to a unit with fewer invasive procedures; but if Ms. N elects to continue working in the ICU, Ms. S is morally required to protect her secret and her job.

Notes

1. Centers for Disease Control, "Updated U.S. Public Health Service Guidelines for the Management of Occupational Exposures to HBV, HCV, and HIV and Recommendations for Postexposure Prophylaxis," 29 June 2001, www.cdc.gov/mmwr/PDF/rr/rr5011.pdf (22 July 2003).
2. For an excellent discussion of rights that are especially important in health care see Baruch A. Brody, *Life and Death Decision Making* (New York: Oxford University Press, 1988), 22–32. For another discussion of the conflict of rights see Norman Daniels, "HIV-Infected Professionals, Patient Rights, and the 'Switching Dilemma,'" *JAMA: Journal of the American Medical Association* 267, no. 10 (1992): 1368–81.
3. Ruth R. Faden and Tom L. Beauchamp, *A History and Theory of Informed Consent* (New York: Oxford University Press, 1986).
4. Franz J. Ingelfinger, "'Informed' (But Uneducated) Consent," *New England Journal of Medicine* 287 (1972): 456–66; Robert M. Veatch, "Abandoning Informed Consent," *Hastings Center Report* 25, no. 2 (1995): 5–12; and Becky Cox White and Joel A. Zimbelman, "Abandoning Informed Consent: An Idea Whose Time Has Not Yet Come," *The Journal of Medicine and Philosophy* 23, no. 5 (1998): 477–99.
5. But compare with Daniels, note 2, above.
6. John R. Tuohey, "Moving from Autonomy to Responsibility in HIV-Related Healthcare," *Cambridge Quarterly of Healthcare Ethics* 4 (1995): 65.

An Ethicist's Analysis

David B. Resnik, JD, PhD

Ms. S, the nursing supervisor in the ICU, faces a difficult management decision: should she recommend that the organization transfer Ms. N from the ICU to another position? From an organization ethics perspective, Ms. S is a middle manager with moral duties to patients, subordinates, and the hospital. This commentary will analyze her decision from each of these perspectives.

Let us consider duties to patients first. Ms. S is responsible for the ICU patients, albeit indirectly via her supervision of other nurses. Since Ms. S has an ethical duty to protect patients from harm and promote their well-being, she should take steps to minimize risks to patients and promote patient safety. Indeed, Provision 3 of the American Nurses Association Code of Ethics requires nurses to protect and promote the health, safety, and rights of patients.[1]

Ms. N represents a risk to patients because she could infect her patients with HIV Disease (HIVD). The health care community became aware of this potential problem when studies confirmed that a Florida dentist with HIVD infected five of his patients.[2] However, a subsequent study of a different dentist with HIVD found he did not infect his patients.[3] A comprehensive analysis of the Centers for Disease Control database of 51 HIVD-infected health care professionals (HCPs) found that none of their 22,171 patients developed HIVD as a result of contact with the infected HCPs.[4] These statistics indicate that Ms. N's risk of infecting patients is real, because professional-to-patient transmission has happened and could happen again. However, the risk is also infinitesimally low and is preventable: effective procedures, such as a strict adherence to universal precautions, can prevent professional-to-patient transmission.

Clearly, Ms. S has a duty to minimize the risk of professional-to-patient HIVD transmission. However, as a representative of her institution, she must weigh this risk against other risks. If Ms. S transfers Ms. N from the ICU, she may have a difficult time replacing Ms. N. Even if she is able to replace Ms. N, Ms N's replacement may have less experience than Ms. N. Ms. S must therefore consider the risks to patients posed by having insufficient or inexperienced staff. Studies have shown that high patient-to-nurse ratios and inexperienced nurses pose risks to patients.[5] For example, one additional patient per nurse was associated with a 7 percent increase in patient mortality.[6] The risks associated with inadequate staffing, also real and preventable, are much higher than the risk of HIVD transmission. When one weighs these different risks, it appears to be much riskier to transfer Ms. N than to keep her in the ICU.

Ms. S also has duties to Ms. N. As her manager and institutional liaison, Ms. S has ethical obligations to promote Ms. N's welfare, to respect Ms. N's dignity, and to treat Ms. N fairly. Transferring Ms. N from the ICU will probably not benefit Ms. N and it may cause her considerable psychological harm, if Ms. N is not satisfied with her new position and becomes angry and resentful. It may also show a lack of respect for Ms. N's dignity by treating her as mere instrument in the service of organizational goals.

If Ms. N becomes angry and resentful, she may impose additional costs on the institution that will affect its reputation, fiscal stability, or even its survival. She may sue the organization for employment discrimination under applicable discrimination law, such as the Americans with Disabilities Act (ADA). The ADA forbids employment discrimination against people with disabilities when a reasonable accommodation will allow an employee to perform his or her job satisfactorily. The ADA defines a disability as a physical or mental impairment that interferes with a major life activity, such as work or socialization, a history of such an impairment, or the perception of such an impairment.[7] Ms. N may qualify as a disabled person under the ADA because HIVD can cause impairments or create the perception of impairment. Although this commentary will not explore these legal issues, it will consider the moral issues that underpin the ADA.

If the organization transfers Ms. N, would this action be unfair? Discrimination in employment can be morally justifiable (or fair) when it is based on a morally *relevant* characteristic. For instance, in deciding whether to hire a nurse to work in the ICU, the organization can fairly discriminate against job applicants that have inadequate education and training on the grounds that these characteristics are relevant to job performance. Unfair (or immoral) discrimination occurs when one discriminates against an employee based on an *irrelevant* characteristic. For instance, the organization should not discriminate against job applicants on the basis of gender or race, because these traits have no relationship to job performance. An organization should also not discriminate against a disabled person if a reasonable accommodation will allow that person to perform his or her job satisfactorily.

Is HIVD a relevant characteristic for discrimination? As we noted above, the risk of professional-to-patient transmission of HIVD is so low that it is close to zero. If Ms. N had a disease (e.g., tuberculosis) which posed a greater risk of infection, then her disease-status would be a relevant characteristic. In this case, it is not. Moreover, reasonable accommodations and institutionally instituted policies, such as strict adherence to universal precautions, can be implemented to virtually eliminate HIV transmission. These considerations support a conclusion that it would be unfair to transfer Ms. N from the ICU.

Finally, one must consider Ms. S's duties to the hospital. In her role as a manager in the ICU, Ms. S has an additional duty to the hospital: to recruit, train, and retain well-qualified employees. Nurses, especially experienced nurses, are in short supply.[8] If the organization transfers Ms. N out of the ICU, she may decide to seek employment elsewhere. Can the organization afford to lose this trusted employee? Even if Ms. S determines that the organization can do without Ms. N's services on the ICU, she still must consider how transferring Ms. N would affect her job satisfaction and continued employment with the organization.

To conclude, Ms. S's moral obligations—to patients, subordinates, and the hospital—favor keeping Ms. N in the ICU while taking steps to prevent HIVD transmission to patients. Though Ms. N poses a very small risk to her patients, transferring Ms. N would create a greater risk, be unfair, and could undermine the organization's goal of retaining qualified nurses.

Notes

1. American Nurses Association, *Code of Ethics for Nurses with Interpretative Statements,* 2001, http://www.nursingworld.org/ethics/code/ethicscode150.htm#prov3 (23 July 2003).
2. Carol Ciesielski et al., "Transmission of Human Immunodeficiency Virus in a Dental Practice," *Annals of Internal Medicine* 116 (1992): 798–805.
3. Harold W. Jaffe et al., "Lack of HIV Transmission in the Practice of a Dentist with AIDS," *Annals of Internal Medicine* 121 (1994): 855–59.
4. Laurie M. Robert et al., "Investigations of Patients of Health Care Workers Infected with HIV," The Centers for Disease Control and Prevention Database, *Annals of Internal Medicine* 122 (1995): 653–57.
5. Linda Aiken et al., "Hospital Nurse Staffing and Patient Mortality, Nurse Burnout, and Job Dissatisfaction," *JAMA: Journal of the American Medical Association* 288 (2002): 1987–93; and A. Morrison et al., "The Effects of Nursing Staff Inexperience (NSI) on the Occurrence of Adverse Patient Experiences in ICUs," *Australian Critical Care* 14 (2001): 116–21.
6. Aiken, see note 5, above.
7. The Americans with Disabilities Act, 42 U.S.C. Sec. 12102(2) (1990).
8. Aiken, see note 5, above.

Further Reflections

Consequences

1. Risk is a function of probability, magnitude, and materiality of harm. If individuals possess wildly different thresholds concerning the risks they are willing to assume, what criterion(a) should hospitals and HCPs use to set policies for notifying patients about the risks associated with disease transmission (including HIVD) from other patients and HCPs? Indicate the language and content of such a policy.

2. To whom does a hospital have greater responsibilities: employees, patients, the community, or its own continued existence? How do the likely effects of a loss of confidence in one's local hospital (should Ms. N's HIVD become public knowledge) affect these responsibilities? Does the increasing ownership of hospitals by corporations with obligations to stockholders alter these responsibilities?

Autonomy

3. Is a patient's signed consent to hospital admission, with its attendant risks, a genuinely autonomous (i.e., informed, understood, voluntary) consent to the risk of infectious diseases?

4. Should all autonomous choices—such as jeopardizing one's overall well-being to avoid a particular unlikely but material risk—be honored?

Rights

5. Should respect for individual rights ever be a function of *how* an individual acquired HIVD? Does infection by an accidental needle stick, for example, provide the infected person (or uninfected coworkers or patients) with different moral claims against others than if the disease were acquired by IV drug use, or homosexual or extramarital heterosexual encounters? Justify your answer.

6. This case takes place in a small community hospital where experienced personnel are in short supply. What role should this fact play in resolving the conflict between Ms. N's right to confidentiality and the rights of others to know their increased risks (if any) from her HIVD? Would the resolution differ in an urban center with more anonymity, job prospects, qualified medical personnel, etc.?

Virtues

7. Nurses often conceive of themselves as patient advocates, using this label more often than any other to define their professional identity and provide a unifying principle that allows for coherent interpretation of the Nursing Code of Ethics. What, precisely, does patient advocacy dictate in this case? What moral and professional principles support your conclusions?

8. Many HCPs try to avoid working with HIVD patients because of the risks of acquiring HIVD (in spite of the use of universal precautions). Is such behavior consistent with professional integrity?

Equality/Fairness (Justice)

9. Justice takes two different forms in this case: (1) an analysis of the nature of the burdens that it is *fair* to impose on patients and HCPs in an environment where HIV is present; and (2) a determination of whether HCPs with HIVD should receive *equal* protections and consideration accorded HCPs carrying other infectious diseases. Specify the burdens fairness or equality require, and suggest a policy that would protect from or compensate individuals for these burdens.

10. Employers are required by the Americans with Disabilities Act to make "reasonable" accommodations for HIV+ HCPs. Discuss what accommodations would be considered "reasonable," including whether "reasonable accommodations" would include preserving confidentiality of HCPs with HIVD.